3.

WD

Contraception Abortion and Sterilization in General Practice

CONTRACEPTION ABORTION AND STERILIZATION IN GENERAL PRACTICE

K. Leslie Oldershaw
MBBS (Lond.), DObst RCOG, MRCGP

Henry Kimpton Publishers
LONDON 1975

ISBN 0 85313 790 0

Printed in Great Britain by
Unwin Brothers Limited
The Gresham Press, Old Woking, Surrey
A member of the Staples Printing Group

CONTENTS

PREFACE

My only excuse for having the cheek to write this book is that I was asked to do so. It was pointed out that although many excellent textbooks on contraception already exist, none has been written from the point of view of the family doctor, who, alone among many competing to give contraceptive care in the seventies, is responsible for the complete spectrum of whole-patient care, day in and day out, possibly for a reproductive lifetime. The responsibility is his to educate, to diagnose, to treat or refer for more expert treatment all his patients, including those using contraception, whether their complaints are due to, associated with, or quite independent of their contraceptive activity. Contraception is, or should be, part of general practice, and this is the theme that runs through this book.

The purists among you may point out that abortion and sterilization are not contraception, and I must agree. They are closely related parts of general practice, however, and of increasing importance today.

Others may point out that the chapter on oral contraception is of disproportionate length. This is as it should be since general practitioners spend more time dealing with patients using oral contraceptives than with those using all other methods put together. Patients question their family doctors very closely as to the effects of the Pill, on themselves and on their relatives and friends. They want to know whether their symptoms could be caused by, exacerbated by or associated with the Pill. They want to check with him the accuracy of reports heard on the radio or television, or of pieces read in women's magazines.

In his turn, the family doctor requires to be very well informed about oral contraception. Women asking to be put on the Pill may have suffered, be suffering, or will suffer while taking it, from any disease in the medical dictionary. The literature relating to oral contraception is now vast: the general practitioner must be able to look up 'The Pill and . . .' rapidly. Hence the section of the index so entitled. On the other hand, the Pill is only one of our contraceptive tools, and in any discussion on the more general aspects of contraception will often require mention. Thus it is inevitable that there is some repetition in this book. I have made little effort to avoid this since I know that the busy family doctor rarely has time to read a book from start to finish. He is more likely to take repeated dips. The repetition may ensure that a particular dip is fruitful.

To some extent therefore, this is intended as a reference book for general practitioners. Most references quoted are to books and journals to which most family doctors will have easy access. Nevertheless it is also intended as a book that can be read: I have eschewed long words, and embraced short ones. This is the only time the word obviate appears on these pages; the typical phraseology of the medical paper is underemployed in these chapters.

This is a time of rapid development in contraceptive matters. Advances in contraceptive knowledge are reported with every issue of the relevant journals. I must apologize if, by the time this book appears in print, some of it is outdated. The reorganization of the National Health Service will bring changes in the administration and delivery of contraceptive services to the community. I am in no doubt as to the part that family doctors should play. Whether they will be enabled to play that part, or whether they will wish to do so, remains, at the time of writing, unclear.

My book owes a great deal to others. I am most grateful to Julian Elias, Research Fellow in Obstetrics and Gynaecology at King's College Hospital Medical School. I am no surgeon, and by kindly reading the sections on intrauterine devices, abortion and sterilization he has enabled me to avoid saying the wrong thing surgically. John McEwan, formerly a general practitioner, but now also a consultant and lecturer in Family Planning at the same hospital, I have been privileged to know for many years. Much of what I have written is the result of argument and discussion with him, and from him I have learnt much. As though this were not generosity enough, he agreed to read the remaining parts of the book and his comments were invaluable.

Finally, without the help of my most patient and long-suffering secretary, June Heron, my scribbles, erasures and alterations would never have progressed to print.

LESLIE OLDERSHAW
London, June 1974

1

THE NEED FOR PLANNING FAMILIES

The need to control the numbers of human beings on this Earth can be looked at from three different but related viewpoints; from the point of view of the individual, when the words 'family planning' are most appropriate; from a national viewpoint, and from an international or worldwide aspect, when the term population control is more appropriate.

FAMILY PLANNING AT INDIVIDUAL LEVEL

Some young people who marry do not want children, ever. There are not many such, but they are helping to overcome the population problem and should be helped by contraceptive advice to avoid pregnancy. Society tends to look askance at such people; to regard them as selfish or peculiar. Unusual they may be, but selfish they are not, and society must change its view.

The majority of young people, however, do want children and, by giving them contraceptive advice, they can be helped to achieve the family size they want, starting their first pregnancy when they wish and spacing their children to their satisfaction.

The timing of the arrival of the first baby may have a very important effect on the quality of the married life of a family, both as regards material possessions, and loving relationships within the family. To acquire a baby before acquiring a home puts the family at an obvious disadvantage. In today's economic conditions, it may be essential that the wife continue to earn for the first few years of married life, but this may be impossible if she becomes pregnant and then has a small child to look after.

The change in the relationship between husband and wife as the result of the arrival of a baby should be for the better, but every family doctor has seen the unfortunate, sometimes disastrous, effect that too early arrival can have. The smart, well-dressed, bright-eyed and cheerful girl may become a hopeless, sullen, nagging drab within the space of a year, and a similar change affects the husband. Because of the baby, the parents have had to accept the first accommodation they could get, possibly living with in-laws.

Living expenses plus the expenses of the baby mean that a vicious circle is created, preventing saving and preventing a move to more suitable accommodation.

They have their name down on the waiting list for local authority housing, but in many areas both the list and the wait is long enough for a host of babies to arrive. Whereas before marriage the couple used to go out together quite frequently they now find the baby prevents this. In former days the wife's mother often looked after the baby on such occasions or while the young wife went to work. Today many older women are at work themselves and anyway 'Mum' may not be near enough to help even if she wished. The husband starts to spend less time at home and more at the pub, and marital disharmony ensues, possibly followed by marital breakdown.

Under these circumstances the baby becomes resented and lacks affection, if not actually neglected or ill-treated, with sequelae, both physical and psychiatric, which last into adult life.

The arrival of further children in quick succession results in a situation that defeats the couple absolutely and condems them to continue in their drab existence, a form of tyranny indeed.

It was freedom from this tyranny of excessive fertility that Sir Dugald Baird had in mind when he advocated a 'Fifth Freedom' in 1965. Freedom from want, from fear, of speech and of worship were the four freedoms for the brave new world envisaged by Franklin D. Roosevelt in 1941.

INFLUENCE OF SOCIAL CLASS

The effects of the tyranny of excessive fertility are least marked in those classified by the Registrar General as belonging to Social Class I and progressively more marked in each succeeding class, reaching a maximum in Social Class V.

People who will suffer most are likely to be those who come from large families have had a poor education, leaving school as early as legally possible, and have then taken dull and repetitive jobs with little or no job satisfaction and low wages.

They tend to marry at an early age, and their knowledge of birth control methods is little or none. If birth control is practised, it tends to be of the least reliable kind, and even then may be practised incorrectly or inefficiently.

THE OLDER WOMAN

Although the problems of the newly married couple are great, this does not mean that excessive fertility may not pose problems for couples who have been married for some years. It is essential that people who have had the number of children they desire should be able to avoid further pregnancies, because if another pregnancy does occur it is often unwanted and abortion is sought.

Apart from the actual occurrence of an unexpected, unplanned and unwanted pregnancy, there is also the worry for the woman that intercourse *may* result in pregnancy. This fear may result in an anxiety state, bringing her to the family doctor complaining of symptoms, often, but not always, related to the genital tract. Her fear of the result of sexual intercourse may produce a revulsion of feeling against the act, and even against her husband, so that sexual problems such as dyspareunia and frigidity may develop in the woman and impotence in the man.

A general practitioner in 1965 suggested that this syndrome be called the 'Sadder syndrome', the name being formed from the initial letters of its cause - 'Sex as a duty due to excessive reproduction'. It is important that family doctors are on the look-out for this syndrome, together with the anxiety and depression it can cause, since it can be cured by efficient contraception.

The social class of the family has a bearing on the problem, in that women of higher social class groups will tend to be using a more effective method than women in the lower groups. But where the extra burden of another child will be seen by the wife of a labourer as mainly financial, with the extra drudgery of household chores, it will appear differently to a woman who, having completed her planned family, has returned to a busy professional or business life. The disruption that an unplanned pregnancy, and the care of the young child will bring to this woman's life, though different in kind, will be just as distressing in degree as for her sister in Social Class V.

The age of the couple certainly does have a bearing since, in general, the older the couple are the less likely are they to welcome the prospect of an unplanned pregnancy, and the more likely it is for termination to be requested. As both pregnancy and termination become more dangerous with age, and there is an increased incidence of such conditions as mongolism in the children of older mothers, contraception has a special importance in the woman over thirty-five.

EFFECT ON THE COMMUNITY

Unplanned and unwanted pregnancies result in problems for the community. Before the Abortion Act one could point to the expense of looking after unwanted babies in homes and orphanages. Since the Act, however, the demand for normal babies for adoption greatly exceeds the supply. It is still difficult to find parents willing to adopt abnormal babies or babies of racially mixed parentage, and the cost of rearing these must be borne by the community.

Unwanted children may not be put up for adoption even though the mother does not wish, or is not able, to care for them. The community has to produce foster parents to look after these children.

Abortion, though eliminating the necessity to consider these problems, brings other problems to the community. Facilities must be provided for the operations; resources, professional and economic, must be diverted.

Without considering the general subject of population growth, which is dealt with in the next section, the purely local effects on a highly industrialised community such as Great Britain of the addition of large numbers of unwanted babies will mean, over the years, more housing needed, more urban sprawl, more roads, less countryside. More people will mean more pollution, more waste to be disposed of.

So far these problems have been considered in a cold and materialistic fashion. There is also of course the emotional side to be considered. The unhappiness of the mother of the unplanned pregnancy has already been mentioned. The unhappiness of the unwanted child must not be forgotten. Even the unhappiness of the gynaecologists and nursing staff who find themselves involved in performing operations that they find distasteful is a factor to remember in assessing the effect on the community of unplanned and unwanted pregnancy.

It is estimated that there are 300,000 unplanned pregnancies in Britain each year.

THE UNMARRIED

In reality marriage is irrelevant in any consideration of contraception. Pregnancy may occur after intercourse in both the married and unmarried, the widowed or divorced. Nevertheless, until about 1969 there was a very obvious reluctance on the part of those providing contraceptive services to make them available to the unmarried.

The failure of the Family Planning Association to provide advice for the unmarried was largely responsible for the formation of the Brook Centres, who specialised in providing advice to young people, married or unmarried.

Ann Cartwright conducted surveys in general practice in 1967–8, and again in 1970–1, in order to ascertain the attitudes of family doctors to contraception. In the first survey, only 51 per cent of the doctors said that they would raise the question of birth control with an unmarried girl who had already had a baby, whereas by the time of the second survey in 1970–1, the proportion of doctors who said they would do so had risen to 73 per cent.

The passing of the Abortion Act without doubt accelerated the change in the attitude of the medical profession, as doctors, both in general practice and especially in hospital gynaecological practice, began to see contraception as a method of preventing abortion, as well as pregnancy.

It has been said that the most effective contraceptive is the ability to say 'No'. This is undoubtedly true, but the modern woman is unwilling to forgo the pleasures of sexual intercourse unless or until she is married.

From the time of puberty, and even before, the young girl is bombarded with advertising directed at persuading her to buy cosmetics, clothes and beauty accessories, the emphasis in the advertizing being that she should increase her sexual desirability.

The money earned by single women, even very young women in their teens, is today sufficient to enable them to become independent of their parents in a way, and at an age, that was impossible before World War II. Parents, faced with the choice of trying to dictate to their children and risking a quarrel and a possible complete break in the family, or of acquiescing in behaviour that to them seems wrong, often choose to aquiesce and remain friends with their child. Parents are no longer certain what is 'right' or 'wrong': the Church, formerly active in laying down moral laws, now seems much less dogmatic, and the beliefs of the parents are referred to by their children as 'square' or old-fashioned.

The influence of pornography, much emphasized by Lord Longford and Mary Whitehouse, is I believe of little importance to the vast majority of young people who are far more interested in living a full life than looking at pictures or reading books about other people's lives.

Of far greater importance is the tendency for young people to move from the family circle into flats and bed-sitters in the great cities, and the virtual disappearance of the chaperone. It is far easier for two young people to be alone together today than in former times. The motor car, already blamed for polluting and destroying, must also be blamed for providing a 'mobile bed-sitter' where two people may escape chaperones.

All this may be very distressing for the older doctor, who, in common with generations before him, may say that he does not know what the world is coming to.

However, he must face up to the fact that the motor car is unlikely to disappear, young people are unlikely to have reduced earnings in the future - rather the reverse, nor are they likely to remain in the family circle until married.

The facts are that pregnancies occurring in unmarried girls are likely to be unwanted pregnancies, and more likely to end in abortion. Over half the abortions performed in England and Wales in 1971 were of single women, and four-fifths of them had no previous children. Almost all were under 25 years old, and more than two thousand of them were aged under 16.

It would be naive to believe that all these unwanted pregnancies could have been avoided merely by offering contraception: the motivation to use available contraception must also be present. But certainly no unmarried girl should have to run the risk of abortion because she was ignorant of the facts of contraception, or because contraceptive advice and supplies were unavailable.

Pregnancy is a most unsuitable punishment for intercourse before marriage.

2

POPULATION

Man first started to cause trouble on this planet about half a million years ago. For the first few hundred thousand years he led the life of a wandering hunter, killing and being killed by the animals and other men he hunted for food. He sowed not, neither did he reap, and during severe winters starvation and extremes of cold took a heavy toll, especially of the very young, the weak and the old. Despite the ability of each female to produce offspring each year, the birth rate under such conditions resulted in little more than the replacement of deaths, and the population grew very slowly.

Eventually, about 2,000 BC, came the agricultural revolution, when man ceased to be a wanderer and lived in one place long enough to plant crops, benefit from their harvest, and store the excess against the winter. More permanent shelter against the elements was provided by the houses he built in the ground, and animals lived with him, relieving him of the necessity to hunt for his next meal. More of his children survived, and the population grew from about five million at the time he abandoned his nomadic existence to about 150 million at the time of Christ.

Birth rates were high but so were death rates, and the average life expectancy was short, about thirty years, but social organisation into larger and more complex units enabled man to become progressively more free of the tyrrany of nature and the population steadily grew at an increasing rate. By the year 1600 AD, the population was about 500 million, and by 1820 AD the number of people in the world was 1,000 million.

At about this time occurred the second great change in the human way of life, the advent of the industrial revolution. Enormous advances in transport, food supplies and manufactured goods, some spread of wealth from the very few to the relatively many, with progress in science, hygiene and medicine resulted in a lower death rate and a longer life expectancy. The year 1800 also saw a storm created in England by the writings of a Surrey clergyman, Thomas Malthus, whose 'Essay on the Principle of Population' had been published two years previously. In it he propounded the theory that population increased geometrically, whereas the world's food supplies increased only arithmetically, and thus there would of necessity be catastrophes such as famine, pestilence and war which would restrain the world's population within the bounds set by nature.

To some extent he was correct, the population having grown not only geometrically but even exponentially since the first thousand million achieved during his lifetime. The next thousand million was reached a century later, and the third followed less than half a century after that. The fourth has now been attained, and by the year 2,000 it is estimated that there will be seven thousand million people on earth. His forecast that natural catastrophes would check increases has not so far come true. The second World War, in which more than fifty million died, provided only a pause rather than a check.

POPULATION: THE BRITISH EXPERIENCE

In 1700 the population of Great Britain was about seven million. By 1800 it had reached ten million, and about twenty million halfway through the century. The thirty million mark had been passed by the time the twentieth century arrived, and at the time of the latest census in 1971, fiftyfour million people lived on this island. Fortynine million of them lived in England and Wales, giving a population density of 323 people per square kilometre, a density greater than that of any comparable country in the world other than Taiwan (Formosa) and Bangladesh.

The latest official projection is that the population of England and Wales in the year 2,000 will be nearly fiftyfive million. For Great Britain the projected population at the same date is over sixty million, and for the United Kingdom over sixtytwo million.

Some indication of the meaning of these figures can be obtained by the realization that to accommodate the six million extra people expected in England and Wales in the year 2,000, ten cities the size of Liverpool in 1972 would be needed. The whole of Greater London in 1972 housed seven and one-third million people.

POPULATION PROJECTIONS

Care must be taken in the interpretation of the figures of population projections for any given year. They are not forecasts, but are forward assumptions taking into account the trends in population change which have been manifest in past years. These trends may continue but they may not. They may even reverse. Hence, although the projection of a population for a short time ahead will be reasonably accurate, the accuracy becomes progressively less reliable as the time span increases.

For example, basing his projections on trends then evident, the Registrar General stated ten years ago that the population of the United Kingdom would exceed 65 million in 1990. Because of alterations in the trends during the last ten years he has had to alter his forward assumptions, so his projection today is that that population will not in fact be reached until twenty years later, in 2010.

Thus when we consider population projections made in 1973 for the year 2000, embodying the passage of twentyseven years during which many of the assumptions regarding trends may be proved wrong, we must not overestimate their accuracy. Panic is not indicated, but neither is complacency.

POPULATION INCREASE

Excluding immigration and emigration, an increase in population will occur when births outnumber deaths each year. This annual increase when expressed as a percentage of the total population represents the annual population growth.

Population growth has varied at different times in history, and in different parts of the world at the same time. In Europe in the nineteenth century the population grew at an annual rate of one-half of one per cent. In the early part of the twentieth century, the rate had increased to one per cent, and today is about two per cent. Population growth rates are higher in developing countries, such as in Africa, Asia and South America, reaching figures of three or even four per cent per annum. By contrast, highly industrialised societies, such as England and Wales, have much lower rates around a half of one per cent.

Because these rates refer to people, who will in their turn reproduce, they are in terms of compound rather than simple interest. With today's high interest rates in the money market, interest rates of two or three per cent seem trivial, but in terms of compound interest the sums involved become enormous. One new penny invested at one per cent per annum compound in the year 0 AD would by 2,000 AD be worth over ten million pounds. Two people alive in in the year 0 AD and increasing by two per cent per annum compound would today number two hundred million billion.

Population growth rates, especially if they increase year by year, of one or two per cent, when applied to millions of people over many years are thus far from insignificant. A one per cent annual increase in the present world population represents one hundred thousand extra new arrivals each day.

Finally we must bear in mind that we are already too late to make plans to reduce growth rates for the next fifteen to twenty years. The babies who will mature over these years to produce the population increases have already been born.

BIRTH RATES

Birth rates are high in undeveloped countries and decrease as an industrialised society supervenes. Rates of thirty or forty per thousand are found among populations in South America and Asia, as opposed to rates of less than twenty in European industrialised nations.

There is always some delay between the emergence of a developing nation and the reduction of its birth rate. Improvements in infant mortality and disease control tend to occur first, and it is during this dangerous interval that explosion is apt to occur.

In England and Wales the birth rate fell from rates of between thirty and forty per thousand births in the years before 1850 to below thirty by 1900 and below twenty by 1950. It thus took a whole century for the birth rate to fall after industrialization in Britain. We cannot afford to wait a century for similar effects to appear in nations developing today.

A falling birth rate does not mean that a population is decreasing, since there may still be an annual excess of births over deaths. Neither does a fall in the birth rate indicate a permanent reduction in the rate of population growth, since it may be due to couples delaying the start of their family. Such a situation was seen during World War II, when birth rates fell to as low as 13.9 only to rise to 19.2 per thousand in 1946.

MORTALITY RATES

Between 1700 and 1900, the infant mortality rate in England and Wales fell from over 200 per thousand to 150 per thousand and then decreased during the present century to about 20 per thousand.

Maternal mortality declined in a similarly dramatic fashion, falling to about 20 per 100,000 pregnancies. Perinatal deaths, that is stillbirths and deaths in the first week of life, have dropped to about 20 per thousand.

The medical profession cannot take credit for the whole of this reduction, for improvements in nutrition and stature, in living conditions and in education, have played a large part.

As a result, more mothers survive childbirth to bear more children and more of the children survive to live through the whole of their adult reproductive life. Improvements in life expectancy at the end of life have little effect on population growth. To increase the proportion of octogenarians in the world certainly brings difficulty to the community, but not because of their reproductive capacity.

EFFECT OF MEDICINE AND SCIENCE

Doctors were able to do very little in the prevention and cure of the killing diseases until the partnership with scientists began in the twentieth century. The growing knowledge of the causes of disease, combined with the development of methods of attack on these causes as well as the treatment of people suffering from disease, has altered the expectation of life of literally millions of people on earth.

Examples of diseases whose effects have been markedly reduced are malaria, bubonic plague, yellow fever, smallpox, typhoid and trypanosomiasis. Malaria is a particularly good example to consider because the attack on this disease demonstrates the interlocking nature of the contribution of the scientist and the medical man, and the way in which the elimination of one disease can result in the emergence of other side-effects - although disasters would probably be a better word.

The invention of DDT provided the means to anihilate the anopheles mosquito which carried the malarial parasite. This function is served well, but as a secondary effect DDT has been found to be a cause of death in birds, whose prey have absorbed relatively large amounts of the chemical.

The formulation of powerful, relatively cheap, antimalarial drugs enabled the disease to be treated in humans. The malarial parasite could therefore be eliminated in both the host and the vector, and at the end of World War II antimalarial campaigns based on spraying with DDT and the identification and treatment of people with malaria were started in various parts of the world.

The island of Mauritius was the site of one such campaign. Starting in 1946, every effort was made to eliminate malaria and by 1948 success had been achieved.

Ten years later, the removal of malaria as a cause of death had resulted in a drop in the infant mortality rate from 150 to 50 per thousand live births, together with a reduction in the death rate from 28 to 10 per thousand, and the population rose by 40 per cent. Mauritius is a relatively small island, and this increase in population resulted in a population density of more than 1,000 people to the square mile, compared with a density of population in England and Wales in 1967 of 828. The lack of housing and employment in a relatively non-industrial country like Mauritius resulted in much misery and unhappiness, culminating in riots and bloodshed.

Such were the unexpected results of removing one of the scourges of mankind. The infant mortality rate fell suddenly in Mauritius mainly due to removal of a disease, but physicians in Europe have been striving to reduce it over a much longer period.

FAMILY SIZE

Another factor influencing population growth is the size of family desired by couples within the population. Once parents are satisfied that they do not have to produce many children in order that few may survive, economic and social factors play a more important part. In the years before World War II, small families were the rule. The parents remembered the effects of the depression, and felt that small families, well-cared for and well-educated, stood a better chance of 'getting on' in later life.

In order to produce zero population growth in England and Wales an average family size of 2.1 children is required. At the moment average family size only slightly exceeds this figure, but there are indications that with increasing prosperity more people consider that more than two children make an ideal family.

SEX RATIOS IN THE POPULATION

More girls are born than boys, but mortality is greater at all ages among males, and so women outnumber men in old age. Improvements in mortality rates have resulted in more males surviving to reproductive age, so that women do not now outnumber men in England and Wales until the age of 35 is reached. The average age at marriage for women is 22, so fewer women are 'left on the shelf' than in former decades and a higher proportion of the women in the population are starting families.

AGE STRUCTURE OF A POPULATION

Diagrams of the age distribution within a population may be constructed, demonstrating the relative numbers of males and females in each age group. Because of their shape, these diagrams are known as 'population pyramids'.

Figure 1 is a pyramid constructed for an imaginary population at an early stage of development. Large numbers of infants are produced but high death rates at all ages result in few surviving to adult life and few reaching old age.

Figure 2 represents an artificial situation where improvements in mortality at all ages are accompanied by no restriction of births. This population will steadily expand, and although more people will reach old age, the main increase is seen among the lower age groups. This is the sort of picture seen in developing countries where insignificant attempts have been made to introduce anti-natal activity.

Figure 3 demonstrates the sort of pyramid resulting from improvements in mortality being balanced by a restriction of births, and is representative of the type of population pyramid seen in advanced countries of the Western World.

It should be noticed that there are dangers at both ends of the scale. A population as indicated in Fig. 1 will be an exploding population with all the disadvantages listed later in this chapter. However, progression further than the situation shown in Fig. 3 will result in a declining population where births

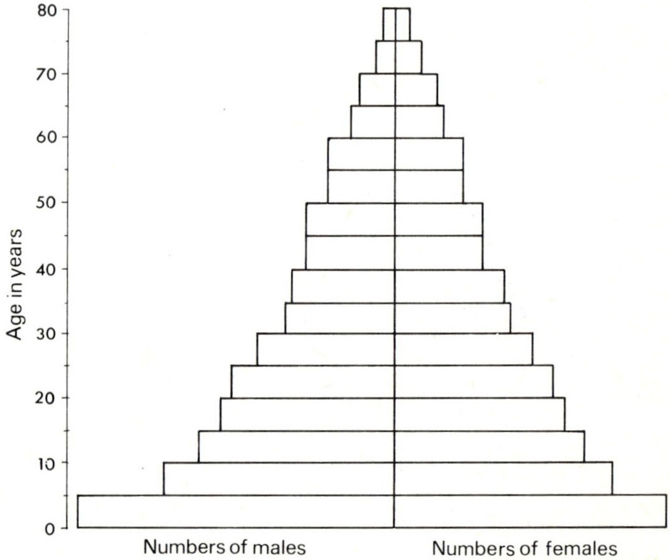

Fig 1.

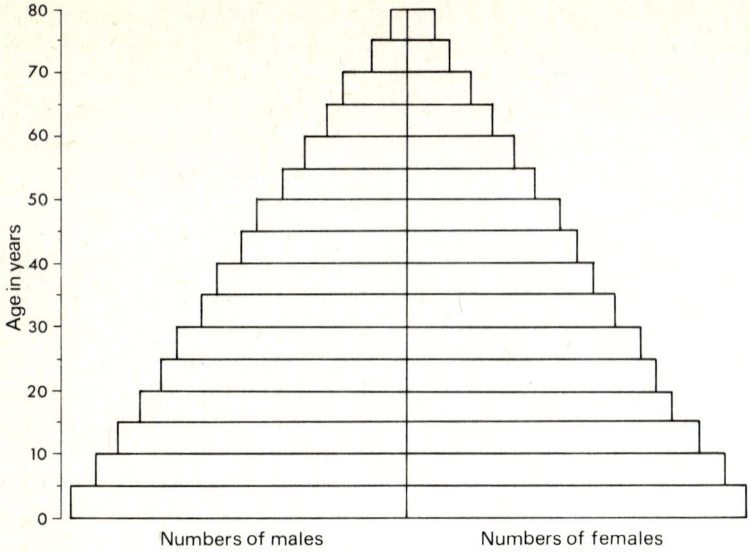
80
70
60
50
40
30
20
10
0
Age in years
Numbers of males
Numbers of females

Fig. 2.

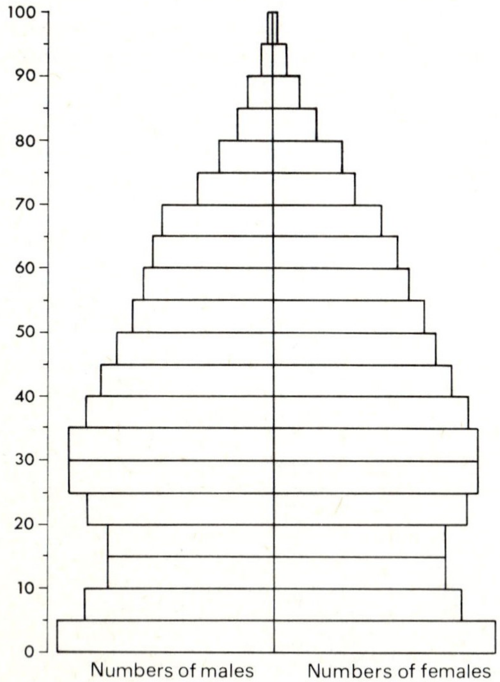
100
90
80
70
60
50
40
30
20
10
0
Numbers of males
Numbers of females

Fig. 3.

are insufficient to replace deaths. The result will be that the proportion of old people in the population will increase. The economic prosperity of a country depends in part on the presence of a working population of adequate size to support those at the extremes of life who do not produce goods or services. Where the numbers of old people greatly outnumber those of working age very great difficulties result, both in the care of the aged and in the ability of the working population to pay for that care.

Hence it is important that in any consideration of population and its growth, the importance of the maintenance of a balance between age groups within a population should be remembered. The birth rate in Britain fell to 14.7 in the first quarter of 1973, and fears were expressed that the balance had been lost and a declining population had arrived.

Rates for one quarter have little significance, of course, but a continuing steady decline in rates quarter after quarter would be quite a different matter.

However, as already indicated, it would seem that the problem of increasing rates is far more likely to be at the root of any population problems we may have in the near future.

RESULTS OF OVER-POPULATION

Too many people mean too little of the world's resources to go round: too little food, too little fuel to produce energy, too little of the raw materials needed to produce manufactured goods. A steadily increasing world population brings increasingly nearer the day when world supplies of commodities such as oil will be exhausted.

More and more people to house means more and more of the world's surface disappearing beneath concrete: more houses, more roads, more urban sprawl. About 60,000 acres of the United Kingdom are covered by building each year. More people mean more pollution, in the ground, in the sea and in the air. Present shortages of schools, hospitals and other services will be aggravated.

Great increases in population in countries still in the emergent stage result in more poverty, more disease. Shanty towns outside Calcutta and in South America stand as ghastly warnings of possibilities to come.

Finally, vast increases in the numbers of human beings result in a reduction of the wild untamed jungles and plains of the world, and decimation and eventual extinction of the animals who live in them. Eight hundred species of animals and birds are today in danger of disappearing. Already one species becomes extinct each year.

The world is rushing towards its own destruction.

So speak the Prophets of Doom. In reply, others point to the fact that the earth is underpopulated in parts: only Man's habit of congregating in large numbers in small areas makes for difficulty. South-Eastern England may be full, but Scotland is almost empty. Food is plentiful and could be more so if advances in technology were universally applied, transport improved and waste eliminated. Raw materials there are aplenty, but are largely used inefficiently and wasted. Pollution is partly a further result of waste and inefficiency and future developments in technology will control it. Energy will be produced by other means, from atomic sources, from the sun, from the centre of the earth.

Poverty and disease in some parts of the world are more the results of unequal distribution of wealth and resources than of overpopulation. One-fifth of the world's population - the developed countries - use and waste four-fifths of the world's natural resources.. Animals are of lesser importance than human beings but, in any case, extinction of wild animals may be avoided by careful animal conservation in selected areas.

And what of the planets? Man may find vast areas of land elsewhere in the universe to colonise.

So speak those who deny the very existence of a population problem. The year AD 2,000 will witness who was right and who was wrong, but it would seem reasonable meanwhile to attempt to avoid accelerating the present rates of population growth.

REMEDIES

This thumbnail sketch of the problem of population growth demonstrates that there are many causes of the phenomenon, and consequently it is reasonable to assume that there may be several ways of counteracting these causes.

1. By increasing mortality rates of children and adults

No sane person would put this forward as a solution, but as a matter of interest, the only person who seriously attempted this method, and who was generally considered to be insane, Adolf Hitler, ran into enormous difficulties in the disposal of the bodies. Students of the macabre are referred to the book 'Treblinka' where the initial experiments were performed which eventually led to the construction of the gas chambers at Auschwitz. Even this madman's efforts removed a number of human beings equivalent only to one month's population increase at today's rate of growth.

2. By increasing mortality rates before birth (abortion)

Abortion has been used in some countries as a method to prevent population growth, the two recent outstanding examples being Hungary and Japan.

Any Hungarian woman in the first trimester of pregnancy may demand abortion, and her doctor may not refuse her. Abortions exceeded births as a result, and the birth rate sank to very low levels.

In Japan in 1948 the Eugenic Protection Law liberalised abortion and over one million abortions annually followed.

Abortion can therefore make a very real impact on population growth. However, religious opposition, especially from the Roman Catholic Church, to the taking of human life, no matter how early, has limited the use of abortion as a method of population control. The safety of the operation, in terms of morbidity as well as mortality, is still being evaluated; the subject is considered in more detail later.

3. **By decreasing conception rates (contraception)**
Both abortion and contraception share the advantage of limiting population growth at the beginning of life, before reproductive activity is reached.

Although contraception does not involve the taking of life, the Roman Catholic Church forbids its followers to use it. Fortunately, other religious denominations do not hold the same view and contraception has been hailed almost universally during the past decade as the solution to the population explosion.

As might be expected with a problem having so many facets, no single solution is likely to effect a complete cure, and it is at last being realised that, on a voluntary basis at any rate, contraception is an ameliorative rather than a cure. Countries which have promoted active contraceptive campaigns using the modern effectve methods best suited to the particular circumstances of the country have been able to show at best a reduction in the rate of population growth, and at worst an actual increase in rate as the population became more prosperous.

4. **By artificial social and economic pressures**
At the moment highly parous women receive admiration, nulliparous women sympathy. This was well brought out on a British radio programme in 1973 when Lady Longford's statement that her grandchildren were now numbered in double figures received huge applause; Malcolm Muggeridge could claim almost double figures and received only slightly less, whereas Robin Ray confessed to no children at all and received no applause at all.

At the moment those who produce large numbers of children receive financial assistance both for the expenses of pregnancy and of confinement, and for more than a decade of the child's life, although those who produce only one child receive less.

In the interests of obtaining a reduction in population growth a reversal is needed. It has been suggested that the production of large families should be regarded as socially irresponsible and undesirable. I think this is unlikely ever to come to pass in a human situation, but I see no reason why those who choose to have large families should be subsidised. Abolition of the allowance for all children after the first, and abolition of the favourable income tax situation for those with children would remove the subsidy now given to population growth. Social security benefits should be available to all needing financial help, without regard to parity.

Such alterations would need a degree of political bravery that is unlikely in the near future, judging from the slowness with which successive British governments have come to realize the necessity for adequate contraceptive services for the population.

However, the appointment in 1973 of the Lord President of the Council, Mr James Prior, as the minister with a special responsibility for population problems, was at least a step in the right direction.

5. **By sterilization**

Voluntary sterilization has limitations in the field of the control of population, since volunteers will come mainly from the group who have already produced children. Nevertheless, as a means of preventing unplanned and unwanted pregnancy it has a definite contribution to make. Perhaps its greatest disadvantage is that at the present time only surgical methods of sterilization are possible which means that where surgical skills are in short supply, as obtains in undeveloped and developing countries where population growth is at its greatest, this method can be little used. In any event, when talking in terms of millions of operations needed every year, only the richest of countries can even think of affording the cost.

The logistics of the problem are daunting, to say the least. The Indian government suggested sterilization of all men who had three or more children. Parkes (1967) calculated that forty million vasectomies would be needed, requiring a thousand surgeons doing twenty vasectomies a day, five days a week, for eight years, by which time there would be more millions who had produced three thildren during those eight years.

Nevertheless, it must be admitted that India has made a gallant attempt to attain her objective. By 1972, eleven million voluntary sterilizations had been performed. The development of more modern, and more rapid operative methods had made possible the performance of four million vasectomies in 1971 and 1972. The gift of transistor radios to volunteers was a method of persuasion well reported throughout the world.

Brazil may be taken as an example of the difficulties in some countries in providing any form of population control requiring medical supervision, whether contraception, abortion or sterilization. In this land of over ninety million inhabitants there is one province containing more than one-and-a-half million people, served only by fifteen doctors. Schoolteachers, of whom there are ten thousand, are being instructed in contraception so that basic information may be given to the inhabitants, but any question of a programme of sterilization to control population is obviously out of the question.

SHOULD ACTION BE TAKEN?

If no action is taken, it would seem that mankind can look forward to an end to civilization on this planet, as at present constituted.The old order will be swept away, since the differing rates of population growth existing among advanced societies and developing nations will result in an enormous increase in population of the latter, with the former becoming relatively fewer and fewer.

Under such circumstances it is possible that famine, flood and war together may result in effective reductions of world populations, especially if nuclear war supervenes. Without this horror, modern conventional warfare does not seem enough. The effects of World War II have already been quoted. In more recent times Bangladesh is a country that has suffered more than its fair share of flood, famine and conventional war, but its population continues to grow at an accelerating rate.

Apart from the solution of nuclear war, it is of course always possible that some dreadful killing pandemic will sweep the world, destroying by the thousands of millions, as the Black Death did in proportionately smaller numbers during the fourteenth century.

Such cures would surely be as bad as the disease, and all possible steps should be taken now to reduce population growth.

WHAT ACTION SHOULD BE TAKEN?

The first line of defence must be education: of governments to persuade them to initiate and carry through planned population policies: of individuals to persuade them that uncontrolled fertility is more vice than virtue, that unplanned and especially unwanted pregnancy is an avoidable tragedy, and to teach them how to use effective methods of contraception and, even more important, to persuade them to make use of such methods.

Education and contraception together constitute the first two lines of defence against excessive population growth. At the moment world-wide education is lacking, our contraceptive methods are not infallible, and we know little of the reasons prompting failure to use them among people who have the knowledge, so abortion must be used as a third line of defence. Sterilization makes a useful fourth in the antinatal partnership.

Changes in social attitudes to sexual responsibility and to fertility, together with economic sanctions rather than rewards in developed countries, may also be promoted as defence mechanisms.

Finally, research to find new and better methods of fertility control, safe medical methods of sterilization and abortion, and new ways in which such methods can be applied in the population at large without the necessity for expensive medical supervision, may allow the human population to turn its own defeat into victory.

Examples of two ways in which the problem may be tackled come from opposite sides of the world, from China and from Aberdeen.

Chinese People's Republic

An interesting example of the way in which the population increase can be contained is provided by Mainland China - with the reservation that no national statistics are available, and conclusions must be drawn from reports culled from localized areas, mostly urban. Probably in the rural areas, different conditions exist.

During the last twenty years the omnipotent government has mounted an attack on each of the aspects of population growth. The minimum legal age for marriage has been raised to 18 years for girls and 20 years for men. At the same time premarital intercourse has been discouraged by making fornication a criminal offence, all the brothels have been closed, and chastity until the age of 25 hailed as a virtue. An intensive campaign has been mounted, using minimally trained non-medical personnel - 'barefoot doctors' - to issue condoms, initiate oral contraception and insert intrauterine devices. Both male and female sterilization are readily available for suitable applicants. Backed up by a liberal abortion law to deal with contraceptive failure, these policies have resulted, in large cities, in a reported crude birth rate of only 7 per thousand, well below the replacement rate (Potts, 1972; Geiger, 1973).

The Aberdeen Experience

An historic paper, entitled 'A Fifth Freedom' was published in 1965. The author, Sir Dugald Baird, Regius Professor of Obstetrics and Gynaecology at the University of Aberdeen, suggested that in addition to the four essential freedoms listed by F. D. Roosevelt in 1941 - of speech, of worship, from want, and from fear - a fifth freedom should be considered, freedom from the tyranny of excessive fertility.

In order to achieve this freedom for the people of Aberdeen all available methods of fertility control have been used. In 1946, twentyfive years before similar action in London, the local authority took over the provision of family planning clinics from the voluntary organizations. In 1966 free supplies were made available for married woman, and in 1968 for the unmarried as well.

Associated with the increase in the availability of contraceptive advice and supplies, was a more liberal attitude on the part of the consultant gynaecologists in Aberdeen towards abortion. Between 1961 and 1963, 203 terminations of pregnancy were performed, and by 1970 there were more than 500 terminations annually.

A greater willingness to sterilize women who had completed their families accompanied contraception and abortion in this three-pronged attack on the 'tyranny of excessive fertility'.

The results have been impressive. Sterilization after desired family size has been reached has resulted in fewer high-risk pregnancies and has contributed to the excellent maternal mortality figures. There were no maternal deaths at all in either 1969 or 1970. Infant mortality has also shown a satisfactory reduction over the years, reaching 12.3 per thousand in 1971, similar to the lowest rates in the world, in Holland and Sweden. Again, at least in part, this low rate reflects the fact that mothers are younger and healthier, due to removal of high-risk pregnancies, the pregnancies are mostly planned and the babies wanted.

Finally, the annual excess of births over deaths in the city has been halved over the decade from 1960 to 1970, approximately twice the reduction of the excess achieved over the same years in England and Wales (Birth Control Campaign, 1973).

THE ROLE OF THE INDIVIDUAL DOCTOR

No doctor may regard his education as adequate unless it includes a rudimentary knowledge of the population problems affecting the world in general and this country in particular.

He must accept that medicine has been and continues to be responsible, at least in part, for some of the problems facing us today, and he must therefore accept some responsibility in the attempt to solve those problems. He thus has a duty to the community.

On the other hand, the doctor's prime duty is the care of individuals. The needs of the patient come first, and no doctor should allow himself to be used by the community as an instrument of population control against the wish of the individual patient.

Finally, each doctor has a responsibility towards his own self-respect, to his own religious and moral beliefs. He must allow neither the community nor his patients to deflect him from his principles. At the same time he must not allow his principles to prevent his acquisition of knowledge of modern methods of fertility control, nor to deprive his patients of access to these methods from sources other than himself.

Few of us are gynaecologists and can perform the surgical procedures involved, but all of us who deal with patients are in a position to help them in the achievement of their desired family size, and no more. We can help our patients to avoid unplanned and unwanted pregnancies and to this end must have a basic knowledge of modern methods of contraception, abortion and sterilization, with a rudimentary knowledge of the sociological background of each, and an awareness of their practical limitations.

REFERENCES

BAIRD, D. (1965). A Fifth Freedom? *British Medical Journal*, **2**, 1141.

BIRTH CONTROL CAMPAIGN (1973). *The Benefits of Birth Control - Aberdeen's Experience 1964-1970*. Birth Control Campaign, London.

GEIGER, J. (1973). Behind the Bamboo Curtain. *World Medicine*, July 25.

PARKES, A. S. (1967). Can India Do It? *New Scientist*, **35**, 555, 186.

POTTS, M. (1972). in *New Concepts in Contraception*. ed. M. Potts and C. Wood. Medical & Technical Publishing, Oxford and Lancaster.

3

CONTRACEPTION AND THE GENERAL PRACTITIONER

I have deliberately chosen the word contraception rather than family planning for the title of this chapter. Certainly the family doctor will help his patients to plan their families, but the major portion of his time will be spent helping his patients to avoid pregnancy altogether. Even contraception is the wrong word, since abortion and sterilization are subjects with which the general practitioner, on behalf of his patients, must concern himself.

Population control is not part of the role of the family doctor, for two reasons. Firstly, the impact that one doctor can make on world population problems is minute, and it is the world problems which are most worrying. The second, and most important reason, is that the primary role of the family doctor is to help his patient. If a couple wish for ten children, then it is the duty of their doctor to help them achieve that number, and any feelings he may have concerning a family of that size in relation to his knowledge of overpopulation must be rigorously suppressed.

However, he can console himself with the thought that by preventing all the unplanned pregnancies that may otherwise have occurred in his practice, he is contributing his widow's mite towards solving at least the problems of the United Kingdom.

THE BRITISH SITUATION

Most women wish to obtain contraceptive advice from their family doctor, and most women do. Despite the noise made by the Family Planning Association and their thousand clinics, two recent studies have confirmed the importance of the general practitioner in this field. Dr Margaret Bone, of the Social Survey Division of the Office of Population, Censuses and Surveys interviewed 3,500 women in England and Wales in 1970, and reported that 62 per cent of them had used or would use their GP, as opposed to only 40 per cent who preferred clinics. In 1972, Dr Mary Brennan offered a multiple choice of sources of contraceptive advice to 1,000 women living in Coventry. The choice included 10 variants of family doctor, neighbourhood health clinic, special family planning clinic, health visitor and the like; almost half the patients chose the two family doctor variants, i.e. either at his surgery or their home.

There is thus a great demand by patients for their GP to provide contraceptive advice and services, and the fact that in 1971 it was estimated that GPs were providing such services to more patients than all other agencies combined shows that family doctors were attempting to satisfy the demand. And this despite competition from local authorities and the Family Planning Association who were providing free advice and supplies which were either free or greatly reduced in price. At the same time, the family doctor was prevented from providing contraceptive supplies on National Health Service prescription and received no payment from the NHS for his services.

In many ways it may be argued that the contraceptive services in this country have been subsidized by the family doctors and their poorer patients, since both reports quoted found that Family Planning Clinics are more favoured by patients of social Classes I and II, and local authority clinics and family doctors by patients of social Classes III, IV and V. Since social Classes III, IV and V are less able to pay for advice and supplies, both reports highlight the mistake of authority in appointing the FPA as their agent in many areas and ignoring the family doctor.

However, before we GPs congratulate ourselves on doing a grand job, we must consider some less favourable findings. Women in Coventry were asked to give four sources from which they had obtained information about contraception. Only 5 per cent had obtained it from the FPA, only 3 per cent from local authority clinics, only 20 per cent from the GP, and 66 per cent from reading, radio, television, family or friends. There is therefore a great need for the family doctor to increase the amount of contraceptive education he gives his patients, and ways in which he can do this are discussed later in this chapter.

Patients felt that GPs did not give enough time to their problems, a feeling that is shared by their family doctors, and in relation to fields other than contraception as well.

Thirty-eight per cent of the women who had not been to their family doctor for contraceptive advice averred that they felt he would show a lack of sympathy for their problems.

Ninety-three per cent of the patients said their GP was male, and some of them found this inhibiting in discussion of contraception.

Since the majority of us are unable to change our sex, it behoves us to attempt to get over to our female patients our willingness to discuss contraception, and our sympathy with their problems.

THE ROLE OF THE FAMILY DOCTOR

The role of the family doctor in ante-natal activity may be considered under the following headings.

EDUCATION - using the word in its widest sense.

1. **Formal sex education in schools**

Some general practitioners, with the skill and the time, may be able to play a part in lecturing to children in secondary schools. All general practitioners can help to encourage the development of such education in their practice area, and can emphasize the need for the children to be taught not only about sex, but about contraception as well. The fact that such education is badly needed is confirmed by the Registrar General's figures for 1971 which showed that over two thousand girls under sixteen underwent abortion in that year - three being aged only eleven.

2. **Education of patients**

Every contact between a patient, of either sex and at any age, and the family doctor is an opportunity for the doctor to educate the patient. The education may concern any aspect of health - smoking, exercise, and eating are three obvious examples. Education about sex and contraception is another aspect that the GP is well placed to deal with.

3. **Education of the general practitioner**

If the GP should make every effort to educate his patients concerning contraception, it is even more necessary that he should ensure his own adequate and continuing education in this field. In past years the training of medical students has been singularly devoid of any instruction: more recently improvements have taken place and most newly qualified doctors have received some tuition in the subject.

It is to be hoped that every general practitioner will be able to attend courses and seminars and obtain practical experience of the various methods by attending teaching sessions. This education should be provided within the National Health Service, with the co-operation of the Royal College of Obstetricians and Gynaecologists, the Royal College of General Practitioners and the Universities.

As well as education relating to knowledge and experience, the GP must educate himself at an emotional level. He must accept that his code of morality may be twenty years out of date in the opinion of his teenage patients. This is not to admit that they are right and he is wrong. The fact is that the patients are the people at risk of unwanted pregnancy, not the doctor - or usually not the doctor. He should not withhold his advice on contraception because he disapproves of the life style of the patient, any more than he would refuse any other type of medical assistance because of his disapproval of the patient's behaviour.

4. **Moral education of patients**

Should the family doctor attempt to educate his patients into the paths of moral rectitude? I think not. I want my patients to come to me for advice without fear of disapproval, or in the expectation of receiving the type of lecture sometimes known as 'a pious jaw'. Anticipation of such a reaction may drive them to seek advice elsewhere or, even worse, not seek any advice at all.

Should a patient indicate that advice on moral questions would be acceptable, then an entirely different situation exists, and the family doctor should not withhold his counsel.

What should be attempted is to instil a sense of sexual responsibility into the patient: to help them to realise that sexual intercourse without consideration of the possible consequences, in terms of unwanted pregnancy or disease, is both immature and foolish, and undesirable both from the point of view of the individual and that of the community.

It would obviously be ridiculous for this subject to be raised at all interviews with all patients, but there are certain situations, and certain types of patient, when to mention it becomes both easy and imperative. Some of these are listed in Table I.

Table I—Situations and types of patient where mention of contraception by the family doctor is both easy and imperative.

Pregnancy and the puerperium.	The new patient.
Post-natal examination.	The adolescent girl.
Abortion—spontaneous or induced.	The adolescent boy.
'Scare' of pregnancy.	The woman with small children.
Gynaecological complaints and sexual problems.	The woman with an anxiety state.

PREGNANCY AND AFTERWARDS

During pregnancy, but even more, during the puerperium, a woman is very receptive to contraceptive advice. But it is important that the doctor initiates the discussion of the matter. Patients in this situation and all the others listed will not usually raise it themselves, however much they want the advice.

The post-natal examination is often quoted as affording a convenient opportunity to discuss birth control. Indeed, after the normal delivery of a healthy baby the GP will often be hard pressed to find any other useful function to fulfil at this examination. Nevertheless, the timing of this interview, usually six weeks after confinement, is far too late to start thinking about contraception. During pregnancy the subject should have been mentioned, and during the first few days after delivery detailed discussions leading to decisions should have occurred. The post-natal examination should be regarded as the longstop to catch those cases missed, for one reason or another, during the preceding months.

Today the majority of babies are born in hospital. After years of indifference to contraception, hospital staff of all disciplines seem to have embraced birth control with the fanatical zeal of all new converts. Patients attending antenatal clinics are bombarded with advice from all directions at almost every attendance, and many of them return to the family doctor somewhat fed up with the contraceptive cacophony. For hospital staff, just as the antenatal clinic is regarded as the only source of antenatal care, so is the 'family planning clinic' of one denomination or another looked on as the only source of contraceptive care.

To counteract this, the family doctor should make the hospital aware of his interest in contraception, and emphasize his desire to look after his own patients. Patients attending hospital obstetric departments remain patients of the GP after all: they are only 'lent' to the hospital temporarily. The patient should be warned that some well-meaning but misguided enthusiast at the hospital will probably direct her to some clinic or other. The fact that the GP will be looking after her following discharge from hospital, and her contraception, and her baby, and the baby's immunization procedures, should be emphasized, both to the patient and to the hospital.

I personally do not like to raise the question of contraception, unless the patient asks me, until the present baby seems well on the way to viability. Accordingly at about twentyfour weeks I raise the subject, without going into details of available methods, and make sure the patient knows that I intend to provide contraceptive care within the practice. Where the mother is to be handed over to the hospital a month or two before the expected date of delivery, I reinforce the information just before the hand-over. The popularity of fortyeight hour discharge results in a GP visiting a happy mother at home several times during the first ten days of the baby's life. The detailed consideration of the contraceptive methods available and their suitability for the particular patient can take place at this time under ideal circumstances. To sit on the mother's bed, stethoscope in one hand and cup of tea in the other, discussing the merits of Pill versus coil, while baby sleeps in the cot and father props up the doorway, is one of the joys of general practice that hospital doctors miss. Following the decision, taken thus *en famille,* arrangements are made for the actual provision of the chosen method.

AFTER ABORTION

A discussion of contraception is obligatory for any girl requesting termination of an unwanted pregnancy and the discussion should take place at the same interview at which termination is requested. Often, insertion of an intrauterine device immediately after evacuation of the uterus is the ideal method, and as today abortions are not performed in general practice, it is right and proper for the hospital to insert the device. The follow-up of the patient afterwards is often best left to the GP.

The letter to the gynaecologist requesting abortion should contain a reference to the contraceptive method suggested to the patient and an indication of the GP's intention to supervise the patient thereafter.

Abortions which appear to be spontaneous should be followed by a discussion of contraception, since a good many are either self-induced or at least viewed as a lucky escape. The exception is of course the girl who has been trying for a baby, but the family doctor can identify these by his questions, or by her tears.

The 'Scare', the period that is late in the girl who fears she is pregnant, and which eventually arrives to her great relief, is another strong indication for contraceptive advice. It is sad that, at the time of writing, pregnancy test kits are not made available to GPs by the National Health Service and in some areas requests to hospital laboratories for tests are restricted to 'medical' rather than 'social' indications.

And this at a time when pregnancy tests are advertised in almost all women's magazines, and available at most chemists. The girl who obtains a negative test result from a source other than her doctor may gain relief of her worry, but may lose her opportunity for contraceptive advice.

URINARY SYMPTOMS

Any young woman complaining of urinary symptoms, especially frequency and dysuria, should be asked whether she has been engaging in sexual intercourse. A young woman, in this context, means any female who appears to have reached the age of puberty. The fact that the patient is wearing school uniform should not prevent the GP asking the question.

Brooks and Maudar (1972) found that a quarter of women with the urethral syndrome related their symptoms to sexual intercourse, and first attacks of symptoms were four times as common in the age group 15–24 years than in other age groups.

The occurrence of the urethral syndrome is very often an indication that sexual intercourse has recently started, and constitutes an opportunity for the family doctor to advise about birth control methods. The complaint of urinary symptoms in boys is very much less common, but when it does occur indicates a similar opportunity. Urethritis with discharge must raise the question of venereal infection as well as of contraception.

GYNAECOLOGICAL SYMPTOMS AND SEXUAL PROBLEMS

A complaint of any of the symptoms usually associated with disease of the genital tract offers an opportunity for the doctor to inquire about contraception. Certain symptoms, notably vaginal discharge and pruritus vulvae in young women, may have a coital origin, and enquiries concerning intercourse and contraception are obligatory. Treatment of the disorder underlying the symptom will not be complete without the offer of contraceptive advice.

When a patient comes to the family doctor complaining of sexual problems it is extremely easy for the doctor to steer the conversation towards a discussion of contraception. This is all the more important because fear of unwanted pregnancy is a potent cause of complaints of sexual difficulties and of other gynaecological symptoms. There is still, even in this so-called permissive age, a remarkable reluctance for patients to take the initiative and ask their doctor for advice about birth control. They do not show the same reluctance to complain of low back pain, painful periods, heavy periods or vaginal discharge. These complaints are brought to the surgeries of general practitioners in large numbers, and offer a splendid opportunity to the doctor for the discussion of birth control.

Quite apart from the simple numerical aspect of the number of opportunities such complaints afford the doctor, there is another aspect which must be considered,and this is the opportunity to test the doctor's attitude which such a complaint will afford the patient. Will the doctor shy away from the subject, evince a general distaste for discussing any genital or sexual matters any further? Will he present an authoritarian and disapproving reaction to any mention of a request for advice on sexual or contraceptive matters?

Even though the patient may know her doctor well, it is likely that previous meetings have been concerned with matters with a content which is obviously medical, so that the patient still cannot be sure that the doctor will react in the same way to a request for birth control as to a request for, say, something for a cough.

If the doctor reacts satisfactorily, if the reaction is neither withdrawal nor obviously disapproving, the patient may be encouraged sufficiently to raise the subject of contraception. But the shy or inhibited patient may still not be able to bring herself to do so, and the experienced family doctor will relieve her anxiety by asking a direct question about the subject, and effectively smash any barrier between them.

It is opportune to mention here that in this sort of conversation medical terminology has limited application only. It is of little use talking to a West Indian labourer about 'erection' or 'ejaculation'. But if the doctor talks about getting stiff, or a hard on, and coming, then the patient will know what he is talking about.

> This can work the other way. I was surprised to find that a youth of seventeen had never heard of a sheath, a condom, nor of a 'French letter'. I embarked on a full description of the method, and produced a specimen of a sheath to illustrate my lecture. He heard me courteously through, and then said, 'I didn't realize you meant one of those: I call them Featherlites' (the proprietary name of a particular make of condom).

The gynaecological symptom produced by the patient may be a 'visiting card', produced to test the doctor's reaction. It may, however, be more than this. Symptoms of a sexual nature, such as dyspareunia, frigidity and impotence may have as their underlying cause the fear of pregnancy, and the provision of adequate contraception will result in relief of the symptom.

Even though a couple are using an apparently adequate method the family doctor should enquire more deeply. Distrust of the efficiency of a method, or dislike of the method itself, may cause the same symptoms.

THE WOMAN WITH AN ANXIETY STATE

General practitioners see many patients suffering from an anxiety state, with or without depressive symptoms, and the vast majority of these patients are women. An attempt will be made to try to identify factors in the patient's life which may be causing or contributing to her symptoms, and the patient will be questioned on her relationships in the family and in the community, her financial situation, her housing conditions and so on.

Among these questions should be some aimed at discovering the degree of sexual satisfaction in the patient's life and her need for contraceptive advice. In some cases the provision of this advice will be therapeutic.

In 1973, a woman aged 35, living in London, complained of headaches, fatigue, loss of energy, and generally feeling unwell. Questioning revealed that she had visited her GP when expecting her third baby, now aged ten months, and had been referred to hospital for booking. A midwife had visited the home and, according to the patient, had persuaded her to have the baby at home. The confinement had been entirely uneventful. Again according to the patient, there had been no mention of contraception by any of her attendants at any time.

She accepted avidly the opportunity to discuss contraception, and chose to try an intrauterine device, which was inserted at her next visit. All the symptoms of which she had originally complained disappeared after her first consultation, and have not reappeared since. No treatment other than contraceptive advice was given.

OTHER OPPORTUNITIES TO DISCUSS CONTRACEPTION

So far this discussion has considered the situation where patients have presented symptoms that the family doctor may use as invitations to discuss birth control.

There are also groups of patients for whom no invitation is needed. The woman with an anxiety state is one example, already considered.

THE NEW PATIENT

Today most general practices employ a receptionist and many have appointment systems. It is possible for patients to register with the practice without even seeing, let alone speaking to the doctor. A unique opportunity exists at this time to practise preventive medicine, and the GP should endeavour to have a few words with the patient bringing the medical cards. A veritable handful of cards leads naturally to comment on the number of children already, whether any more are desired and what contraceptive steps, if any, have been taken. When more modest numbers of cards are produced, enquiries regarding general health can be followed by enquiry about contraception. Even the single card donor, especially the bed-sitter girl in the big city, should prompt the enquiry. If mother produces cards among which are those belonging to her teenage children, she may welcome the suggestion that the children might be told that the 'new doctor' says he would be very happy to see them if they have any problems regarding sex or birth control. The experienced family doctor will be able to assess whether this suggestion will be welcome or not: certainly many parents in this day and age feel that their children ought to be receiving advice, find difficulty in giving it themselves, and are not certain to whom they ought to refer them. To be able to place upon the doctor the responsibility both for giving the advice and for mentioning the subject in the first place, often makes it easier for the parent to initiate the subject in conversation in the family.

This interview when the patient joins the list need take only a minute or two. If advice is found to be needed an appointment is made for a full discussion at a later date.

THE ADOLESCENT GIRL

If all girls in a general practice were told at the time they started going out with boys that contraceptive advice and supplies were available from the family doctor, then none of these girls should later suffer an unwanted pregnancy due to ignorance. There are many other causes of unwanted pregnancy, but ignorance of the existence of contraception, or ignorance of where to obtain contraception, could be completely eliminated.

It would be possible to use the age-sex register of the practice to write to all girls reaching a chosen age, but this impersonal approach is to be deprecated, if only because any age chosen is likely to be either too early or too late for many girls. The doctor must see the girl and, from her appearance, her degree of sexual development, her mode of dress, and her behaviour he will be able to assess whether she is likely to be sexually attractive to the males in the neighbourhood. Her age in years is of little importance in this assessment.

Whenever the doctor feels that his patient has reached this stage and whatever the reason for her visit to him, he should ask her if she knows what is meant by birth control. Thanks to the increasing amount of sex education in schools, she usually does, and he should then indicate his willingness to advise her on the subject if and when she needs it.

This advice, to talk about contraception with nearly every young female consulting the family doctor, may seem somewhat daunting, and I must confess that when I first started doing this some years ago I approached the task with considerable trepidation. Would I get my face slapped? Would there be tears and hysterics? Even worse, would Mum arrive after surgery to attend to me with a rolling pin? Happily the answer to all these questions turned out to be in the negative. It may be helpful to outline the procedure I have developed in my practice.

After dealing with the problem that has brought the patient to me, the sore throat or the cough, and the ritual of prescription and certificate writing is over, I scrutinize the medical record card and say,

'By the way, how old are you now?'

The patient may say she is fourteen or fifteen, or may amaze me by saying she is twelve. Having made certain that she knows what birth control is, I then continue,

'I'm trying to make sure that you and all the other girls of fourteen (or whatever age she has given) in the practice know that if at any time you should ever want any advice about birth control, you will be very welcome to come and see me about it. So don't forget, the offer's there, and I'll be pleased to see you'.

The response of the patient is always to thank me for the information. Sometimes they add that they are not in need of advice and I reply, 'Fine, but if ever you are, you know where to apply'. Sometimes they tell me that they are thinking of getting engaged soon and intend to come to see me then. And sometimes they say 'I'm glad you raised the subject, doctor. I've been sleeping with my boy friend for some months now, and have been thinking I ought to go somewhere'.

I have yet to have my face slapped. No one has swooned with horror. And far from coming round with a rolling pin, several mothers while consulting me for their own problems, have thanked me for 'talking to' their daughters.

However desirable it is to mention the subject of contraception to these girls, it would obviously be most undesirable to continue to mention it on every occasion they visited the doctor. A mark should be placed on their card to indicate that the interview has taken place. A variety of marks is possible, but I personally place my initials in red ink in the margin against the date.

THE ADOLESCENT BOY

In theory, an identical procedure should be adopted with all the boys as with all the girls. In practice, there is only one mechanical male method of contraception, the condom, available to boys. They tend to learn of its existence by conversation among themselves and (at the time of writing) do not need to see a doctor to obtain it.

It is also arguable that as the female is the one at risk from unwanted pregnancy and abortion, the contraceptive effort should be directed at her rather than at the male.

Nevertheless, the family doctor should indicate his willingness to provide contraception to the adolescent males. In my experience they rarely come back to me for advice themselves, but occasionally send, and may even bring, their girl friends along.

THE WOMAN WITH SMALL CHILDREN

In this day and age it is most unlikely that a woman appearing in the surgery with one or more infants will not have been offered contraception. Most will be using a method already. However, there will be some who are not satisfied with their method, or may already have abandoned it either from dislike or inertia. Occasionally a young mother will be found who is still in the process of making up her mind as to which method to use, even though the baby is many months old.

To raise the subject of contraception with these women is easy, and can reinforce advice given elsewhere.

WILL THE GP HAVE THE TIME?

I can imagine many doctors reading the preceding pages will feel that my suggestions imply a considerable extra work-load, which in the context of crowded surgeries and a general shortage of doctors seems an impossible proposition. Let me say straight away that on a Monday evening in the winter, with patients outnumbering available appointments by two to one, the telephone ringing incessantly, and the doctor himself fighting the effects of a feverish cold, there is simply no chance of practising preventive medicine of any kind.

But not all days are hectic, and there are many days in a year, and the years follow each other with remarkable rapidity. As available opportunities are taken, the vast crowd of patients at risk of unwanted pregnancy may be offered advice one by one, and the crowd dwindles eventually to manageable proportions. Priority may be allocated to one or more of the groups I have described and the other groups neglected until time allows.

In addition, the process involves not only a spending of time; there is a parallel saving of time as well. One short interview offering contraceptive advice to a young single girl may save many longer interviews dealing with an unwanted pregnancy. An anxiety state due to fear of pregnancy or dissatisfaction with a contraceptive method may result in frequent appearances of a patient complaining of many symptoms. Both attendances and symptoms may cease following solution of her contraceptive problems.

In 1968, Dr J. Eric Murphy, a general practitioner, investigated the surgery attendance records of women in his practice who had recently started to use a reliable contraceptive method, the combined Pill. 184 women, who had taken the Pill for at least three cycles, and whose records were available and believed to be complete, constituted the group.

Attendances for repeat prescriptions for the Pill were not counted, but, if the patient complained of symptoms at that attendance, then it was counted.

Murphy reported that the surgery attendances of the average patient corrected to one year had dropped from 4.8 for the period before using the Pill to only 1.8 for the period after starting the Pill. He went on to calculate that if the annual reduction of three attendances were applied to each of the 322 woman taking oral contraceptives in his practice, then the total saving in surgery time would amount to 161 hours in a year.

Although it should be noted that this investigation related specifically to the Pill, I think it likely that a similar effect will be produced by any reliable method of contraception which is acceptable to the patient.

As regards abortion, figures from my own practice reveal that, with the exception of 1970, the year of the 'Oestrogen Scare', the number of requests for abortion has remained steady year by year since 1968, despite the enormous increase in the number of abortions performed in England and Wales over the same period. The number of criminal abortions known to me and the number of 'spontaneous' abortions in the practice have also diminished.

REFERENCES

BONE, MARGARET (1973). *Family Planning Services in England and Wales.* HMSO, London.

BRENNAN, MARY *et al.* (1973). Demand for family planning advice among patients in a District Maternity Hospital. *British Medical Journal,* **3**, 19, Suppl. 4.

BROOKS, D. and MAUDAR, A. (1972). Pathogenesis of the urethral syndrome in women and its diagnosis in general practice. *Lancet,* **ii**, 897.

4

MEASUREMENT OF THE EFFICIENCY OF CONTRACEPTIVE METHODS

One of the recurring questions put to the family doctor is 'How safe is this method?' Sometimes the patient has in mind the risk of death or disease following its use, but more often she is requesting information as to the efficiency of the method at preventing pregnancy. (I believe efficiency, efficacy and effectiveness have the same meaning when used in a contraceptive context).

There are several ways of measuring contraceptive efficiency. The simplest is to report the pregnancy rate among the users. For example, of 100 women using a certain method, five became pregnant, a pregnancy rate of five per cent. This takes no account of the length of time for which the method was used, and in 1932 Raymond Pearl of Baltimore introduced his formula for calculating contraceptive efficiency. Known as the 'Pearl Index', this calculation expresses a pregnancy rate among users of a method measured in pregnancies per 100 women-years.

PEARL INDEX

$$\frac{\text{Number of pregnancies x 1200 (the number of months in 100 years)}}{\text{Total number of months of use of the method}} = \text{Pregnancy rate per 100 women-years}$$

For example, 200 women used a method for two years (i.e. 200 x 24 months) with four pregnancies reported during that time:

$$\text{Pearl Index} = \frac{4 \times 1200}{200 \times 24} = 1.0 \text{ pregnancies per 100 women-years.}$$

Using this index one can compare the relative efficiency of two methods, even though the number of women using each method and the length of time for which they use the method differ.

Method A 50 women used the method for 5 years with 10 pregnancies resulting:

$$\frac{10 \times 1200}{50 \times 60} = 4 \text{ pregnancies per 100 women-years.}$$

Method B 200 women used the method for 1 year with 5 pregnancies resulting:

$$\frac{5 \times 1200}{200 \times 12} = 2.5 \text{ pregnancies per 100 women-years}$$

Method B can therefore be said to be more effective than Method A, provided other variables were standardized for both trials. Both can be said to be highly efficient methods, since various studies have indicated that without any form of contraception approximately 50 pregnancies per 100 women-years may be expected.

The Pearl Index calculations are sometimes modified for reports concerning trials of oral contraceptives, where patients use the tablets during cycles of 28 days. As there are then 13 cycles in each year, the figure of 1300 is substituted for the 1200 in the calculation. Similarly women-cycles of use are substituted for women-months.

VARIABLES AFFECTING EFFICIENCY IN USE

Unfortunately there are many other variables difficult to standardise which make the Pearl Index a crude indicator. Some variables relate to the population studied and some to the method under investigation.

Age and parity

The age and parity of couples using the method may influence the results obtained. A high proportion of nulliparous women in a trial may produce an inaccurate assessment, due to the possibility that many infertile women are included. This factor may assume increased significance when attempting to compare a method such as the Pill, used mainly by nulliparous women, with another method, such as the intrauterine device, used mainly by parous women. However, it may be argued that women of previously proved fertility may still suffer secondary infertility. To avoid these difficulties, results in parous and nulliparous women should be assessed separately.

Frequency of intercourse

Another factor of obvious importance is the frequency with which intercourse takes place. A husband away at sea for months at a time or a commercial traveller home only at weekends is hardly comparable with the newly-wed husband enjoying his role every night.

Degree of motivation

The degree of motivation of the couple is also significant. Those highly motivated in their desire to avoid pregnancy will produce fewer accidental pregnancies than those without such motivation, even when using the same method. The intelligence and education of the couple using a method may influence the results obtained. A method beyond the control of an unintelligent couple, such as the intrauterine device, may in practice be far more effective than a method under their control, be it simple like the Pill or needing relatively complicated calculation, like the rhythm method.

Method failure

Contraceptive methods properly used may have a very low failure rate, but nevertheless their use may in practice result in large numbers of unwanted pregnancies, either because patients fail to use them correctly, or because they cease to use them. Both these factors affect the results of oral contraceptives, where missing Pills may result in pregnancy and where, during epidemics of adverse publicity, many women stop taking them altogether. Similarly, using a sheath every time is associated with very low failure rates; most failures occur in couples who occasionally omit the sheath.

Attempts have been made to differentiate between 'method failure', i.e. failure of a method properly used, and 'patient failure', i.e. failure of the patient to use the method properly. This distinction is of interest only to the protagonist of a particular contraceptive method; both types of failure result in unplanned pregnancy.

The influence of the family doctor, instructing and supervising the contraceptive care of his patients, must not be minimised. The doctor who ensures the patient is adequately instructed in the use of a method and that the patient has ready access to him in case of side-effect, real or imaginary, or in case of anxiety due to adverse publicity, will meet fewer failures than his colleague who omits instruction and supervision. This applies particularly to oral contraception, and the rhythm method, but to a lesser extent to all methods. An enthusiastic family doctor tends to produce patients enthusiastic in their use of a method but more technical considerations may apply in some types of contraception. Unplanned pregnancy following the insertion of an intrauterine device may be the result of lack of expertise or inexperience on the part of the medical attendant.

Differing failure rates for users of the same method may be related to coincident use of another method, at all times, or on occasions. For example, women fitted with conventional intrauterine devices may be advised to use chemical contraception in addition during the early months after insertion, or they may not. Sheath users may insert chemical spermicides into the vagina on some or all occasions, or they may never do so. Results for couples using two methods simultaneously should not be included in an assessment alleged to be of a single method.

Acceptability

Lastly, one must consider the concept of 'acceptability' when considering the effectiveness of any method. Absolute abstinence from all heterosexual activity is a method of unparalleled effectiveness, but of such low acceptability that few patients would agree to start using it, and even fewer to continue for any length of time. This rather extreme example also illustrates the point that the degree of acceptability for a method may be different at the beginning of use, when compared with the degree of acceptability after long periods of use. Few patients will agree to commence using the cap, but if they do they tend to continue its use for many years. Many patients will agree to start the Pill but few continue to use it regularly for many years. Acceptability is affected by experience; an unplanned pregnancy in a cap-user may make the method unacceptable thereafter. The experience of others influences acceptability: if Mrs Jones suffered dreadful troubles from her intrauterine device, then her nextdoor neighbour, Mrs Smith, may find the same method quite unacceptable. A newspaper report of the sudden death of a young woman taking the Pill may make many other couples decide not to use it.

Personal and psychological factors also affect acceptability. One woman will recoil with horror from the idea of 'having something put inside her womb' but will cheerfully take a Pill by mouth. For another woman the reverse will be true. Some men will use a sheath quite happily, whereas others will refuse to use it. In addition to the differences between individuals as regards the acceptability of any particular method, there are differences between educational, socio-economic and racial groups.

THE LIFE TABLE METHOD

In an attempt to remove the effect of some of these variables, and to demonstrate the effectiveness of a method not only in terms of accidental pregnancies, but also in relation to unwanted complications and continuation of use over a period of time, Potter and Tietze in the United States have suggested the use of the life table method, similar to that used by insurance companies in assessing risks.

Occurrences during use of the method are classified either as events or closures, the latter being an event which is not followed by a resumption of use of the method. The events which are recorded will vary for the method under investigation; pregnancies, removals for bleeding or pain and expulsions usually being considered the significant events for users of intrauterine devices, whereas for users of oral contraceptives pregnancies and changes of formulation are considered significant.

Rates per 100 women are computed for events and closures for a stated length of time. In addition the percentage of the number of women commencing who continue with the method at the end of that time is computed as the continuation rate for the method, and this rate gives a valuable indication of its acceptability to the patient.

This method of assessment is suitable for doctors wishing to make accurate comparisons, and particularly useful for the comparison of results obtained after insertion of intrauterine devices. Examples of tables demonstrating cumulative events and closures rates are illustrated in the chapter devoted to these devices.

THE PROTECTION RATE

Another method of measuring the efficiency of a method of birth control is to compare the pregnancy rate within the same population before and after the introduction of the method. The rate per hundred women-years during use of the method is then deducted from the rate before using it and, expressed as a percentage, is known as the 'protection rate'.

For example, a study was performed in 1965 of the use of the condom by couples who already had four pregnancies. Between them, before starting to use the method, the couples had managed 315 pregnancies during 517 years at risk, a pregnancy rate of 60.9 per 100 women-years. Using the method, the pregnancy rate dropped to 3.1. The difference between these rates, 57.8, expressed as a percentage of the original rate of 60.9, indicated that the protection rate of the condom, in the circumstances of that study, was 95 per cent.

This method is obviously limited to studies of groups who have a previous reproductive history: it is valueless in an investigation which includes large numbers of women who have not experienced intercourse at all before starting to use the method, as may be the situation in trials of oral contraceptives.

TALKING TO PATIENTS

For the average patient who asks her doctor whether a certain method is

Table II Comparative 'safety' of commonly used methods of contraception

Method	*Pregnancy rate*
Withdrawal Rhythm method Spermicides alone	20
Cap Condom	10
Intrauterine device Progestogen-only Pill	2·5
Combined Pill	0·25

'safe', complexities such as life tables or protection rates would result in confusion and far more satisfactory is to give her figures illustrating the approximate pregnancy rates for each method expressed as pregnancies per 100 women-years. Such a table, for the use of doctors talking to patients, appears opposite. A more detailed consideration of the effectiveness of each method and the factors influencing it appears under the appropriate heading in the chapters which follow.

5

COITUS INTERRUPTUS

This, as the name implies, involves the interruption of the act of sexual intercourse by the removal of the penis from the vagina shortly before ejaculation. It is also known as withdrawal, and 'My husband is careful'.

Once Man had realised that the ejaculate contained the seed to fertilize the female, then only motivation to avoid pregnancy was needed for this form of contraception, and so it is not surprising that this is one of the earliest methods known, its use being widespread throughout the world before the arrival of more sophisticated methods. Even in 1970, a study in Hull (Peel, 1972) and another in the same year by the Medical Care Research Unit (Cartwright, 1970a) revealed that about 45 per cent of the couples interviewed had used withdrawal at some time. The method is used least by couples in Social Class I, and is increasingly used in succeeding groups, reaching a maximum in Social Class V.

The advantages of this method are that it costs nothing, and no premeditation in the way of buying supplies or taking pills is required. In fact, anyone performing coitus at any time, anywhere, can practice coitus interruptus.

There are two disadvantages, a high failure rate and an adverse psychological effect on the woman.

FAILURE RATE

Reported failure rates show remarkable variation. In an analysis of ten reports published between 1938 and 1965, rates of between 10 and 38 are quoted, the average of all ten being 18.7 pregnancies per 100 women-years of exposure.

The reason for the high pregnancy rate is not difficult to find. During intercourse fluid seeps from the penis for some time before ejaculation and spermatozoa can sometimes be demonstrated in it. Thus even if withdrawal is practised according to plan, the possibility of impregnation exists.

If the man has been drinking, or if orgasm occurs unexpectedly rapidly, the intended withdrawal may not materialize, and the woman is particularly unprotected in this respect, as she is relying entirely on her partner in a way that she does not have to when using female methods.

With a failure rate of about 20 per hundred women-years and such widespread use of the method, one would expect that women requesting abortion would number among their ranks many who had become pregnant due to failure of coitus interruptus. In fact this does not appear to be so.

Diggory, in 1969, found only 4.8 per cent of his patients requesting abortion had used withdrawal as a method on the occasion they became pregnant, and the Birmingham Advisory Service reported only 5 per cent in their series in 1968. In my own series of patients in general practice only 4 per cent alleged pregnancy occurred despite using withdrawal, and the majority of these admitted the withdrawal had been late on the presumed occasion of the conception.

The method seems in fact to result in unplanned pregnancies rather than unwanted ones, an important distinction. Those who use the method do so from choice rather than from ignorance, and its use is often associated with a desire to delay pregnancy or make it unlikely, rather than to avoid pregnancy altogether, as evidenced by the fact that the stimulus of pregnancy may be needed before couples will abandon coitus interruptus.

Cartwright (1970b) found that 60 per cent of women abandoning the method did so because they had discovered its unreliability. In Hull, the main reason for using it seemed to be dislike, not ignorance, of other methods.

For many women the possibility of pregnancy adds spice to intercourse. They therefore do not find a high pregnancy rate unacceptable, unless and until they feel that one more child would be an intolerable burden.

PSYCHOLOGICAL EFFECTS

For the male, coitus interruptus carries no danger of psychological trauma, providing he has a willing and cooperative partner. Usually he will complete his orgasm by ejaculating on the abdomen of the woman, often assisted by the caresses of her hand on his penis.

For the woman there is a danger. If he reaches orgasm more quickly than she does, then withdrawal will leave her 'in mid-air', unhappy and unsatisfied. If he then turns over and goes to sleep, the sound of his snores will add anger and resentment to her unhappiness and, after a time, frigidity, an anxiety state, and depression may well follow. Masters and Johnson (1966) describe two main patterns of orgasm in women, the one consisting of multiple small frequent orgasms, and the other of large infrequent (although perhaps repeated) climaxes. Women in the second group are those most likely to suffer from premature withdrawal.

Eventually, unless the man is completely insensitive, he will realise her lack of sexual enjoyment, if she has not already attempted to relieve her feelings by aggressively telling him of his inadequacy as a lover, and the end result is lack of erection or premature ejaculation in the man.

These are very real dangers, which the doctor advising on contraception will hear about from patients coming for advice.

However, it must be realised that these are the results of errors of sexual technique in association with coitus interruptus and not dangers of the method itself, properly used.

If the man can produce and maintain a good erection and delay orgasm until after that of his partner, then withdrawal can be highly satisfactory for both, as evidenced by the number of couples who still practice the method today.

Couples seeking medical advice on contraception are almost never advised to use withdrawal, presumably because of the high theoretical failure rate. However, where a couple have chosen to use the method, understand that unplanned pregnancy is possible, and both find sexual satisfaction in its use, the doctor should encourage them to continue to use it.

Coitus interruptus is better than nothing, and for any particular couple, may be better than anything else.

A patient requesting abortion in 1970 told me that since the birth of her third child, she and her husband had used withdrawal, contentedly and apparently efficiently, since no pregnancy had resulted for eight years. She then read in a book that 'withdrawal was bad', and despite her husband's opposition insisted on changing to a chemical pessary. Within three months she was pregnant.

REFERENCES

CARTWRIGHT, ANN (1970a). *The Medical Care Research Unit National Survey.* Routledge & Kegan Paul, London.

CARTWRIGHT, ANN (1970b). *Parents and Family Planning Services.* Routledge & Kegan Paul, London.

DIGGORY, P. L. C. (1969). *Lancet*, **i**, 873.

MASTERS, W. H. and JOHNSON, V. E. (1966). *The Human Sexual Response.* Little Brown, Boston.

PEEL, J. (1972). The Hull Family Survey II. *Journal of Biosocial Science,* **4**, 333.

6

THE RHYTHM METHOD

The idea behind this method is to avoid intercourse at and around the time of ovulation in order that conception will not occur.

Ovulation occurs 14 days before the next menstrual period. The rhythm method is thus based on forecasting that something will happen on a certain date in the future. If the date forecast turns out to have been wrong, then all calculations based on this date will also be wrong. Hence it must be said at the outset that the rhythm method is a very inaccurate method with a high failure rate, but since it is the only method looked on with favour by the Roman Catholic Church it behoves family doctors to know something about it in order to be able to advise patients who enquire.

Let us consider the somewhat unusual woman who menstruates regularly with a cycle length of exactly 28 days. Ovulation will usually occur on the fourteenth day, but may on occasions be a day or two earlier, or a day or two later. The ovum remains capable of fertilization for only 24, or at most 48 hours. Spermatozoa are believed to be capable of fertilizing the ovum for up to three days after their arrival in the vagina. The sum of these possibilities is illustrated below, remembering that one is counting backwards from 28 to 14 all the time. Thus the days between which fertilization of an ovum produced at or about the fourteenth day are possible are from the nineteenth day before the next period to the tenth day before it, i.e. from the ninth day of the cycle (28-19) to the eighteenth (28-10).

These ten days are the only fertile days in the cycle. The days before (cycle days 1 to 8) may be regarded as safe, although somewhat marred by menstruation, and the days after (cycle days 19-28) are also to be regarded as safe, the combination (cycle days 19 - 8 of the next cycle) being known as the 'safe period'. Immediately after a short menstruation, when the endometrium has been seen to be shed, is obviously safer than immediately before a menstruation that may never appear.

Difficulties can be seen to arise if menstruation lasts for many days or if the cycle length is short, as in either case the safe period dwindles.

Further problems will arise if the woman menstruates irregularly. In such a case it is advised that a record be kept of cycle length for six months, or even a year. The length of the longest and the shortest cycle during that time gives the maximum cycle variation.

Hopeful day of ovulation			14			days before period
Allowance for early or late ovulation		+2		−2		
Ovum persists for 48 hours					−2	
Sperm persists for 3 days	+3					
Totals:	14 + 2 + 3 = 19					14 − 2 − 2 = 10
i.e. Cycle day 9 (28 − 19)			to			cycle day 18 (28 − 10)

Fig. 4. Dates on which ovulation can occur in a 28-day cycle

To calculate the safe period in such a woman, 19 is deducted from the number of days in the shortest cycle and 10 from the number of days in the longest cycle.

For example: Longest cycle recorded 33 days
Shortest cycle recorded 27 days

$$27 - 19 = 6 \text{ and } 33 - 10 = 23$$

Safe period = before cycle day 6 and after cycle day 23.

Readers may care to practise their arithmetic working out the safe period for women with really irregular cycles. An unfortunate whose cycles vary between twenty and forty days, for example, is theoretically in the safe period on the day she starts to menstruate, and then not until after day 30, a lapse of more than four weeks.

An attempt may be made to identify the date of ovulation with greater accuracy by recording the woman's body temperature. Rising levels of progesterone following ovulation produce an elevation of temperature of about a half of one degree Fahrenheit. If intercourse is avoided until three days after the rise in temperature, then the ovum should be no longer capable of fertilization.

Efficient use of this refinement of the rhythm method demands considerable time spent by the doctor in the instruction of the patient. She should be told to go to a chemist and buy herself a thermometer with markings that she can clearly see. There is remarkable variation in the clarity of the markings on thermometers marketed in the United Kingdom, and markings adequate for the professional, i.e. the doctor, may be useless for the patient. An appointment is then made at which the doctor, by means of large diagrams drawn at the time, demonstrates the markings, the degrees, the fifths of degrees, and the meaning of the black or red arrows found on various specimens of thermometers. (Despite decimalization, no patient has as yet brought me a Centigrade thermometer to explain). Care must be taken that the patient understands that each small division represents 0.2F. Fractions and decimals may have played a very small part in her life. After explanation, the patient is presented with the thermometer shaken by the doctor to various levels and asked to give her readings of it. Once both are confident that she can read it accurately, the mercury should be raised in the thermometer (a very quick dip in the sterilizer works wonders) and she should be shown how to shake it down. 'Like cracking a whip - but don't let go whatever you do!'

Finally it is pointed out that it has to be shaken down before the reading disappears, and therefore can be read with equal success either at the time, or later - a matter of considerable import to a girl rushing against the clock in the mornings.

The thermometer should be placed under the tongue in the morning, before getting out of bed, having a cup of tea, smoking a cigarette or doing anything else. To place it in the rectum is an extra refinement that I have never found necessary to inflict on my patients. It should be left under the tongue for double the time advised by the manufacturer, then placed on the bedside table to be read when the eyes are clearer later in the day.

The reading should be entered on a chart. Suitable charts are available commercially to give to patients, who should be instructed to bring them back for perusal by the doctor for two or three months before deciding that they may be relied upon.

Not all patients produce the nice clear temperature rise illustrated in the textbooks. Sometimes a double rise occurs, in which case the patient should be told to abstain for three days after the second rise. Sometimes a zig-zag pattern is produced which is completely unhelpful, and of course, sometimes no rise is detectable, indicating possible infertility.

Paradoxically, failure of ovulation due to a reduced total progesterone level may be associated with an ovulatory type of temperature chart. Finally the patient must be warned that a sore throat or other infection may also produce a temperature rise. Such an episode can usually be easily identified provided it occurs at a time well away from the expected date of ovulation.

Other methods for the detection of ovulation are of course available, but none are suitable for patient use, with the possible exception of the method recently reported from Australia. Patients were taught to recognize the increase in quantity and decrease in viscosity of both the cervical and vaginal secretion produced at the time of ovulation. Some women could recognize the sensation of increased moisture in the vagina; some could detect that the mucus was less tacky when manipulated between finger and thumb. Initial

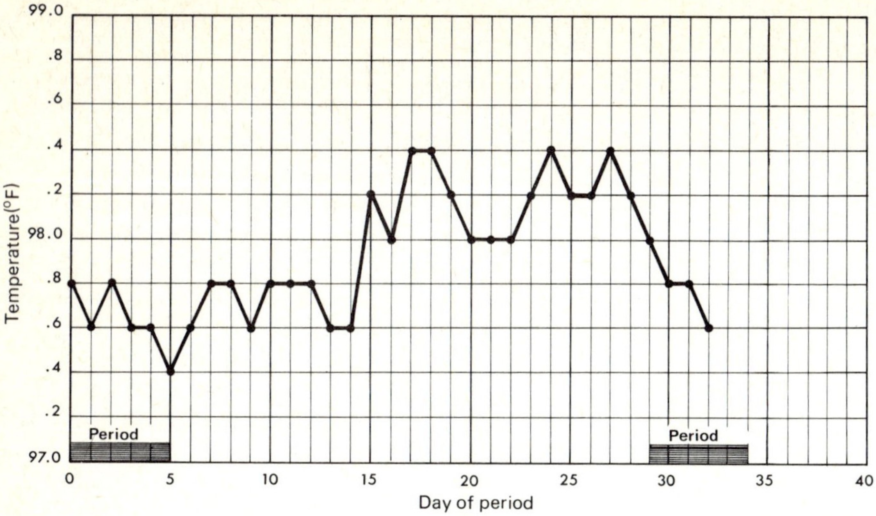

Fig. 5 A patient's temperature chart

reports have indicated considerable success with this method, but I have no experience of using it.

It is possible that at some time in the future an accurate method by which patients may recognize ovulation will be evolved. Until then it must be stated that the rhythm method is most unsatisfactory. In the puerperium, menstruation may be delayed for months especially if the mother is lactating, and the rhythm method is useless at this time. For women with very irregular cycles and women at the menopause it is almost useless. Women having anovular cycles who follow this method will, of course, be avoiding intercourse at the time of greatest safety.

FAILURE RATES

Provided a useful temperature chart is produced, giving clear evidence of the day of ovulation, and providing intercourse is restricted to the time after the rise in temperature, failure rates as low as six per 100 women-years have been reported. If intercourse also takes place before the temperature rise, in that part of the safe period following menstruation as calculated by the formulae given above , then the failure rate is at least trebled. For women using the rhythm method without the refinement of temperature-taking, rates as high as 40 per hundred women-years have been reported.

A factor which may be operating to produce these high rates is that there is some evidence that ovulation may be induced at times other than mid-cycle in response to unusual stimulation. Pregnancy has followed rape performed during the safe period. Where the date of impregnation can be assessed with considerable accuracy, as obtains in the wives of soldiers or sailors home on leave for a strictly limited time, conception can not infrequently be shown to have occurred at a time which should have been safe. That coitus-induced ovulation occurs in the animal kingdom is a known fact. The suspicion exists that it may under certain conditions occur also in the human animal. However, the suspicion must also exist that some of the women may have had their reasons for misleading others as to their dates.

ACCEPTABILITY

Few couples are willing to accept a method involving such suppression of their natural desires, coupled with such gross inefficiency. It is not a method to be considered unless both partners are willing to use it. A relatively high degree of intelligence is required to make the necessary calculations. Some couples find that in addition to the disadvantage of being unable to make love at certain times, there is also the disadvantage that making love is almost obligatory at others.

The few advantages of the method are that it costs nothing, needs no equipment (other than monumental self-control) and has the blessing of the Papal Encyclical of 1968 in which it is stated that recourse to the infecund periods is considered licit.

USE IN THE POPULATION

The Second Hull Family Survey (Peel, 1972) and the Medical Care Research Unit Study (Cartwright, 1970a) found that only 15 per cent of patients reported ever using the rhythm method. General practitioners who are not themselves Roman Catholics will find that they very rarely receive requests for advice about the rhythm method. Most Roman Catholics who want such advice go elsewhere, either to family doctors of the same religion or to such organizations as the Catholic Marriage Advisory Council.

Couples who have strong religious motivation and regular cycles, do use the method with persistence and relative success, although Cartwright (1970b) found that 82 per cent of patients giving up the rhythm method gave as their reason its unreliability. It is noticeable in general practice that as their family size increases, so women become increasingly unwilling to continue using 'Roman Roulette'.

Couples with strong religious motivation and very irregular cycles may be helped, by a doctor whose tongue must be firmly in his cheek, in the regulation of their menses by the use of synthetic progestogen and oestrogen tablets.

REFERENCES

CARTWRIGHT, ANN (1970a). *The Medical Care Research Unit National Survey,* Routledge & Kegan Paul, London.

CARTWRIGHT, ANN (1970b). *Parents and Family Planning Services.* Routledge & Kegan Paul, London.

PEEL, J. (1972). The Hull Family Survey II. *Journal of Biosocial Science,* **4**, 333.

7

SPERMICIDES

Throughout recorded history more or less disgusting material has been inserted into the female vagina in an attempt to prevent conception by killing spermatozoa. The Kahun Papyrus of ancient Egypt, dated at about 1850 BC, gives a prescription detailing the use of crocodile dung for this purpose. Later elephants were substituted for crocodiles, any increase in efficiency being due not, as might be imagined, to an improvement in the memory of the user, but to a decrease in the pH of the excreta.

Jumping 3,000 years to 1850, Kölliker in Germany carried out tests with acids, alkalis and cyanides, assessing their efficiency in killing sperm. Less dangerous materials were used by subsequent workers, and Rendell in 1885 produced a pessary containing quinine sulphate as the spermicidal ingredient. Since then many other chemicals have been used and many variations developed of the vehicle carrying them.

Today four groups of spermicidal chemical vaginal applications can be listed.

1. **Pessaries**

These may have a water soluble gelatine base or a water insoluble oily base. There is a time-lag between insertion in the vagina and completion of melting at body temperature. Insertion at or near the cervix cannot be guaranteed.

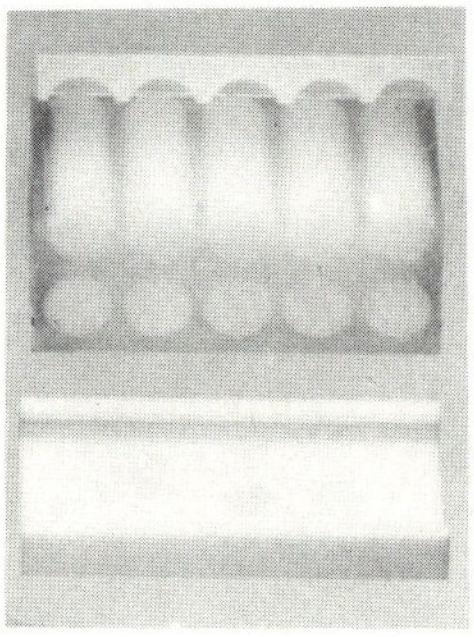

Fig. 6. Pessaries.

2. **Creams, pastes and jellies**

The difference in the consistency and appearance of these products relates to

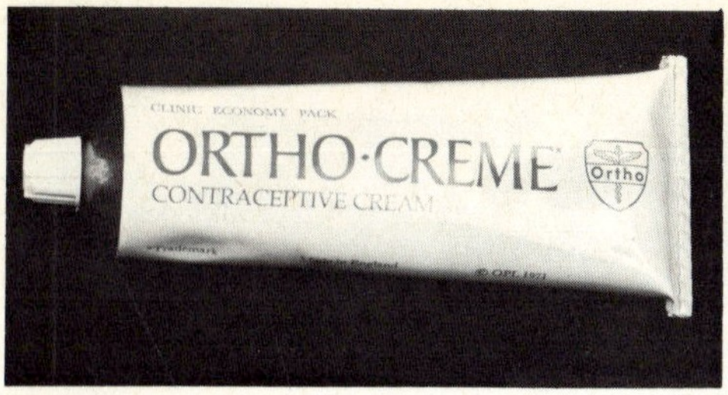

Fig. 7. Contraceptive cream.

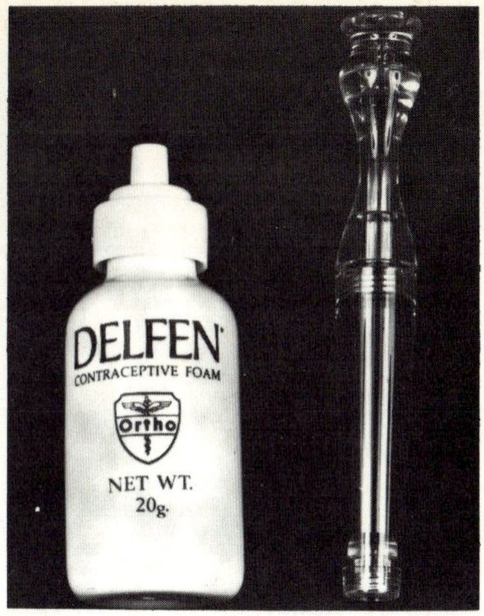

Fig. 8. Contraceptive foam and applicator.

the type of base used, jellies containing water soluble or miscible bases, creams an emulsion of water insoluble oils. All types may be inserted by means of a syringe introducer.

3. **Foaming tablets**

Containing sodium bicarbonate and tartaric acid these tablets react with water to produce a foam, which carries the spermicide throughout the length and breadth of the vagina. They should be dipped in water before being inserted in the vagina.

4. **Aerosol foams**

The contents of the aerosol are released into a plastic syringe which is then inserted into the vagina. Pressure on the plunger results in transfer of the foam to the upper part of the vagina.

A fifth type, 'C-film', consisting of a small square of soluble plastic material in which is incorporated a spermicide, may be placed either over the external cervical os or over the meatus of the penis prior to its introduction into the vagina. The effectiveness of this type of application seems no greater than that of other chemical methods.

Among chemicals used as spermicides are phenyl mercuric acetate, boric acid, and various chemical variations of phenoxypolyethoxy ethanol.

ADVANTAGES

Chemical contraceptives do not need a prescription and can be obtained over the counter in chemists' shops. Jellies, and to a lesser extent creams, assist in vaginal lubrication. All types can be used in combination with other methods, indeed their use is obligatory with diaphragms or caps. It is possible that in addition to killing spermatozoa, vaginal contraceptive chemicals may also kill, or at least inhibit, the growth of Trichomonas vaginalis and Candida albicans.

DISADVANTAGES

The slow dissolution of pessaries has already been referred to, and their use should probably be discouraged. The general disadvantages that the method requires forethought, the purchase of supplies, and the possibility of running out at a critical moment applies to chemical contraception as to other mechanical methods.

The suspicion has recently been voiced that spermatozoa may be damaged rather than killed by spermicides, resulting in congenital deformity in the baby. At the moment such a cause for abnormal babies remains a suspicion only, but further investigation is obviously indicated.

A great disadvantage is the fussiness and messiness involved, which many women find unacceptable. Cartwright (1970) found that 46 per cent of women abandoning the method gave as their reason the fact that they found it unpleasant to use. A further 37 per cent gave it up because they found it unreliable, and this must be regarded as the greatest disadvantage of this method when used without the addition of mechanical barriers.

FAILURE RATES

It is difficult to give an accurate figure for the effectiveness of a method which depends so much on the way in which the patient uses it. Failure rates reported vary from as little as 2.2 pregnancies per 100 women-years to as much as 23.1 for the same preparation. For all types of preparation failure rates as high as 35 can be found in the literature but rates of between 5 and 20 may be taken as representative of most recent studies.

USAGE

The choice of contraceptive methods today is so great that few couples use chemical contraception, other than in addition to other mechanical methods. Consideration of recent publications indicates that probably only about ten per cent of the population of the United Kingdom has ever used it as their sole contraceptive method.

THE FAMILY DOCTOR'S ROLE

There is no doubt that the use of a chemical contraceptive on every occasion would be followed by fewer unwanted pregnancies than would follow the use of no method at all so the method may be said to be better than nothing. Hence couples of low fertility who have used and are using the method with apparent success should not be dissuaded from continuing to do so. Couples who have not yet achieved their desired family size may find the high failure rate acceptable, but once it has been achieved some more effective method should be advised.

Spermicides

The use of chemical contraceptives in addition to mechanical barriers is discussed in the chapters on condoms and diaphragms. Except when advising in such circumstances it is doubtful whether the family doctor should ever suggest to his patients that they should use a method known to be unacceptable to so many people and associated with such a high failure rate.

REFERENCE

CARTWRIGHT ANN (1970). *Parents and Family Planning Services*, Routledge & Kegan Paul, London.

A Selection of Chemical Contraceptives

Type	*Brand name*	*Manufacturer*
Pessaries	Genoxol	Rendell
	Ortho-forms	Ortho
	Rendells	Rendell
	Staycept	Syntex
Creams	Antemin	Coates & Cooper
	Delfen	Ortho
	Duracreme	London Rubber
	Genoxol	Rendell
	Ortho Creme	Ortho
	Rendells	Rendell
	Staycept	Syntex
Jellies	Duragel	London Rubber
	Orthogynol	Ortho
	Preceptin gel	Ortho
	Staycept	Syntex
	Volpar	British Drug Houses
Paste	Volpar	British Drug Houses
Foaming tablets	Gynomin	Coates & Cooper
Foam	Delfen	Ortho
	Emko	Gerhardt
Soluble film	C-Film	Potter & Clarke

8

DIAPHRAGMS AND CAPS

For many centuries attempts have been made to occlude the upper part of the vagina and so prevent conception. Among methods used were the insertion of sponges or pads, with or without hopefully spermicidal compounds such as vinegar, wine, or olive oil. The discovery of the process of vulcanization of rubber enabled the diaphram to be developed in Holland, whence originates the name 'Dutch cap'

In reality, mechanical exclusion of bodies as small, motile and numerous as human spermatozoa by a diaphragm is mere wishful thinking. Modern vaginal occlusive appliances are used as carriers for spermicidal substances, either creams, jellies or foams, all of which are equally effective. The choice is largely a matter of patient preference. A spermicidal pessary may be used with a diaphragm or cap, but takes rather longer to dissolve and spread than other forms of chemical contraceptive.

TYPES OF VAGINAL OCCLUSIVE DEVICE

1. The vaginal diaphragm

This is the most frequently used type of device, consisting of a dome of rubber with either a flat watch spring or a coil spring enclosed around the base. The smallest size is about 50 mm in external diameter, the largest about 100 mm.

Diaphragms when in use lie with their anterior margin behind the symphysis pubis, and their posterior margin in the posterior fornix. They remain in place because of the balance between the spring pushing outwards and the tone of the vaginal walls and surrounding musculature pushing inwards. Because of this, they are *unsuitable* for the patient with lax vaginal walls, poor musculature, or actual prolapse of the uterus.

2. The cervical cap

Shaped like a cup, the cervical cap has a dome which fits closely over the cervix. The thickened rim of the cap encircles the cervix, lying in the vaginal fornices. The smallest is 20 mm in external diameter, the largest, 30 mm. A cervical cap should fit snugly, and so create a suction effect, which keeps it in place. Extraction of a well-fitting cap can be difficult, so a thread or loop is incorporated by means of which the device can be pulled out.

A cervical cap is suitable only for a patient with an ideal cervix, which in this context may be defined as not too short (or the base of the cap will not grip properly), tubular rather than conical (or the cap may slide off), and is neither eroded, infected, nor grossly torn. Ideal cervices (like ideal women) are not too common.

3. The vault cap

A hemispherical device, similar to a diaphragm, but without a spring in the thickened base, and available in sizes 50 - 75 mm in external diameter.

This device fits in the vault of the vagina, and again is held in place by a vacuum or suction effect. It is useful where the diaphragm is unsuitable because the vaginal walls are lax or there is minor uterine prolapse, or where the cervix is conical, torn or otherwise unsuitable for a cervical cap.

However, if the cervix is unusually long, the vault cap will be like a bowler hat placed over the ferrule of a walking stick and will not fit.

4. The vimule

The vimule is designed to fit the long cervix, being in essence a flanged vault cap at the base, providing the suction, with a cervical cap rising from it to accommodate the long cervix. Vimules are made in sizes 40 - 55 mm in external diameter.

Caps and vimules are made of plastic or of rubber.

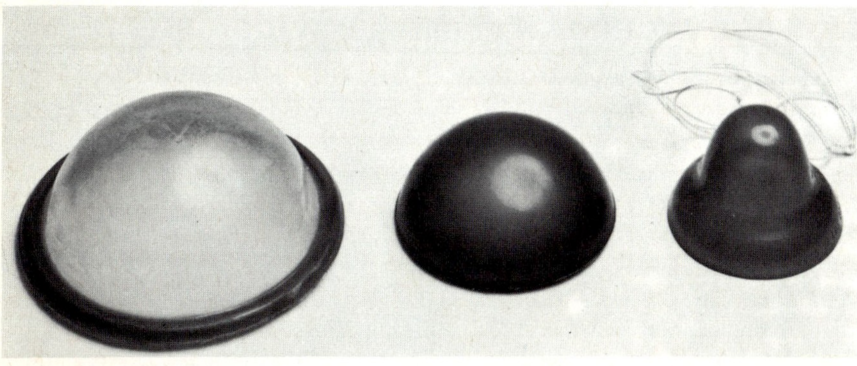

Fig. 9. Diaphragm, vault cap, vimule.

DIAPHRAGMS

Fitting a diaphragm

The first visit of the patient is a useful opportunity to perform any general screening procedures such as urine testing, breast examination or Papanicolou smear, which the patient has not undergone recently. A full bimanual pelvic examination, including speculum examination of the cervix, is in any event necessary before making a decision as to which type of device will best suit the patient.

During vaginal examination the extended examining fingers are thrust into the posterior fornix, and the position of the posterior margin of the symphysis pubis, in relation to the fingers, indicates the size of diaphragm required. A suitable diaphragm is squeezed flat and passed into the vagina, angling it against the posterior wall so that it reaches the posterior fornix.

The anterior rim is then pushed up behing the symphysis and, if correctly positioned, the cervix can be felt through the dome of the diaphragm. There should be no stretching of the vaginal walls if the size chosen is correct, nor should the device move if the patient is asked to cough or strain down.

The patient herself is asked to feel the position of the diaphragm in the vagina, particularly noting the cervix palpable through the diaphragm and the retropubic position of the anterior rim. She is then asked to remove it, by disengaging the device from behind the pubis with a finger and pulling it out. Next she must practise insertion for herself. To do this some women prefer to squat, some to put one foot upon a chair, and others to lie down with their knees drawn up. Those who are accustomed to inserting tampons at the time of the menses may be encouraged to use the same position for inserting the diaphragm. Some women find the spring of the diaphragm liable to twist out of their grasp: holding it between thumb and second finger with the index finger inside the spring may be easier for them.

After a couple of successful self-insertions, and when the woman is quite certain she knows when she is feeling her own cervix ('it feels like the tip of your nose'), she is sent away with a diaphragm to practice with and an appointment to return in a week, with the diaphragm *in situ*, so that its fit and position may be checked. It is not uncommon to find the fit too loose, indicating that the patient was nervous and tense at the first visit. A larger diaphragm is then substituted.

After this she is provided with a diaphragm of her own, and a tube of spermicidal jelly, if she wishes extra lubrication, or cream if she does not. She is shown how to squeeze a small sausage of it, about an inch long, into the dome and another onto the dome. Whether the diaphragm is inserted dome up or dome down then makes no difference, and both penis and cervix are presented with a spermicidal barrier. It is unnecessary to smear the chemical all over the device; this merely makes it more messy and difficult to hold without increasing its efficiency.

Although ideally a week's practice should precede use of the cap for the first time during coitus, if the girl is already having intercourse it is obviously safer to compress the two consultations into one and check the situation hopefully a week later.

Correct use of a diaphragm

The diaphragm should be inserted up to two hours before intercourse. If a longer time elapses, or if intercourse occurs more than once, extra contraceptive chemical should be applied. Insertion immediately before intercourse is contraceptively satisfactory, but the wife who says to her husband, 'Hold everything, while I find my cap' is liable to find his ardour dissipated on her return. Even worse, he may verbally apostrophize the thing, and press on regardless. Hence the wise wife should adopt the motto of the Boy Scouts and insert the diaphragm routinely before going to bed.

The fact that spermatozoa are persistent little blighters, capable of fertilizing her ovum many hours after their arrival in the vagina, must be explained to the patient. She should be advised to leave the diaphragm in place until the next morning or, at the very least, for six hours after intercourse.

If the enthusiasm of the husband demands it, a diaphragm can be left in place for twentyfour hours, provided it is removed for cleaning daily and additional spermicide added as required. Menstruation commencing with a diaphragm *in situ* causes no harm of course, but women are sometimes very worried about this possibility and need reassurance.

Care of a diaphragm

The device should be washed with soap and water, dried, and dusted with talcum powder. It should never be lubricated with petroleum jelly, left in sunlight, nor stored near a source of heat, all of which encourage the material to perish. The patient should be advised to hold it up to the light every so often to detect any weaknesses appearing, and particularly to watch for any puckering around the rim, indicating that the device is reaching the end of its useful life.

Follow-up of the patient

The size of the vagina alters after initial experience of regular intercourse, after confinement, or after gaining or losing a considerable amount of weight. Where these conditions apply, the patient should be told to report to the doctor to have the fit of the diaphragm checked. Otherwise, a 'social' visit annually, to confirm that all is well, receive complaints or comments, and perform any screening procedures due is all that is required.

CAPS AND VIMULES

Vault or cervical cap and vimules

Basically the procedure is the same as for the diaphragm, the doctor selecting the best type for the patient, assessing and inserting the correct size, and supervising its correct use by the patient. All these varieties of occlusive device are made in plastic as well as rubber, which is of use in women who are allergic to rubber.

Contemporary usage

To use a cap successfully, a woman must be both intelligent and possessed of a high degree of motivation. The contrast between the ritual described above, and the ease with which a Pill may be swallowed is so marked that comment is superfluous. Because of this 'fiddling about with the cap', as so many patients describe it, the use of the cap has declined as the use of the Pill has increased.

The Hull Family Survey in 1970 (Peel, 1972) and the Medical Care Research Unit study in the same year (Cartwright, 1970a) both showed that only about one-sixth of couples had ever used the diaphragm as their chosen contraceptive method, as compared with one-half who had used the Pill.

Women choosing the diaphragm tend to be of a higher social class, of greater intelligence, and more highly educated than those using other methods. They also tend to go to clinics rather than to general practitioners, but even so, of new patients attending the clinics of the Family Planning Association in 1971 five women asked for the Pill for each one who asked for a diaphragm or cap.

The small part played by family doctors in the provision of this method may be easily understood. Until recently neither appliances nor creams were provided nor was any payment made by the National Health Service. Numerically, the type of patient who wished to use a cap constituted a minority in most general practices, and consequently there was little demand for the service. The medical content of the service was small, and indeed in most clinics a good deal of patient instruction and supervision was performed by the clinic nurse: until recently nursing assistance was a rarity in general practice. In most neighbourhoods clinics existed where charges to the patient were low or non-existent. And finally, the efficiency of the cap as a contraceptive device was far from a hundred per cent: many doctors at a time when abortion was illegal did not wish to be faced with a patient who accused them of supplying and supervising the method which had resulted in the unwanted pregnancy.

EFFICIENCY OF METHOD

A survey of seven series reported between 1938 and 1962 (Oldershaw, 1968) revealed wildly varying pregnancy rates, averaging 11.8 pregnancies per hundred women-years. Diggory (1969) found that almost one patient in four requesting abortion asserted she had been using the diaphragm as her chosen contraceptive method at the time of conception of the unwanted pregnancy.

Despite these disparaging figures, every doctor knows of women who happily use this method for years, with conspicuous success. Probably there is no other method in which motivation to use, and efficiency and regularity in use, are so important.

The diaphragm has certain disadvantages. Cartwright (1970b), questioning women as to their reason for abandoning the use of the diaphragm, found that 64 per cent alleged it was unpleasant to use and 18 per cent said they found it unreliable. Sometimes the male objects to the rim of the diaphragm which, if the vaginal musculature is firm, may obtrude during intercourse.

On the other hand the method has certain advantages, particularly in women who are spacing rather then preventing pregnancies, in whom the failure rate is of less importance. Chief among these is the absence of any medical complications - other than rubber sensitivity - and thus immunity to periodic 'scares'. It is also completely under the control of the female, which advantage can be used both to prevent unwanted pregnancies, and to produce 'accidental' wanted pregnancies.

Finally, for those couples whose delight is to sample the more athletic suggestions in the Kama-Sutra, it must be confessed that the diaphragm or cap is liable to become dislodged in the more unusual positions.

REFERENCES

CARTWRIGHT, ANN (1970a). *The Medical Care Research Unit National Survey.* Routledge & Kegan Paul, London.

CARTWRIGHT, ANN (1970b). *Parents and Family Planning Services.* Routledge & Kegan Paul, London.

DIGGORY, P. L. C. (1969). *Lancet* **i**, 873.

OLDERSHAW, K. L. (1968). General practitioner group trials of oral contraception, *Clinical Trials Journals,* **5**, 131.

PEEL, J. (1972). The Hull Family Survey II. *Journal of Biosocial Science,* **4**, 333.

9

THE CONDOM

The condom is a very thin membrane, tailored to fit tube-like closely over the erect penis, to be worn during sexual intercourse and ejaculation and to collect within it the ejaculate, thus preventing spermatozoa entering the vagina or cervix.

Alternative names are a sheath, a rubber, a prophylactic, a preventive, a protective, and a French letter. This compliment is returned by our Common Market cousins in France who refer to a condom as an English overcoat (une capot anglaise).

Condoms have been in use for centuries, and legend has it that they were invented by one Dr Condom, a courtier in the reign of Charles II. That Merry Monarch made free use of the invention and, as a token of his appreciation, dubbed Dr Condom knight in recognition of his service to King and country. Unfortunately, Dr Condom seems to be no more than a legend. However, that other male exponent of sexual prowess, Casanova, certainly did exist and was reputed to be much favoured by his paramours because of his use of condoms manufactured from animal intestines.

The process of vulcanization of rubber, invented in the middle of the nineteenth century, enabled the hand-made animal sheaths to be replaced by mass-produced rubber condoms, at first crepe rubber, later, in the 1930s replaced by latex, and in the 1960s challenged by the production of plastic disposable condoms.

I remember reading in the press in 1952 of the discovery of some early animal condoms, made about the year 1800, and found in an old country house in England. The thickness of the material of which they were manufactured was about 0.04 mm, as compared with the thickness of the modern latex rubber condom which is about 0.05 mm, and that of the new plastic condom, 0.03 mm.

In the United Kingdom today, condoms are usually white, grey, or flesh-coloured, have a teat at their distal end to collect the ejaculate, and are packed in sealed foil within discreetly elegant outer wrappings. Elsewhere in the world plain-ended items are more popular and gay colours are favoured, both for the condoms and their packaging. Recently manufacturers in this country have attempted to package their wares more attractively to appeal to female purchasers in chemists' shops.

Pre-lubrication has been a great advance, the silicone lubricant being applied during manufacture. This has greatly assisted the introduction of the condom-covered penis into a vagina with poor natural lubrication as may occur not only in anxious women or after amputation of the cervix - and also reduces the chance of the condom being torn by rough hands or finger nails or by friction against the outer side of the labia majora.

Washable varieties are available, which may be used more than once. These are manufactured of rather thicker latex and are not pre-lubricated.

METHOD OF USE

The condom is supplied rolled from the proximal towards the distal end. It should be positioned over the glans of the erect penis and rolled downwards towards the pubis. Some authorities advise the application of an elastic band around the base of the condom in position on the penis. This is not usually necessary, but in men whose ability to maintain erection is poor, the interference with the venous return caused by the band may help them to do so.

It must be applied before any contact between the penis and vulva occurs: the pre-ejaculate may contain some spermatozoa, albeit few in number. Ideally the teat should be applied collapsed, in order that no bursting strain should result from the addition of the ejaculate. In practice this is unnecessary for normal ejaculate volumes.

After ejaculation the condom should be held at the base with the fingers as the penis is withdrawn to avoid it slipping off the diminishing penis and spilling its contents in the vagina. Withdrawal before the penis is completely flacid is essential, or spillage is very likely.

To improve the efficiency of the method, in case of bursting or tearing of the condom, and also to improve lubrication, a spermicidal chemical, either a pessary, jelly, or foam, should be used in addition.

After removal of the condom, the penis should be carefully wiped dry before the couple lie together in any position where penis and vulva are in apposition.

The final and most important instruction for efficient use of the condom is that it must be used at each and every act of intercourse.

ADVANTAGES OF THE CONDOM

1. **A male method, par excellence, enabling the male to retain control over fertility.**

But not exclusively male, since the application of the condom may be performed by the female and, in happy and successful users, this act may constitute an enjoyable part of regular sexual foreplay. By such action the female may ensure that the condom is in fact used on every occasion.

2. **Lack of side-effects.**
There are no complications, side-effects or contra-indications with this method, other than the rare instance of dermatitis due to rubber sensitivity. In such cases plastic condoms provide the answer.

3. **Availability.**
Women may buy sheaths from chemists, men from the barber's shop, and both by post from mail order firms. Even bashful doctors may read the FPA advertisement in the *British Medical Journal* and order impersonally by post.

Neither visits to clinics nor doctor's surgeries are necessary to obtain supplies, making it the ideal method for the young unmarried man who does not wish to advertise his hope that he might get the opportunity to use it. Condoms may be available from slot machines placed in private places such as gentleman's toilets, ensuring absolute anonymity for the bashful male.

Vending machines as distribution outlets for condoms have great advantages, and it is to be hoped that their numbers will be increased. Unfortunately, some out-of-date local bye-laws specifically prohibit them in public places.

Unfortunately also, it is a standing joke – in rather poor taste – that such machines will provide a constant source of income even if the contents are never replaced, since few males using them will be willing to beard the owner to get his money back.

That this is very true was brought home to me in a restaurant on a Motorway last summer. There was a condom vending machine in the toilet, but when I looked in the crowded cafe it served there was not a single male member of staff in evidence to whom an unsatisfied customer could have addressed himself, and only one female member one could have spoken to with any degree of privacy. As she appeared both formidable, menopausal and slightly deaf, considerable courage and a loud voice would have been necessary.

4. **Occasional suitability**
For the individual, male or female, who expects to have intercourse on infrequent occasions, this is a very suitable method. To take the Pill every night or to wear an IUD, with the possible side-effects of both, when one's consort is a seaman or with the Army in Northern Ireland, is plainly carrying contraception too far.

For the young man indulging in occasional intercourse the condom is again ideal, and Peel and Potts (1969) make the comment that it is 'a satisfactory receptacle for wild oats'. Alex Comfort (1963) has suggested that a young man of chivalry may today be defined as one who invariably carries a condom about his person.

5. **Possible combination with other methods**
The condom can be used as well as chemical contraceptives, or during the 'waiting days' after vasectomy or when starting the Pill, or during the other

waiting days after missing a Pill or Pills. It can be used during the first few weeks after insertion of an IUD when pregnancy is most likely. Combination with the rhythm method is possible, using it during the unsafe period, although care must be taken to be as accurate as ever in the arithmetic of the safe period. Its use can be combined with the diaphragm in the hope that the total reliability of the two methods combined will be near 100 per cent. Such a combination is rarely the result of professional advice, but has been used by some of my patients anxious to avoid both pregnancy and the side-effects of the Pill.

6. **Protection against venereal disease**

It is doubtful whether much protection is in fact provided by the use of a sheath, although Potts (1973) states that in Sweden the increased sales of condoms as part of a contraceptive campaign in that country was associated with a decrease in numbers of cases of VD. Obviously a condom would provide no protection against infection from parts of the body other than the penis or vagina.

Secondary syphilis has long been known to produce infective lesions in the mouth. The relatively recent discovery that the gonococcus can be isolated from the tonsils, taken in conjunction with the frequency of inter-oral and oro-genital contact during sexual intercourse, explains to some degree the frequent failure of the condom to protect against infection.

Nevertheless, some degree of protection from vaginal infection may be expected, and certainly my prostitute patients are convinced of the value of the condom for this purpose. Certainly also one of my patients has had no recurrences of a previously troublesome recurrent non-specific urethritis since starting regular use of the sheath.

7. **Effectiveness**

The effectiveness of the sheath as a method of contraception has tended to be underrated. Most failures occur because of failure to use it on every occasion, the chances of rupture of modern lubricated sheaths being very small.

If used regularly, pregnancy rates of only one per hundred women-years have been reported. The second Hull Family Survey (Peel, 1972) reported a failure rate overall of 3.9 pregnancies per hundred women-years, of which the majority were due to occasional failure to use the sheath.

Peel (1969) reported the results of a trial lasting from March 1965 to April 1968. Only couples who had had at least four pregnancies, the last less than twelve months previously, were recruited to the scheme. Condoms were issued without charge by a social worker visiting the home at the beginning of the scheme and sent by post after one year. At the end of April 1968 the 53 couples then in the group had used the method for 1,548 months, with only four accidental pregnancies resulting, a pregnancy rate of 3.1 per 100 women-years.

Thus, properly used, the condom is comparable in effectiveness with the intrauterine device or the progestogen-only Pill.

DISADVANTAGES

The main disadvantage of the condom lies in its mode of action, being a barrier, both physical and psychological, between male and female at intercourse.

The pause necessary to apply the condom results in an interruption of penile stimulation, which may in turn lead to loss of erection. There is a diminution of the sensation transmitted to the penis during coitus, including a reduction in the transfer of heat from the vagina. Both result in a lessening of stimulation and may in turn result in loss of erection. Once this has occurred it may be difficult to apply physical stimulation to regain erection without removing the condom, and there may be such a blow to the male pride that psychological inhibition of erection ensues.

Conversely, this diminution of stimulation may be helpful in men who achieve orgasm too quickly, slowing them down to a speed more satisfactory to both partners.

Both men and women complain that the presence of a sheath separates them both physically and emotionally. They are not having sex with a person, but with a thin bit of latex material. Couples who hold strongly to this view are particularly liable to agree some excuse for not using the method on occasions, with consequent failure.

Further disadvantages of this method when compared with others are that use of equipment is necessary at the time of intercourse, some forethought is needed to ensure adequate supplies are available, and supplies may become exhausted if intercourse is repeated.

Disposal of the condom after use poses no problem when used in the home, but there can be no doubt that used condoms abandoned in public places present a sorry appearance and invite the disapproval of the later passer-by. Such disapproval is reflected in the public image of the condom as a method of birth control which is 'not quite nice', and may even have contributed to the negative attitude of general practitioners to their involvement in the distribution of condoms.

USAGE

The condom is a very widely used method, the total annual demand in the United Kingdom being about 150 million. The Hull Family Survey reporting on recently married couples found that 63 per cent had used or were using this method. The Medical Care Research Unit Study (Cartwright, 1970a) of the same year reported a similar figure, 68 per cent. Bone (1973) found that one-third of the married women at risk who were using contraception used the condom as a method.

The Hull survey produced an interesting profile of the sort of married couple likely to be using the sheath. Unlike most other forms of contraception, the sheath transcends the barriers of class, all social classes making equal use of it. Users include all religious groups, but are likely to have fewer children than couples using other methods, and are also more likely to take risks, i.e. fail to make use of the method on all occasions, than are other method users. The inference is that as this risk-taking results in an increasing family size, couples change to methods they feel will be more reliable, such as the Pill.

Questioning women as to why they had given up using the sheath as their contraceptive method, Cartwright (1970b) found that 25 per cent gave as their reason that it was unreliable.

Thus despite the effectiveness of the method when properly used at every intercourse, most patients regard it as an unreliable method. This is partly because, if used for long enough, most couples will be faced with a situation where they will have the choice of abstaining or taking a risk and, given the frailty of human nature, they feel they would probably take the risk. However, there is no doubt it is also due to the attitude of both general practitioners, who favour the medical, prescribable Pill or the medically inserted intrauterine device, and of the Family Planning Clinics, who have favoured pills, IUDs, and diaphragms. Of recent years the clinics have looked on the condom with more favour, and local authorities providing free family planning supplies now tend to supply condoms as well as other methods.

Regrettably general practitioners still regard providing condoms as an activity in which they will take no part. Among their reasons are that the method has 'no medical content' and a fear that if condoms were to be available on NHS prescription, doctors would be compelled to provide vast quantities for large numbers of patients, under Terms of Service that include penalties and were never designed to apply to such an activity. Although there is some force in the second argument, the first seems to me to be quite invalid. Lack of medical content infers a complete lack of side-effects and complications, a circumstance which should endear the method to the physician.

It is to be hoped that in the future a doctor who feels that the condom would be the most suitable method to advise for the particular patient in his surgery will be able, but not compelled, to prescribe it.

At the present time there is no doubt that few requests for advice or supplies of condoms are addressed to the family doctor.

Properly used by patients who find it a satisfying method of birth control it can be a very effective method, and doctors should encourage such patients in its use rather than attempt to persuade them to change to more complicated methods of greater medical content.

REFERENCES

BONE, MARGARET (1973). *Family Planning Services in England and Wales.* HMSO, London.

CARTWRIGHT, ANN (1970a). *The Medical Care Research Unit National Survey.* Routledge & Kegan Paul, London.

CARTWRIGHT, ANN (1970b). *Parents and Family Planning Services.* Routledge & Kegan Paul, London.

COMFORT, A. (1963). *Sex in Society.* Duckworth, London.

PEEL, J. (1969). Male-orientated fertility control. *Practitioner*, **202**, 677.

PEEL, J. (1972). The Hull Family Survey II. *Journal of Biosocial Science,* **4**, 333.

PEEL, J. and POTTS, M. (1969). *Textbook of Contraceptive Practice.* Cambridge University Press.

POTTS, M. (1973). Family Planning. *Community Health,* **4**, 185.

10

ORAL CONTRACEPTION

The knowledge that ovulation could be inhibited by the administration of progesterone, or of oestrogen, dates back to the nineteen-twenties. Both substances were extremely costly to extract from animal sources, and their low potency when given by mouth, coupled with the short time for which they produced an effect when injected, made them unsuitable for any practical use as a contraceptive.

In 1938 diethyl-stilboestrol, usually called stilboestrol, was synthesised. During the nineteen-forties this compound and other related compounds developed by the chemists were used to treat dysmenorrhoea by suppressing ovulation. The possibility that long-term administration of stilboestrol to suppress ovulation could be used as a method of birth control was considered and tested during this decade, but it was found that bleeding was irregular and sometimes heavy, and after several cycles the pituitary 'escaped' from the inhibiting effects of the oestrogen.

Russell Marker, in 1943, produced a synthetic progestational compound in commercial quantities, using as his source a chemical diosgenin, found in a type of wild yam growing in Mexico. Although very much cheaper than progesterone obtained from animal sources, it still was necessary to give it by injection.

In 1951, Carl Djerassi synthesised norethisterone, which was both extremely potent and effective when given by mouth.

Another synthetic progestational compound - for which the generic name 'progestogen' is now accepted - was produced at about the same time in the laboratories of G. D. Searle in Chicago and was named norethynodrel.

By the mid-1950s, therefore, there were available both synthetic oestrogens and progestogens which could be taken orally, and the stage was set for clinical trials of combinations of these products for contraception.

Just as an oestrogen alone had proved unsatisfactory, so a progestogen alone seemed equally unsatisfactory because of irregular bleeding - 'breakthrough bleeding' - during therapy. The addition of an oestrogen to the progestogen avoided this difficulty.

The compounds used in the original Pill, Enavid, marketed by G. D. Searle & Co in 1957, were norethynodrel as the progestogen and the 3-methyl ether of ethinyl oestradiol (mestranol) as the oestrogen. Clinical trials of these compounds were carried out in 1956 in the United States and, on a large scale, in Puerto Rico.

Clinicians involved in these studies included Dr Gregory Pincus - later to achieve fame under the title 'The Father of the Pill', Dr John Rock, Professor of Gynaecology at Harvard, Dr Min-Chueh Chang, working with Pincus at the Worcester (Massachusetts) Foundation for Experimental Biology, and in Puerto Rico and Latin America, Dr Edris Rice-Wray.

Since the early trials of the Pill, the dose of progestogen has been progressively reduced and newer progestational compounds have been developed. Only two oestrogens have been used, but their dosage has also been reduced.

STEROID CHEMISTRY

For a detailed discussion of this subject the reader is referred to specialist textbooks.

Basically a steroid molecule consists of rings of carbon atoms joined together, with side chains arising from them. There is a convention for numbering the carbon atoms according to their positions on the rings or the side chains (Fig. 10).

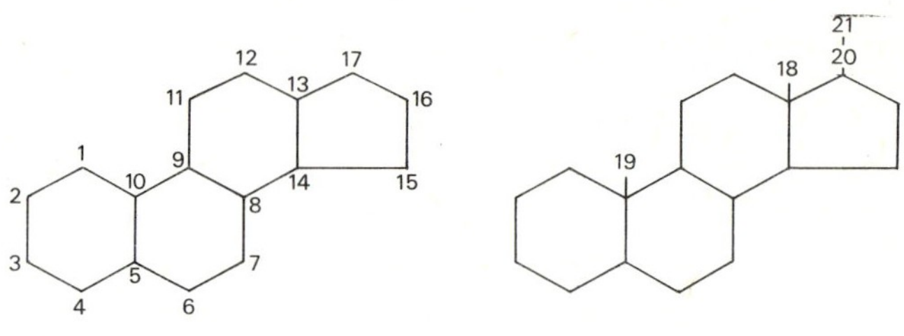

Fig. 10.

These drawings of the steroid molecule should really be three-dimensional. The valency bonds of the side chains may project upwards from the page towards the reader - in which case they are labelled β - or downwards and away from the reader - in which case they are labelled α. β bonds are represented by unbroken lines, α bonds by dotted lines.

Oestrogens have a total of 18 carbon atoms, testosterone has 19, and progesterone 21.

Oestrogens

There are only two oestrogens used in oral contraception, ethinyloestradiol and mestranol.

Ethinyloestradiol

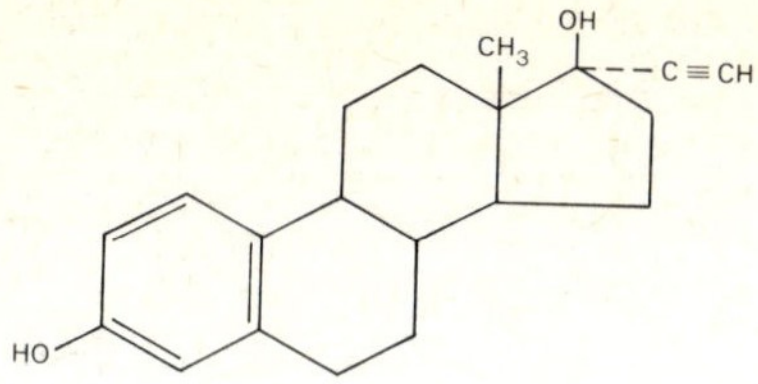

Fig. 11.

This compound has an OH group at carbon 3.

Mestranol

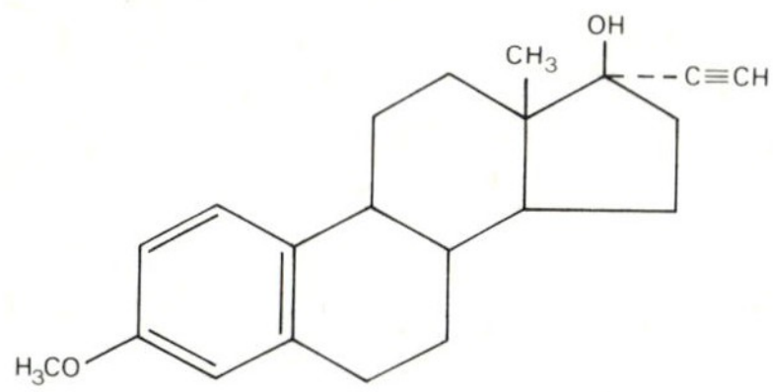

Fig. 12.

The only difference between this compound and ethinyloestradiol is the substitution of a methyl group (CH_3) for the hydrogen atom in the OH group at carbon 3.

Ethinyloestradiol is said to be oestrogenically 1.8 times more powerful than mestranol.

Progestogens

There are many different progestogens, but all can be assigned to one of only two groups.

1. Those related to 19-nortestosterone (the 19-norsteroids).

e.g.

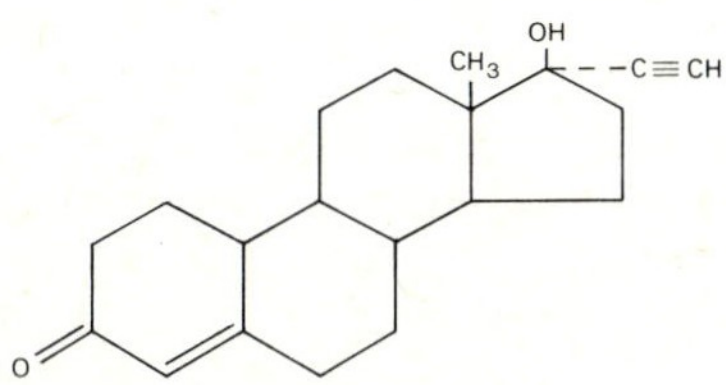

Fig. 13 Norethisterone.

2. Those related to 17α - hydroxy progesterone

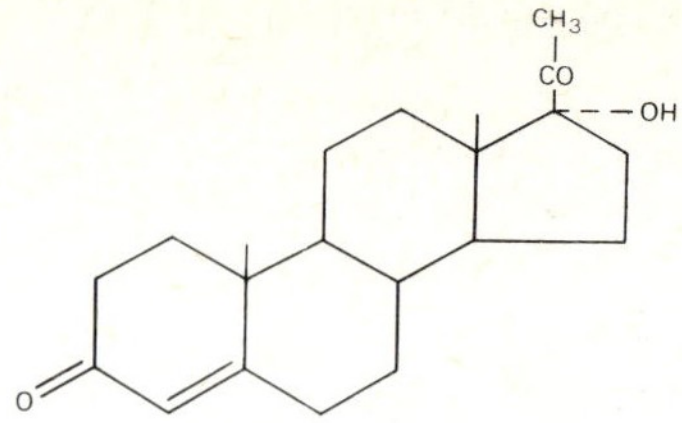

Fig. 14 17α-hydroxyprogesterone

Megestrol acetate is an example of a progestogen in this group.

TYPES OF ORAL CONTRACEPTIVE

1. **The combined Pill**

Containing both a progestogen and an oestrogen, this is the type of Pill most commonly used. The original 'Pincus Pill' was one of this group.

Some types of combined Pill, although containing a progestogen as well, are referred to as 'low-oestrogen Pills'. The dosage of oestrogen in most oral contraceptives was reduced to 50 microgrammes as a result of the Scowen report, and attempts to reduce the oestrogen still further, e.g. to 30 microgrammes, have been successful.

Combined oral contraceptives are usually taken daily for twentyone days, with no tablet being taken for the succeeding seven days, making a twenty-eight day 'cycle' in all. One manufacturer produces a pill that is taken for twentytwo days, followed by six days with no tablets, again making a twentyeight day cycle.

There are several combined products which are designed to to be taken continuously, inert tablets being taken on days when no medication is required. The thinking behind this scheme is that women find it easier to remember to take a tablet every day, rather than stopping and starting. In practice, women who remember tablets at all remember either method with equal ease. In fact some women prefer to 'have a rest' from tablet-taking.

Some manufacturers have produced preparations substituting iron-containing tablets for the inert ones. This would seem to be somewhat superfluous, as few women taking combined oral contraceptives are anaemic.

2 **Progestogen-only Pills**

Colloquially known as 'the Minipill' or 'POP Pills', these tablets contain no oestrogen. They are taken every day, continuously.

3. **Sequential Pills**

Goldzieher, in 1963, reported a sequential method of hormonal contraception, consisting of the administration of oestrogen for fifteen days, followed by a further five days when a progestogen was added to the oestrogen.

This method was originally thought to have advantages, but for reasons which will be discussed later is little used today.

4. The 'Morning-after' Pill

Large doses of oestrogen or progestogen alone, taken within 72 hours of intercourse, have been shown to have a contraceptive action. This Pill, as such, is not marketed in this country.

A list of names and contents of oral contraceptives obtainable in the United Kingdom, 1974

A. Combined oral contraceptives.

(note: E.E. = ethinyloestradiol M. = mestranol)

Proprietary name	*Progestogen and dosage*		*Oestrogen and dosage*
Anovlar	Norethisterone acetate	4 mg	E.E. 0.05 mg
Conovid	Norethynodrel	5 mg	M. 0.075 mg
Conovid-E	Norethynodrel	2.5 mg	M. 0.1 mg
Demulen	Ethynodiol diacetate	0.5 mg	M. 0.1 mg
Demulen-50	Ethynodiol diacetate	C.5 mg	E.E. 0.05 mg
Eugynon-50	dl-Norgestrel	0.5 mg	E.E. 0.05 mg
Eugynon-30	dl-Norgestrel	0.5 mg	E.E. 0.03 mg
Gynovlar 21	Norethisterone acetate	3 mg	E.E. 0.05 mg
Lyndiol 2.5†	Lynestrenol	2.5 mg	M. 0.075 mg
Microgynon	d-Norgestrel	0.15 mg	E.E. 0.03 mg
Minilyn†	Lynestrenol	2.5 mg	E.E. 0.05 mg
Minovlar	Norethisterone acetate	1 mg	E.E. 0.05 mg
Minovlar ED*	Norethisterone acetate	1 mg	E.E. 0.05 mg
Norinyl-1	Norethisterone	1 mg	M. 0.05 mg
Norinyl 1-28*	Norethisterone	1 mg	M. 0.05 mg
Norlestrin 21	Norethisterone acetate	2.5 mg	E.E. 0.05 mg
Orlest 28*	Norethisterone acetate	1 mg	E.E. 0.05 mg
Orthonovin 1/50	Norethisterone	1 mg	M. 0.05 mg
Orthonovin 1/80	Norethisterone	1 mg	M. 0.08 mg
Orthonovin 2	Norethisterone	2 mg	M. 0.1 mg
Ovran	de-Norgestrel	0.5 mg	E.E. 0.05 mg
Ovranette	d-Norgestrel	0.15 mg	E.E. 0.03 mg
Ovulen	Ethynodiol diacetate	1 mg	M. 0.1 mg
Ovulen-50	Ethynodiol diacetate	1 mg	E.E. 0.05 mg
Volidan	Megestrol acetate	4 mg	E.E. 0.05 mg

Products marked † are taken for 22 days in each 28-day cycle.
Products marked * are continuous 28-day regimens, seven of the 28 tablets being inert.

Con-fer	Norethisterone acetate	1 mg	E.E. 0.05 mg

is also a 28-day regimen, each of the seven contraceptively inert tablets containing 75 mg ferrous fumerate.

Conovid is packed in batches of twenty tablets.

B. Progestogen-only oral contraceptives.

Proprietary name	*Progestogen and dosage*	
Femulen	Ethynodiol diacetate	0.05 mg
Micronor	Norethisterone	0.35 mg
Noriday	Norethisterone	0.35 mg

C. Sequential oral contraceptives.

Proprietary name	*Contents of tablets and regimen of use*
Ovanon	Seven tablets containing mestranol 0.8 mg, followed by fifteen tablets containing Lynestrenol 2.5 mg and mestranol 0.75 mg. followed by six tablet-free days.
Serial 28	Sixteen tablets containing ethinyloestradiol, followed by five tablets containing megestrol acetate 1 mg and ethinyloestradiol 0.1 mg, followed by seven inert tablets.

All oral contraceptives marketed in United Kingdom are provided with some method of identifying the day of the week on which a particular pill was taken. Most are in 'push out' plastic packs, some in more elaborate containers. Considerable market research has been carried out to make the packaging attractive to women.

EFFECTS OF THE PILL ON THE HORMONAL CONTROL OF THE MENSTRUAL CYCLE

Opponents of oral contraception often remark that the exact mode of action of the Pill is unknown. This is true only inasmuch as there is a good deal of ignorance concerning the ultimate details of the normal physiology of the pituitary and hypothalamus, and therefore anything that affects their action and interaction - as the Pill undoubtedly does - can be understood only as completely as our incomplete knowledge of the underlying normal physiology will allow. A great deal of research is taking place all over the world in an attempt to unravel the normal psychological actions of the pituitary-hypothalamic axis, and certainly the investigation of the action of the Pill has been more thorough than the investigation of any other drug.

The sum of the knowledge gained from this research is most impressive, but is of little importance to the general practitioner in his everyday work. Indeed, without the special training of the endocrinologist, the reproductive physiologist, the gynaecologist, and the biochemist, it is difficult for the average doctor to follow the experts in their exposition of the mode of action of the Pill. The description which follows is a simple one, a skeleton to which those interested may add the detail from reading elsewhere.

Menstrual cycle (Fig. 15)

The cycle begins on the first day of menstrual bleeding, when the en-

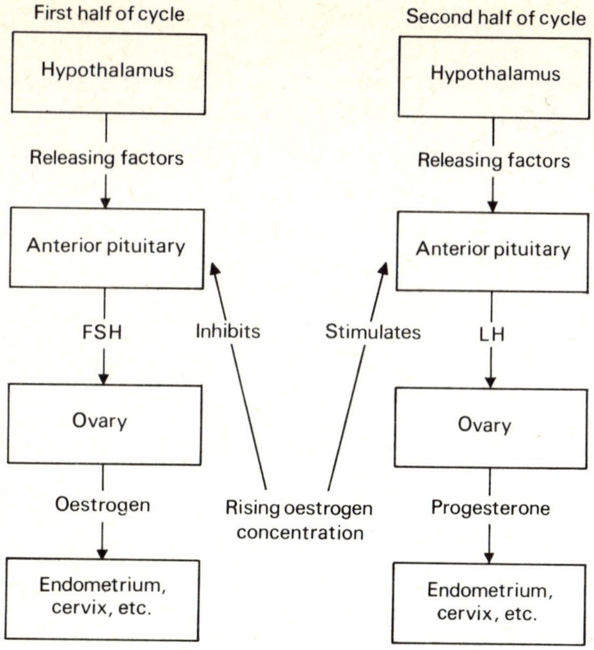

Fig. 15 Hormonal influence on menstrual cycle.

dometrium is shed, leaving a basal layer in which are the remnants, the bottom ends, of the glands. From the margins of these remnants the epithelium grows to cover the rest of the surface, until by about the fourth day the interior of the uterus is covered with cuboidal epithelium, into which open the mouths of the glands. Proliferation then occurs, the epithelial cells growing taller until they become tall columnar epithelium, their nuclei showing more mitoses as growth proceeds. The glands grow taller also, assuming the shape of a test-tube, the stroma becomes more oedematous, and blood vessels grow in.

This is the proliferative phase, lasting to mid-cycle when ovulation occurs, and takes place under the influence of oestrogen, produced by the granulosa cells of the developing Graafian follicle in the ovary, the development of which is in turn being stimulated by follicle-stimulating hormone (FSH) from the anterior pituitary. The FSH level in the blood reaches a peak during menstruation, and then a 'feed-back' mechanism comes into effect, the rising concentration of oestrogen inhibiting further FSH production, and stimulating the production of luteinising hormone (LH) from the anterior pituitary, which reaches its peak at about the time of ovulation.

When ovulation occurs, the endometrial glands grow faster than the stroma and so become coiled and tortuous. Secretion starts below the nuclei, forming subnuclear vacuoles, and then pushes past them to appear in the lumen of the gland, giving the post-ovulatory phase the alternative name, the secretory phase. At the same time the stroma becomes more oedematous and the arterioles become more numerous and spiral. Towards the end of this phase the stroma becomes infiltrated with leucocytes, and after this degeneration of the endometrium leads to menstruation.

The secretory phase is controlled by progesterone from the granulosa lutein cells and the paralutein cells of the theca interna of the corpus luteum. Oestrogen is also produced by the corpus luteum, and it is the combination of the correct amounts of both oestrogen and progesterone that produce the normal menstrual changes.

Development of the corpus luteum and production of these hormones is dependant on the increasing production of LH from the anterior pituitary, and also on the production of luteotrophic hormone, or prolactin, produced from the same source.

There is again a feed-back mechanism, the rising concentration of progesterone inhibiting the production of both LH and prolactin.

The production of the gonodotrophins, FSH, LH and prolactin, from the pituitary is controlled by releasing factors produced in the hypothalamus and carried to the anterior pituitary by a portal system of blood vessels.

Circulating levels of oestrogen can be assessed by estimation of the quantity of total oestrogens (oestrone, oestradiol and oestriol) in the urine. Normally an ovulatory peak is demonstrable at mid-cycle, and a smaller luteal peak a few days before menstruation. Circulating levels of progesterone can similarly be assessed by the quantity of pregnanediol in the urine which reaches a peak in the last week of the menstrual cycle. Direct estimations of the blood levels of progesterone are now possible.

The cervix

Cyclical changes take place in the cervix under the influence of oestrogen and progesterone. During the first half of the menstrual cycle the rising level of oestrogen stimulates the cervical glands to produce mucus, which at the time of ovulation is profuse, clear, watery and readily penetrable by spermatozoa. If some of this mucus is mixed with a drop of normal saline on a slide and allowed to dry, crystallization occurs in a distinct pattern known as 'ferning'. The concentration of sialic acid in cervical mucus rises at the time of ovulation, and there appears to be a critical level at which sperm penetration can occur. Progesterone alters the character of the cervical mucus so that it becomes thick and tacky, ferning no longer takes place, and spermatozoa cannot penetrate.

MODE OF ACTION OF VARIOUS TYPES OF ORAL CONTRACEPTIVE

1 Progestogen-only Pill

There is a consistent effect on cervical mucus. Normal ovulatory mucus does not appear and ferning cannot be demonstrated. The sialic acid content is raised to several times the normal ovulatory level and Eckstein (1972) suggests that this may be the reason that spermatozoa cannot penetrate the mucus.

On the endometrium the effect is less marked than with the combined type of Pill, both proliferative and secretory changes being identifiable. The endometrial appearances are difficult to correlate with the irregular cycles that are prone to occur on this type of therapy, but it is likely that the changes in the endometrium are sufficient to interfere with implantation of the ovum.

Ovulation inhibition was thought not to occur in patients taking progestogen-only contraceptives. This opinion was based on the more normal pattern of hormonal excretion found in these patients, as compared with those taking combined Pills. However the patterns are altered, and it is probable that ovulation inhibition is dose-related, the preparations containing a larger dosage, or compounds of greater potency producing their more satisfactory antifertility effect (and their less satisfactory effect on the regulation of vaginal bleeding) by inhibition of ovulation.

In addition, there may be an effect on ovum transport due to the influence of the progestogen on tubal motility.

2. Sequential preparations

The initial administration of unopposed oestrogen in the first half of the cycle minimizes the effect on both cervical mucus and endometrium, the latter showing almost normal proliferative and secretory changes. The endometrium does not become atrophic with long-term therapy.

Ovulation inhibition occurs more regularly than with compounds containing only progestogen, but less regularly than with combined Pills.

3. The combined Pill

The changes in cervical mucus already described as occurring in patients taking progestogen-only Pills occur equally in patients taking combined oral contraceptives.

Endometrial changes are most marked. During the first cycle or two of therapy, the normal proliferative changes seen in the oestrogenic phase of the cycle do not develop fully, and the endometrial glands rapidly assume the appearances of the secretory phase. After several cycles, however, the vaginal blood loss during the days when the Pill is omitted may be scanty, or even absent. Currettage of the uterus of a patient who has taken combined oral contraceptives for many months produces only tiny fragments of endometrium.

Ovulation is suppressed in most cycles in women taking combined Pills. The fact that not all cycles were anovular was suspected from the clinical observation that dysmenorrhoea reappears in occasional cycles in women who have taken the Pill for years. Peel and Potts (1969) quote breakthrough ovulation as occurring in 2 to 10 per cent of cycles.

The mechanism of ovulation suppression has excited much intensive investigation. Diminished pregnanediol excretion and diminished excretion of total oestrogen was early evidence that ovarian function was suppressed, but whether by direct action of the Pill upon the ovary, or whether by indirect action on FSH and LH, which in turn suppressed ovarian function was not clear. The confusion was due to the inexact methods of assaying LH and FSH, which did not distinguish clearly the effects of each.

It is now considered that the ultimate action of the combined Pill is to inhibit the production of gonadotrophin-releasing factors from the hypothalamus. As as result there is a constant inhibition of pituitary LH production. Suppression of FSH production sometimes occurs also but is of lesser importance.

The rapidity with which ovulation returns after stopping combined oral contraception provides presumptive evidence that ovarian function itself is not suppressed. Evidence from experimental animals supports this, since the ovulation-inhibiting effect of oestrogen and progesterone can be cancelled by administering gonadotrophins as well.

Finally, ovum transport may also be influenced by the combined oral contraceptives.

4. Post-coital contraceptives

Large doses of oestrogen (e.g. 50 mg stilboestrol daily) are given for four or five days after intercourse. Implantation of a fertilized ovum is prevented, possibly by accelerating the tubal transport of the ovum, possibly by interfering with implantation.

Progestogen alone may be used in place of oestrogen.

Side-effects of combined oral contraceptives

A. BENEFICIAL SIDE-EFFECTS

Quite apart from the peace of mind that an efficient method of contraception brings there are certain side-effects which are welcomed by many women.

1. Regulation of the periods

For the woman whose periods have been irregular, the change wrought by the combined Pill can be little short of miraculous. Many patients can forecast exactly not only the day on which bleeding will occur, but the exact hour of the day.

2. **Diminution of blood loss**

Due to the atrophic endometrium which develops after a few months use of the combined Pill, especially the more progestogenic types of Pill, the amount of blood lost at a period may be very much reduced. The woman who bled for seven or eight days may bleed for only two or three, and the number of pads or tampons used daily may be reduced to a similar degree. As a consequence, iron deficiency anaemia has become very rare among patients taking the combined Pill in my practice.

A girl aged 25 took the combined pill for three years after marriage, while she continued to work full-time. She bled for one hour at 2.0 p.m. every fourth Monday. As she was a physical training instructor at a girl's school she found this pattern most convenient.

3. **Relief of pain**

Blood escaping from the ruptured follicle at the time of ovulation and causing peritoneal irritation can result in the sudden onset of lower abdominal pain at mid-cycle. This pain is known as ovulation pain, or Mittelschmerz, and can vary from a mild ache on one side to agonizing pain with collapse due to several pints of blood in the peritoneal cavity. Although the more severe examples of Mittelschmerz are rarely encountered in general practice, it is not uncommon for women to present with the milder forms.

Pain at or before the periods, dysmenorrhoea, is also reported to be associated with ovulation. Primary spasmodic dysmenorrhoea occurs in nulliparous women, typically begins a day or so before the menstrual flow, rises to a crescendo on the first day of bleeding, and then fades away as the period is established. In general, childbirth seems to lessen a patient's liability to this type of pain, but many parous women continue to have some pain with their periods nevertheless.

As one of the actions of the combined Pill is to inhibit ovulation, it is not surprising to find that both ovulation pain and dysmenorrhoea are relieved by this therapy. The relief may be complete, but may be only partial. Although difficult to quantify, my impression is that the relief obtained has been lessened by the introduction of the lower dose of oestrogen. The fact that ovulation is not suppressed in all cycles is evidenced by the occasional recurrence of ovulation pain or dysmenorrhoea, or both, in some patients, irrespective of the length of time they have taken the Pill.

For the patient who needs contraception, the combined Pill is of great value, since the pain is relieved at the same time. I do not believe that the young girl with dysmenorrhoea who does not need contraception should be given the Pill as a first treatment, because of the complications of oral contraception considered elsewhere. Simpler measures should be tried first, and only if they fail should the Pill be considered.

4. **Relief of the pre-menstrual syndrome**

Many women feel bloated, depressed and irritable for several days before their periods, with pains and distension of the lower abdomen, tenderness of the breasts, headaches and general malaise. Some women complain of aching in the legs. It has been shown that during this time both physical and intellectual performance are diminished and, because of the depression, attempts at suicide are more common.

All these symptoms may be lessened or abolished during therapy with the combined Pill.

5. **Ability to delay periods**

By continuing to take the Pill beyond the end of the course, the withdrawal bleed may be delayed. This facility is much appreciated so that bleeding may be avoided at times when it would be inconvenient, as at holiday times or weddings, for example.

Certain points must be explained carefully to the patient, however. Firstly, it is obvious that only continuation of Pills containing the active ingredients will delay the period. Hence women taking courses of tablets containing placebos or iron must be warned to take extra tablets before, not after, the placebos. Secondly, experience shows that the longer the attempt to delay the period lasts, the greater the chance that breakthrough bleeding will occur. This was so even with the higher dosage Pills used in the mid-1960s, and is even more true with modern low-dosage tablets. In general, an attempt to delay the period for one to two weeks will be successful in almost all women. To delay beyond this becomes increasingly likely to be unsuccessful.

The amount lost at the delayed bleed may be rather heavier than usual, but not invariably so.

After taking extra tablets, if she takes them out of her next pack, the woman will be left with an incomplete pack. The wise family doctor will have a store of spare packs in his desk, so that he may supply the extra Pills needed. The presentation of these Pills makes an acceptable holiday gift - or wedding present.

6. Effect on the breasts

It may seem surprising to include it under this heading but in general practice today this side-effect attracts more laudatory comment from patients than the reverse.

In pregnancy, oestrogen and progesterone build up the breasts, the ducts responding particularly to the action of oestrogen, and the glands to both oestrogen and progesterone.

During the first few cycles, the patient taking a combined Pill notices changes very similar to those in early pregnancy, the breasts enlarging, becoming firmer, exhibiting slight tenderness on palpation, and discomfort on movement. Irritation, or 'tingling' of the nipples may develop. Dilatation of the veins over the breasts may be in evidence.

These changes may disappear completely after the second or third month of therapy, but in most women, although the tenderness and discomfort goes, the enlargement and firmness remains, much to their delight.

We live in a breast-conscious society. The complaint of inadequate breast size or unsatisfactory shape is not at all uncommon among women consulting their family doctor. Often it is not simply a question of vanity but a deep-seated anxiety, exaggerated by the consort's obvious appreciation of other girls with large busts, or of photographs in magazines where flat-chested models simply do not appear.

A sympathetic approach by the GP is essential; reassurance that her breasts are within normal limits is simply not enough.

The many advertisements in women's magazines extolling methods of increasing breast size bear witness to the fact that women worry about the matter enough to spend money on it.

The help of the plastic surgeon is indicated in some cases of minute breasts, but such operations rightly have a low priority on National Health Service waiting lists, and most patients cannot afford the private fees. Silicone injections had a vogue, but in view of reports of mastectomies following ulceration after repeated injections, should not, in my view, now be considered.

Topical oestrogen ointment does produce some enlargement, but also an exaggerated pigmentation of the nipple and areola and an unpleasant nodularity of the breast tissue, to which the patient and her consort object.

The arrival of the combined Pill has enabled the family doctor to suggest a method of treatment when contraception is also required that may produce very good results. Indeed, the fact that the Pill has this effect on breast size is well known in the female population at large, and the suggestion often comes from the patient.

Where improvement of breast size and contour does occur, the effect is maintained, without further increase in size, for as long as the Pill is taken. If no effect is noticed, changing the progestogen, on an empirical basis, may produce the desired result, as may increasing the dose of progestogen. Changing or increasing the oestrogen does not seem to have much effect. Progestogen-only Pills seem to have less effect than the combined Pill.

7. Relief of acne

Acne may be improved by taking a combined oral contraceptive.

Preparations containing larger doses of oestrogen are more likely to produce improvement; progestogen-only preparations are least likely. Pre-existing acne may show an exacerbation on first taking the Pill, but will settle within a few cycles.

A very few women develop acne for the first time when taking oral contraceptives of any type. The acne responds to long-term treatment with tetracycline, but it is obviously preferable to change to another method of contraception if possible.

8. **Increase in libido**
As with all reliable methods of contraception, there may be an increase in libido where fear of pregnancy has caused a previous diminution. However, there are women who report increased sexual desire when taking the Pill, even though no previous fear of pregnancy existed.

9. **A feeling of well-being**
Some women declare they feel better on the Pill than they have ever felt before.They may request a continuous method of tablet-taking as a result, and it is interesting that such women can detect 'dummy' tablets. If complications occur in these women it is sometimes difficult to persuade them to abandon oral contraception. Similarly some women insist on continuing the Pill even though intercourse is not even remotely likely, simply because they feel so much better.

B. ANNOYING SIDE-EFFECTS OF ORAL CONTRACEPTIVES

Before consideration of this subject, we should consider the significance of complaints of any symptom in patients taking the Pill.

1. If patients are warned before taking the Pill that certain side-effects may be expected, then they will oblige and develop the expected symptoms.

Pincus and Paniagna in Puerto Rico told women they were being given the Pill but gave lactose tablets instead, with warnings of possible unpleasant side-effects due to the therapy. Another group were given genuine Pills but with no warning concerning side-effects. Both groups were protected by another contraceptive method in addition. Seventeen per cent of the 'warned' group developed unpleasant side-effects while taking placebos, whereas only six per cent of the 'un-warned' group taking the Pill did so.

Goldzieher asked women wearing intrauterine devices whether they suffered from symptoms usually attributed to oral contraceptives. As many women in this group complained of such symptoms as in another group asked the same questions who were using oral contraception.

2. At the follow-up, the GP should never ask whether the patient has suffered a particular symptom, but should always use an enquiry phrased in general terms; for example, 'Have you noticed any troubles since I last saw you?' It must be remembered that one of the most important therapeutic agents any doctor prescribes is himself. Suggesting possible symptoms must be avoided.

Dr Eric Murphy, a Northampton GP, made the shrewd comment in 1968 that to a large extent, patients suffer the side-effects their doctors deserve.

3. Any investigator who is particularly interested in any particular symptom will tend to find a higher incidence of this symptom.

This was graphically shown in clinical trials conducted by general practitioners of products manufactured by G. D. Searle & Co Ltd where it was found that for any particular symptom, the difference in reporting between GPs was greater than the difference between the incidence of the symptom for each of the different products on trial.

Randomised, double-blind, cross-over trials against a placebo would eliminate the influence of these factors in assessing side-effects due to oral contraception. Ethically, to give a placebo to women requiring contraception is obviously unjustifiable. This difficulty may be overcome by arranging for all the women in the trial to use an entirely different type of contraception in addition to the Pill.

One such trial has been reported by Goldzieher and others (1971). A sequential Pill, two combined Pills, a progestogen-only Pill, and a placebo were used. All were placed in capsules to look alike, and packaged alike in strips. Patients were unselected and randomly allocated to one of the five types of Pill. It was arranged that all patients allocated to the placebo group used a vaginal contraceptive cream in addition, but so also did ten per cent of the subjects in each of the other four groups. Use of the vaginal cream thus did not identify the placebo users.

A cross-over was planned at three points in the study, half the placebo users being transferred to combined Pills after four cycles, and half to progestogen-only. Those taking one of the combined Pills were switched to progestogen-only, and those taking progestogen-only were switched to one of the combined. All these changes were incorporated in the sets of Pills made up for each patient in advance, so that they were unknown either to the patients or the investigators.

And then, when only four-fifths of the planned number of patients had been enrolled, the investigation had to be abandoned because of reports of breast tumours in beagles treated with the progestogen contained in the progestogen-only Pill being used in the trial. This episode in itself was a very neat example of the effect that publicity may have on users of oral contraceptives.

Nevertheless, sufficient data was available for statistical analysis and some most interesting conclusions resulted.

1. With the exception of nausea and vomiting, the incidence of all symptoms as recorded during the pre-treatment cycle was diminished markedly by treatment with the placebo.
2. Placebo users suffered more symptoms than women taking genuine Pills.
3. A significant increase in the incidence of nausea, vomiting, headache and nervousness could be demonstrated only in the first treatment cycle with high-oestrogen preparations.
4. There was no evidence at all for the association of depression with four of the five compounds used. With the fifth, there was contradictory evidence.

5. There were no significant changes in blood pressure.
6. There was no significant difference between the weight changes seen in patients in the placebo group and the contraceptive groups.

From these results it would seem that symptoms usually attributed to the use of oral contraceptives (headache, nervousness, depression, and weight gain) are complained of with some frequency in women not using oral contraceptives - if they are asked. There is therefore probably considerable over-reporting of such symptoms as being due to the Pill. Many studies have used the incidence of symptoms in pre-treatment cycles as controls: others have compared Pill users with women using other methods, or even randomly chosen women using no method. These types of investigation are not equivalent to controlled trials against a placebo in women using oral contraception.

The results of this trial do not demonstrate that side-effects never occur in women on the Pill. They do suggest that the true incidence of side-effects actually due to the Pill is probably considerably lower than reports so far indicate.

In the discussion of side-effects which follows I have where possible avoided giving numerical estimates of the incidence of side-effects and used general terms such as 'common' or 'rare', basing my assessment on the frequency with which I have been faced in general practice with patients complaining of the particular symptom. The various methods of relieving symptoms which I suggest are methods which I have found helpful. If it is suggested that many of my suggestions are probably more psychotherapeutic than anything else, I would wholeheartedly agree. Most of the treatment given in general practice is psychotherapy: none the less it is therapy for all that and, by and large, efficient, satisfying and safe.

1. **Nausea and vomiting**

Slight nausea is common in the early stages of taking the Pill, usually for a few days at the beginning of each of the first cycle or two, rarely longer. Vomiting is rare, but can be very severe and enough to prevent the patient continuing with the method. It is also important, since if the vomiting happens soon after swallowing the Pill, the Pill may be returned and the contraceptive action is lost. Most modern Pill packages contain a warning that vomiting due to any cause, such as gastroenteritis, may result in loss of efficacy unless another Pill is swallowed.

As the Pill is often taken before going to bed, nausea is common in the morning on rising. Some patients find that altering the time the Pill is taken - for example, taking it after breakfast, or taking it with food - will avoid trouble.

The oestrogen is to blame for these symptoms and, where they are severe enough to warrant action, changing to a preparation containing the other oestrogen will usually relieve them.

Rarely women are unable to tolerate either oestrogen, with really incapacitating nausea and vomiting. Unless they fall into this group, women starting oral contraception in the puerperium never complain of these symptoms. There seems to be no relationship between the occurrence of nausea and vomiting in pregnancy and the occurrence of the same symptoms in the same woman when taking the Pill. For a list of preparations classified by the type of oestrogen contained see Table III

Table III. Classification of oral contraceptives by oestrogen contained

Preparations containing Ethinyloestradiol	*Preparations containing Mestranol*
Anovlar	Conovid 5
Demulen 50	Demulen
Eugynon 30	Lyndiol 2.5
Eugynon 50	Norinyl 1/28
Gynovlar	Orthonovin 1/50
Microgynon 30	Orthonovin 1/80
Minilyn	Orthonovin 2 mg
Minovlar	* Ovanon
Norlestrin	Ovulen
Orlest 28	
Ovran	
Ovranette	
Ovulen 50	
*Serial 28	
Volidan	

**Sequential regimen

2. **Breakthrough bleeding**

Occasionally a woman will bleed while still taking the course of Pills, before the days without the Pill - or the days on the dummy tablets - are reached. This is more likely to happen during the first cycle or two during which this form of contraception is used, in recently confined women, and with preparations containing the lower dosages of progestogen, or very large women where the dosage is relatively low.

If the bleeding is enough for the patient to notice, but not enough for her to wear a pad or a tampon, then by convention it is known as 'spotting'.

Breakthrough bleeding or spotting, occurring shortly after starting the Pill, lasting for only a day or two, or only small in quantity, may be dealt with by reassuring the patient that the symptom will disappear in the next few cycles. The chart that the patient keeps can be of use, as the doctor can demonstrate that the number of bleeding days is decreasing month by month.

If the bleeding is heavy, or if it does not show signs of disappearing, a change to a preparation with a larger dose of progestogen will usually prevent it. Several manufacturers make Pills containing increasing quantities of progestogen but with the same amount of oestrogen (Table IV). It should never be necessary to increase the number of Pills taken daily, as formerly advised, as this also increases the oestrogen.

Bleeding or spotting occurring in a woman who has taken Pills for many cycles must be viewed with suspicion. There may be several explanations.

(i) She may have forgotten, or been late taking, one or more tablets. The GP may then inform her that the bleeding is merely the wages of sin and remind her of the possibility of pregnancy.

(ii) The bleeding may be a reaction to emotional stress. The stress involved may be major, such as the illness of her child, or ridiculously minor as, for example, going on holiday. If due to such a cause, the bleeding will not recur in subsequent cycles.

(iii) There may be an underlying cause, carcinoma of the genital tract being obviously the most important.

It cannot be too strongly emphasized that unexplained spotting or bleeding in a woman established on oral contraception must be investigated. In this connection it may be noted that a negative Papanicolou smear is not enough.

Breakthrough bleeding in a woman in the puerperium can be a difficult problem for the general practitioner. There is a vogue at the present time for hospitals to initiate oral contraception before the patient leaves for home, which may mean within 48 hours of delivery. When bleeding follows it is impossible to decide whether it is due to the oral contraceptive or to retained products of conception. (See also under 'Oral contraceptives after pregnancy or abortion,' p. 113).

Table IV. Preparations containing differing dosages of the same progestogen, without alteration of oestrogen dosage

Maker	*Progestogen*	*Dosage*	*Preparation*
Ortho	Norethisterone	1·0 mg	Orthonovin 1-50
		2·0 mg	Othonovin 2 mg
Schering	Norethisterone-acetate	1·0 mg	Minovlar
		3·0 mg	Gynovlar
		4·0 mg	Anovlar
	d-norgestrol	0·15 mg	Microgynon 30
		0·25 mg	Eugynon 30
Searle	Ethynodiol-diacetate	0·5 mg	Demulen 50
		1·0 mg	Ovulen 50

3. **Weight gain**

This symptom looms large in the mind of all women about to take the Pill, and questions concerning weight gain are those most commonly asked of the doctor. The oestrogen component of the Pill invariably produces a transient fluid retention, resulting in a gain of a few pounds in weight, associated with a bloated feeling. This effect wears off in almost all women by the third month of therapy. The progestogen component seems in some few women to produce an increased appetite and an anabolic effect which results in a steady, progressive increase in weight.

It is useful to warn women that they may feel bloated to begin with, and essential that their weight before starting therapy is recorded in order to demonstrate that they may temporarily feel fatter without being fatter.

If a genuine progressive gain in body weight is demonstrated, dietary measures should be started immediately. The consumption of carbohydrate is too great in most people in the United Kingdom, and restriction of carbohydrate is usually all that is required.

Using no other measures, the average weight change in 350 of my patients observed over 3,000 cycles was a slight weight loss rather than gain.

However, in the patient where weight gain persists despite genuine efforts at dieting, a change to a less progestogenic preparation, or a change to an entirely different progestogenic compound, may solve the problem. On rare occasions the method may have to be abandoned, often at the insistence of the patient.

4. **Leg cramps**

The patient complains of pains in the legs, and the main importance of this symptom is that the doctor must, by the history and examination, distinguish between leg pain due to cramp and pain due to venous thrombophlebitis or arterial blockage. Typically cramp pain occurs at rest, particularly at night, and complaints are more common in summer than in winter. An increased salt intake during hot weather often relieves the symptom altogether. Failing this, changing to a less progestogenic compound will usually result in disappearance of the cramps. Complaints of cramp are not very common and will rarely trouble the patient sufficiently to make her abandon oral contraception.

5. **Headache**

That all symptoms in users of oral contraceptives are not induced by warnings given by the medical attendant is evidenced by the fact that I have never yet warned a woman that she may suffer headaches but, despite this, complaints of headaches occur regularly in my contraceptive practice and can be a very difficult symptom to deal with.

Young women on oral contraceptives may present to their family doctor with headaches due to a variety of causes, and to list these causes would be to duplicate the function of a textbook of general medicine. From a clinical point of view, however, it is possible to identify certain groups of patients complaining of headache.

(i) *Headache associated with oral contraception, but not directly caused by it.*

The patient who fears the rare and dangerous complications of the Pill; and the patient who takes the Pill to avoid the pregnancy she cannot, for socio-economic reasons, embark on, but who desperately wishes she could - both these are examples of the sort of situation that can cause a girl using oral contraception to complain of headaches.

They are part of the symptomatology of an anxiety state, sometimes with depressive features, and usually show the characteristics of 'tension headaches' - pain at the top of the head, going down to the back of the neck and shoulders, and do not occur cyclically, but may be worse at period times.

Such patients require time to elucidate the cause and appropriate treatment, which may include the use of mild tranquillisers.

A 23-year-old married woman complained of severe vertical headache, starting shortly after beginning oral contraception, and worrying her almost every day at varying times during the day, sometimes keeping her awake. After long discussion she eventually admitted that although she desperately wanted a baby, her husband had convinced her that it would be madness to start a pregnancy in their present financial circumstances - large mortgage, huge hire-purchase debts, etc. A meeting between husband, wife and GP was arranged and a date was fixed when the strain of the financial situation could be expected to have eased, and the Pill would - come what may - be abandoned. The headaches disappeared after the meeting.

(ii) *Headache due to oral contraception*

In this category there are three types; the rare headache due to a cerebral vascular castrophe, the common 'Pill headache' and migraine.

(a) *'Pill headache'*. Usually, but not invariably, this shows itself during the first few months of oral contraception. It starts a day or two after finishing a course of Pills and goes shortly after the next course is begun. With sequential preparations it appears during the time 'dummy' tablets are taken, even though the patient is unaware the tablets contain no active substance. The headache is usually frontal, is often described as throbbing, and is lessened by analgesics but not completely relieved. The intensity may vary from mild to very severe.

Changing the progestogen may bring relief, but may bring worse headache with other symptoms in addition.

After reassurance that although due to the Pill, the headache does not indicate serious disease, the choice of remedy should be left to the patient: either to continue therapy and take household analgesics as necessary - a course which is usually chosen by patients with mild Pill headaches - or try a change of progestogen but with no guarantee of success. This solution is usually adopted by patients with more severe headaches. At least two cycles on the new preparation are necessary to assess improvement, if any. If there is none, then another switch to a different progestogen is indicated.

No guidance as to which progestogen will prove to be of benefit can be given, as the headaches seem a specific reaction of the individual patient rather than the effect of a particular preparation.

After several changes with no improvement, both patient and doctor are usually happy to change to another contraceptive method. The GP should state his willingness to supervise this change at the outset, or he may find the patient abandons all contraception altogether.

Another method of dealing with the problem is to cut out the tablet-free days for two or three months, or until breakthrough bleeding happens - whichever is the sooner, thus reducing the frequency of the headaches. Not all patients are willing to go for much longer than a month without bleeding, so patients must be chosen carefully.

(b) *Migraine*. Menstruation and migraine are often associated in women not taking oral contraceptives, and the migraine may be relieved by progesterone. Oral contraceptives contain synthetic progestogens, whose actions are not precisely similar to naturally occurring progesterone. It is therefore not surprising to find that it is unusual for pre-existing migraine to be relieved by the Pill, although it is reported that it sometimes is. It is more commonly made worse, and may begin for the first time when a woman starts the method.

Treatment with ergot preparations relieves the migraine in Pill-users as efficiently as in non-users. In patients where the Pill seems to have started or worsened the migraine, it is bad treatment to give one drug to relieve the symptoms of another, so that an alternative method of contraception should be chosen.

Attempts have been made to correlate the level of mono-amine oxidase and the development of the arterioles in the endometrium with the occurrence of headaches, but no definite conclusions are as yet generally accepted.

(c) *Severe headache due to a rare complication of oral contraception.* The sudden onset of severe headache may indicate a cerebrovascular thrombo-embolism, and in such cases oral contraception should be stopped immediately. Headache may also be a symptom of hypertension due to the Pill.

6. Amenorrhoea

This subject is best considered under three headings:

(i) Absence of bleeding between packs of Pills.
(ii) Menstruation delayed for less than ninety days after ceasing oral contraception.
(iii) Prolonged or permanent delay after ceasing oral contraception.

(i) *Failure to bleed between packs of Pills*
Active tablets are taken for 21 or 22 days, and there follows a period of 7 or 6 days when either no tablets or 'dummy' tablets are taken. During these days without therapy, most patients experience a bleed, which they refer to as a period. Occasionally there is no bleeding, especially if the patient is taking Pills containing low doses of progestogen. A patient who fails to bleed in one cycle may bleed in the next and subsequent cycles. Cycles without bleeding tend to recur in the same patients, who may develop a pattern of one bleed every three or four months. Sometimes many months pass without any bleeding, but stopping the medication results in a return to normal menstruation very quickly.

> A married woman of 34 had no vaginal bleeding for ten months while on the Pill. She moved from London to Brighton and during the next six months enjoyed the beach and the sun, unworried by menstruation. She attended hospital for an unconnected reason and was advised to stop the Pill immediately. Menstruation returned after three weeks and she suffered two further periods before defying her medical advisor and insisting on returning to the Pill - and freedom from bleeding.

A woman who had regular periods, with a normal or heavy loss at each period before she started oral contraception, can be reassured that to miss one monthly bleed is of no significance. The wise GP will examine her and perform a pregnancy test before reassuring her, in order to reassure himself as well.

Very strong reassurance may be needed. Women tend to regard several days blood loss as healthy and a very scanty, or absent loss as a sign of something wrong. Patients quite often say. 'Where does the blood go then?' Or, 'My mum says it will go to my brain and send me mad.'

The GP must remember that the patient may have not the remotest idea of what normally happens inside her, and a simple statement that absence of bleeding does not matter is not going to put her mind at rest. Unless she is completely reassured she will go elsewhere - with consequent loss of face for her own doctor - or she may abandon oral contraception altogether, with pregnancy ensuing.

Particularly dangerous is the girl who fails to start her next pack of Pills, but waits to see if she bleeds. She almost invariably does bleed, but when she eventually starts her next pack she is no longer protected. Unless she uses another method for the first fourteen days of the new pack, she is liable to become pregnant.

I have found that the following simple explanation, although not entirely accurate from a physiological point of view, is enough to reassure almost all girls, even those with absolutely no knowledge of how their body works.

'Every month, when you are not on the Pill, you produce an egg, and the womb builds up a lining like a thick eiderdown, so that if the egg is fertilized it can bed down comfortably in it and grow to be a baby. It is this unused lining coming away that is a period, and is a complete waste of iron, minerals and so on. If you're on the Pill there is no egg, so after a bit the womb no longer bothers to build up a thick eiderdown, but merely a thin sheet instead. Hence the periods when you take the Pill become scanty. Sometimes the sheet is so thin there is virtually nothing to come away at all and so there is no period. But the minute you stop the Pill, the womb will start forming an eiderdown again and the usual type of period - and the possibility of pregnancy - will return. Meanwhile, far from being harmed by seeing no bleed, you are benefitting by retaining all the iron and minerals which would have been wasted at the period. Which is why people who take the Pill are pink and healthy people.'

Just occasionally the doctor's reassurance is insufficient to overcome Mum's continuing prophesies of doom, and in such patients the substitution of a more oestrogenic compound will result in the appearance of a heavier loss.

The really important thing is that the patient noticing any bleeding abnormality feels free, and has the opportunity, to discuss matters with her doctor BEFORE she stops taking the Pill.

(ii) *Menstruation delayed for less than ninety days after ceasing oral contraceptives*

After using oral contraceptives of the combined type there may be a delay in the establishment of normal menstruation. Pincus, in his original clinical trials, found that this delay could be as long as ninety days. Since then, it has become evident that the delay may in rare cases be much longer.

From the point of view of the general practitioner, it is convenient to regard delays of up to ninety days as falling within his province, whereas delays longer than this should indicate referral for special investigation.

Clinically, the patient completes her last packet of Pills, the usual withdrawal bleed follows, and she expects to bleed again one month later. This she may do, but in the majority of women there is a delay of a few days, commonly about two weeks, before the first spontaneous menstruation.

If the GP is aware that his patient intends to stop the Pill, he should always warn her that her next period may be a couple of weeks late, otherwise she may believe herself to be pregnant and announce the fact to her relatives, or even worse, may go elsewhere seeking abortion.

As well as warning her of the possible delay, I also advise patients to avoid becoming pregnant until they have bled twice after stopping the Pill. I emphasize that no harm will result if they do not wait, but that the date the baby is due will be uncertain, and most women agree that they much prefer to avoid this uncertainty. The precision with which ultrasound can estimate the age of an early pregnancy may make this advice superfluous in the near future.

If the first spontaneous period following the withdrawal bleed after the Pill is delayed for a month or more, patients often ask their doctor for 'something to bring the periods on'. There are several preparations available to treat secondary amenorrhoea (Menstrogen, Primodos, Amenorone) but their action is, like the Pill, on the hypothalamic-pituitary axis, and although they may produce a bleed, are also likely to delay spontaneous ovulation still further.

The GP should resist invitations to use these preparations in these circumstances and content himself and his patient with physical examination, a pregnancy test on the urine, and reassurance.

Secondary amenorrhoea lasting more than six months after oral contraception is very rare, but in practice, especially if pregnancy is wanted, women will demand referral to a gynaecologist before this. It would seem wise for the GP to fix an arbitrary time limit of three months and then to refer these patients for a second opinion.

(iii) *Prolonged (more than ninety days) secondary amenorrhoea after use of oral contraception*

If menstruation has not returned six months after stopping oral contraceptives, the patient should be referred to a specialist. Such causes as adrenal tumours, pituitary tumours, hypothyroidism, or the Stein-Leventhal syndrome must be excluded before attributing the condition to the Pill.

Secondary amenorrhoea may occur after taking the Pill for only three months, or after many years of use. It is more common in women whose periods were scanty or infrequent before using the Pill, and so careful consideration should precede the use of this method in such patients. As yet prolonged amenorrhoea has not been reported following progestogen-only contraceptives, but it may follow both combined and sequential types.

Golditch (1972) reported the crude incidence of the condition among nearly 20,000 women who had taken the Pill as being 2.2 per thousand. However as the incidence of secondary amenorrhoea from all causes in the population of the United Kingdom is unknown, it is difficult to produce an exact figure for the true incidence due to the Pill.

Galactorrhoea may occur in association with amenorrhoea after normal childbirth, and is then known as the Chiari-Frommel syndrome. A similar condition may follow oral contraception.

The Pill is assumed to cause oversuppression of hypothalamic function, either because of hypersensitivity of the hypothalamus in the individual patient, or because pre-existing hypothalamic dysfunction is exacerbated by oral contraceptive usage. Possibly an abnormal feed-back mechanism plays a part in causation in some patients (Arrata and De Alvarez, 1972).

Treatment, after excluding other causes, is with clomiphene or pergamol and chorionic gonadotrophin where necessary. Resumption of ovulation follows in the majority of treated women, and pregnancy has followed this in about half, although Steel *et al.* (1973) reported twelve pregnancies following treatment of nineteen women.

'Having a rest from the Pill'
Even today, patients tell me that their friends have been advised by their doctor to 'have a rest' from the Pill for a few months every year, or every two years, or every three years. Cartwright and Waite (1972) found this practice to be widespread among GPs.

The rationale behind this advice seems to be that the pituitary ovarian axis will recover from repeated short courses of oral contraceptives more quickly and more completely than from long courses.

This is simply not so. Secondary amenorrhoea has followed only three months oral contraception, as has galactorrhoea also.

When patients used to the efficiency and convenience of the Pill are advised to 'have a rest', the result of the rest is very likely to be a pregnancy.

The GP will serve his patients better by advising against starting oral contraception in women with scanty. infrequent periods, but continuing to prescribe the Pill to those who need it for as long as they need it.

7. **Depression**

Almost every patient consulting a general practitioner can be persuaded to complain of one or more of the multitude of symptoms characterizing depression. Indeed, at some time or other, most family doctors have depressive symptoms themselves. Given that depression is such a common clinical entity in general practice, and given that about two million women in Britain use oral contraceptives, it is inevitable that the two will be frequently associated. Bearing in mind that women may choose the reliable contraception provided by the Pill because their life pattern is such that an unplanned pregnancy would be a disaster, to compare women using the Pill with those using other methods is not entirely satisfactory, since the life pattern itself may predispose to anxiety and depression.

Other factors may complicate the elucidation of the problem. These include the emotional make-up of the patient, the possibility of inducing symptoms in susceptible patients, and the timing of the interview in the menstrual cycle, since many women feel depressed pre-menstrually anyway. Some compounds or combinations of compounds used in oral contraception may be more likely than others to produce depression.

Finally, depressed patients – and their doctors – may blame a depression on the Pill, even though the real cause lies elsewhere.

The impression that among the many patients with depression while taking the Pill were some with depression due to the Pill has been strengthened and quantified by Brenda Herzberg and her colleagues (1971). Biochemical changes which may be the cause of the depression have been identified in some of these depressed women by workers in Professor Victor Wynn's department (Adams *et al.*, 1973) and a rational method of treatment suggested.

Depression due to the combined Pill appears to be characterized by lethargy, irritability, pessimism, anxiety, weepiness and a lack of interest in sex. The sleep disturbances so characteristic of other forms of depression do not occur.

About five per cent of women using the Pill develop these symptoms, as opposed to about two per cent of women who become depressed when using other methods, although the interim report of the RCGP study (1974) assesses the risk of depression attributable to oral contraception at the slightly lower figure of 2.2 per hundred takers per year. The depression may begin immediately the method is started, but the longer a patient has been on the Pill, the more likely she is to be depressed. The depression in these long-term patients may have a different origin, the patient often saying she is simply fed up with taking pills, or is depressed by the inevitable regularity of her cycle, or by the fact that she 'feels sterilized'.

Patients with a previous history of depression are more likely to become depressed when using the Pill.

As regards the composition of the Pill, it has been suggested that compounds with a more progestogenic effect were most likely to cause depression, and sequential preparations were less likely. Since the reduction in the total number of preparations available and the virtual disappearance of sequential products, these differences have become less clear-cut, and it is more likely that differences in susceptibility between individual patients is of more importance than differences between contraceptive Pills.

Support for this view has been provided by the observation that 80 per cent of women taking combined oral contraceptives can be shown to have abnormal tryptophane metabolism. Half of these women can be shown to have chemical evidence of pyridoxine (Vitamin B_6) deficiency.

The assumption is that in some women the abnormal tryptophane metabolites may exert a chemical action on the brain, producing depression. Similarly in some women, pyridoxine deficiency may alter the metabolism of tryptophane in the brain, thus producing depression.

Administration of pyridoxine to women with pyridoxine deficiency and depression results in alleviation of depression and, after one month's treatment, the benefit continues for a further two months.

Clinical implications

Careful consideration is needed before prescribing oral contraceptives to a patient whose past history includes episodes of severe depression. Where alternative methods of fertility control, including sterilization, are acceptable, oral contraception with combined compounds is probably best avoided. However, the risk of precipitating further depressive episodes in the individual patient must be weighed against the risks of an unwanted pregnancy, which in turn may produce depression. Careful follow-up of such patients to detect early symptoms is essential.

A simple test by means of which the GP could detect pyridoxine deficiency would be most helpful. As none is as yet available, the approach must be empirical. Addition of pyridoxine to the diet of all patients on the Pill is not without danger, but it might be of value to give pyridoxine intermittently. Trials are proceeding along these lines.

Meanwhile, my own approach to the problem is as follows.

An attempt is made to identify reasons other than the Pill that may have caused the depression, and if such reasons exist, treatment is given as for any patient not taking the Pill. If no such cause can be identified, then the patient is given pyridoxine tablets 20 mg twice daily for one month. If improvement results, and usually it can be detected after two weeks, then the patient finishes the course of pyridoxine and is told to return immediately for a further supply at the first suggestion of symptoms returning.

If pyridoxine alone produces no benefit within two weeks, then a tricyclic antidepressant is substituted. Nortryptylline tablets, 10 mg three or four times daily, usually relieve the symptoms within two weeks, and should be continued until one month after the patient feels completely back to normal. Repeated courses are in practice rarely necessary.

Since sleep disturbance is not a problem in these patients, amitryptylline, with its marked sedative action, is best avoided. In my view it is unjustifiable to use MAO inhibitors, with their own possible severe side-effects, to treat side-effects of the Pill.

The danger for these depressed women is that they will abandon oral contraception and not use any other method, returning only when pregnant. Accordingly, the aims and expectations of giving the tablets are explained to the patient and she is told that if treatment fails, or if she decides to abandon oral contraception, the family doctor will be very willing to help her change to another method.

Experience shows that patients feel that the doctor will be 'cross with them' if they abandon oral contraception, and it is most important to correct this impression. Some patients will remain feeling below par despite pyridoxine and antidepressants, and a change of contraceptive method then becomes obligatory.

8. Lack of libido

There is no way in which libido can be measured, so that increases or decreases are equally difficult to assess. Even the patient's own assessment may be misleading.

> A young coloured man complained that his 'sex life was no good any more'. Questioning revealed his complaint to be that the lapse of time between his first ejaculation and the next had lengthened from ten to fifteen minutes. He was strongly (and admiringly) reassured.

Pincus *et al.* (1959), in early reports of patients using the Pill, found coital frequency increased. Guttmacher (1965), reporting findings in a large group of women who had taken the Pill for more than two years, found that only 3 per cent complained of reduced libido, which was exactly balanced by 3 per cent who reported increased libido. Herzberg *et al.* (1971) reported a progressive decrease in libido in women taking the Pill, especially if they stopped or changed Pills, when compared with women using the IUD. The interim report of the RCGP (1974) found that Pill-takers complained of diminished libido four times more often than non-takers.

Diminished sexual desire is a not uncommon complaint, and as with other symptoms previously discussed, women on the Pill are likely to blame the Pill. Some women certainly feel relief at the prospect of 100 per cent freedom from anxiety about pregnancy: others find the complete removal of the risk makes sexual intercourse less exciting.

The fact remains that the family doctor will be faced in his surgery with a patient who says that her husband has insisted that she tell the GP that since being on the Pill she has become 'frigid'. Enquiries about sexual activities in general are worthwhile as occasionally it transpires that although frigid with her husband she is far from frigid with the boy-friend, and in such cases the Pill can be exonerated completely.

In practice, the best way to deal with this problem is by a therapeutic test in reverse. Stop the Pill, making sure an alternative relatively efficient method is used in its stead, and see what happens. Only a minority of patients will find their libido returns to normal, but in these the Pill must be assumed to be to blame and oral contraception abandoned. The exception is where the couple find all other methods of fertility control unacceptable, and then switching to a combined Pill with different constituents, or to a progestogen-only Pill, may result in improved libido. There are no rules to follow when switching; some patients do better with one Pill and some with another. Once again the reaction of the individual patient seems more important than the constituents of the Pill.

The majority of women find that stopping the Pill for three months makes no difference to their sexual performance. They are then able to admit to themselves that the Pill is not to blame and in consequence are able to examine other possible causes. They can be assisted in this by the GP or, if he is fortunate enough to have access to a psychiatrist interested in sexual problems, reference to such a specialist will often produce excellent results. Meanwhile, oral contraception can be resumed.

> An unmarried girl of 23 complained that since returning to the Pill after an interval of six months, her libido had decreased so much that she was unable to attain orgasm, which had been regularly possible in the past. She stopped the Pill, but found no improvement. It then transpired that as well as a new Pill, she had a new boy-friend who, unlike previous ones, did not practice pre-coital play. Education of the boy-friend resulted in a return of orgasm and a satisfied resumption of oral contraception.

Thrombo-embolism and Oral Contraception

The question most commonly asked by a patient considering oral contraception is 'Will it make me fat?' The second commonest is 'What about clotting?'

The story of 'clotting' and the Pill is one of particular interest to general practitioners, who were deeply embroiled in the battle without knowing whether there was a battle going on or not. On the one hand were those who were convinced that thrombo-embolism was more common in those using oral contraceptives, but, until the late 1960s, could produce no concrete evidence. On the other hand were those who maintained that oral contraceptives were used by millions of women, and it was no more than coincidence that a common condition such as thrombo-embolism occurred in some of them.

The organisation of the family planning services in the United Kingdom delayed the decision between these two points of view. Family doctors working in their surgeries had long-term care of their patients, and almost invariably knew of any complication or catastrophe affecting those taking oral contraceptives. Unfortunately, liaison between clinics and family doctors was so poor that the GP had no idea of the total number of his patients receiving oral contraceptives, because so many were being given them from other sources. Even had this difficulty not existed, the family doctor, working with small numbers of patients taking oral contraceptives, could not amass sufficient data for statistically significant conclusions in a reasonably short time.

This difficulty did not apply to the clinics, where large numbers of patients were available but most of whom looked to their family doctor or the hospital to deal with complications or catastrophes following the use of the Pill. The follow-up of patients defaulting from clinics was virtually non-existent, so the clinic doctors remained in blissful ignorance of most of the troubles occurring as a result of their treatment.

Unless of course a death occurred, when the news media paid it great attention, even though the far more numerous deaths from other causes, such as road traffic accidents, were ignored completely.

The first report of pulmonary embolism in a woman taking the Pill was by W. M. Jordan, a general practitioner in Suffolk, in 1961. But his letter to the *Lancet* made it clear that the medication had been for treatment of disease, not contraception, and large doses of both progestogen and oestrogen had been given.

Further reports appeared in both medical and lay press of cases of thrombo-embolism in patients taking contraceptive doses only.

In 1963 a Committee of the Food and Drug Administration of the United States of America issued a report in which the conclusion was drawn that there was no significant increase in the risk of death from thrombo-embolic disorders in women taking oral contraceptives, but further study was required.

A World Health Organisation Scientific group made a similar report.

These reports reassured family doctors and their patients, but the reassurance wore off as the months went by, and reports of disasters in women taking the Pill continued to appear.

Representatives of drug firms visiting doctors in their surgeries were very persuasive, stressing the lack of any definite evidence of the danger of their products. Conversations with individual hospital consultants, who described cases seen in hospital, tended to make the family doctor less certain that he was benefiting his patients by prescribing the Pill.

In 1966 a lone doctor stood up before several hundred medical men and women at a symposium on oral contraception held at Folkestone and stated categorically that he, personally, would never prescribe an oral contraceptive to a patient with a history of previous thrombo-embolic disease. This statement was a bomb-shell, since the speaker was Dr Celso-Ramon Garcia who, with John Rock and Gregory Pincus, had been involved in the early work on oral contraception in the mid-1950s.

For some reason this pronouncement received little publicity and general practitioners had to wait until 1967 for an authoritative answer to their doubts and worries. This took the form of the publication in the *British Medical Journal* of a preliminary report by a sub-committee to the Medical Research Council.

Three separate investigations were reported:

1. In 1965, a pilot survey involving sixty family doctors was carried out under the auspices of the Royal College of General Practitioners.

The conclusion drawn was that the risk of developing venous thrombosis or pulmonary embolism was increased threefold in women taking oral contraceptives.

2. In 1966, Doll and Vessey studied twentynine women admitted to seven London hospitals with a diagnosis of venous thrombosis or pulmonary embolism. They found that the proportion of women who had been taking oral contraceptives during the month before their admission was higher in those admitted for venous thrombosis or pulmonary embolism than in a control group of women who had been admitted because of other diseases.

3. The Committee on Safety of Drugs carried out an investigation of the records of women who had died in 1966 of pulmonary embolism, coronary thrombosis, or cerebral thrombosis.

There seemed no evidence of any relationship between coronary thrombosis and oral contraception, but a relationship was found between the use of oral contraceptives and death from pulmonary embolism and possibly cerebral thrombosis.

Thus these three studies all gave a similar answer: the risk of death from thrombo-embolism appeared to be increased in women using oral contraceptives.

Risks of thrombo-embolic disease in women using oral contraceptives

A further report by Inman and Vessey in 1968 enabled family doctors to assess the risks run by their patients taking the Pills in use at that time.

Table V Annual mortality per 100,000 users of oral contraceptives compared with that of non-users in Great Britain.

Age	*Users*	*Non-users*
20–34 years	1·5	0·2
35–44 years	3·9	0·5

The risk of death from thrombo-embolism in a woman taking the Pill is about seven times greater than in her sister who does not take it. The magnitude of the risk varies with the age of the patient, being more than twice as great in the women over thirtyfive. There is no relationship between the length of time for which the Pill has been taken and the likelihood of thrombo-embolism.

Later work showed this risk varied with the blood group of the patient, the woman whose blood was Group O being three times less likely to develop venous thrombo-embolism than a woman whose blood was of other blood groups.

Although of academic interest only to most clinic doctors, this is a factor of importance for the family doctor who often has the blood group of the patient recorded in her notes, especially, of course, in puerperal patients.

Morbidity

Although rarely seeing the patient who dies from thrombo-embolic disease, the family doctor sees a good many women in his surgery with lesions due to the same cause but not constituting a risk to life. Attempts to quantify the numbers of such patients have been made.

Incidents of thrombo-embolism seen by GPs were recorded in a study organised by the Royal College of General Practitioners in 1967. Oral contraceptive usage of patients admitted to hospitals in Great Britain because of venous thrombo-embolism between 1964 and 1967 was also studied (Inman and Vessey, 1968) and comparisons made of the risks in Pill-users as compared with non-users (Table VI).

Table VI Annual morbidity from thrombo-embolism per 100,000 users of oral contraceptives compared with that of non-users in Great Britain.

Age	*Users*	*Non-users*
15–49	450	130
16–40	50	6

These studies indicated that the risk of a patient needing to consult her GP because of a thrombo-embolic episode was more than three times greater in Pill-users and the risk of hospital admission more than eight times greater.

However, both these studies were made at a time when combined oral contraceptives containing more than 50 microgrammes of oestrogen were widely used. The thrombo-embolic episodes reported from general practice were chiefly leg vein thromboses, predominantly superficial, but some deep. The hospital figures included deep vein thrombosis of the legs, venous pulmonary embolism and arterial cerebral thrombosis, although it is generally agreed that the pathology of arterial thrombosis differs from that of venous thrombosis.

Later reports have attempted to examine the incidence of thrombo-embolism in specific systems of the body, and to examine the effects of variations in oestrogen dosage.

Significance of dosage of oestrogen

Inman *et al.* (1970) analyzed the reports received by drug safety committees in the United Kingdom, Sweden and Denmark. The number of reports of thrombo-embolism attributed to each product were compared with the numbers that would have been expected from a market research estimate of their relative sales, assuming that all products carried the same risk.

The figures showed this assumption to be unlikely, and a positive correlation was found between the dose of oestrogen and the risk of pulmonary embolism, deep vein thrombosis, cerebral thrombosis and also, for the first time, coronary thrombosis in the United Kingdom. There was a similar correlation for venous thrombosis and pulmonary embolism in Sweden and Denmark.

With regard to dosage, it appeared that preparations containing more than 75 microgrammes of oestrogen (whether mestranol or ethinyloestradiol was the oestrogen made no difference) carried three times the risk of causing death from thrombo-embolism. Sequential preparations carried precisely the same risk as combined preparations.

It was suggested that if all women using oral contraceptives were in future to take only preparations containing less than 75 microgrammes, mortality in Pill-users should be reduced by half and morbidity by a quarter.

Unfortunately, the contents of this report were published in the lay press before family doctors were informed, and the immediate result was that many women ceased to take their Pills, even Pills containing a suitable dose of oestrogen, and many unwanted pregnancies and requests for abortion ensued.

However, also as a result of this report, oral contraceptive preparations containing more than 50 microgrammes of oestrogen virtually ceased to be prescribed, partly as a result of the action of the manufacturers withdrawing products or altering the amount of oestrogen in them; partly by a change in prescribing habits of doctors, but also because of quite remarkable insistence by patients that they wished to take the lower oestrogen dosage.

In the years following this report, the clinical impression in the surgery was that morbidity from thrombo-embolic disease had certainly diminished.

To back this clinical impression, evidence came in 1974 with the interim report of the prospective study of the Royal College of General Practitioners. Although deep vein thrombosis of the legs was found to be five times more common in Pill-users than in non-users (a figure rather higher although of the same order as the 1968 estimate from the same source), the risk was calculated to be reduced by about 25 per cent if the Pill used contained less than 75 microgrammes of oestrogen. The risk of deep vein thrombosis of the leg attributable to the use of the combined Pill was 81 per 100,000 users annually if the Pill contained less than 75 microgrammes, as opposed to 112 per 100,000 users annually if the Pill contained a higher dosage.

As regards mortality, a letter sent by the Committee on Safety of Medicines to all doctors in May 1973 reported a substantial fall in the number of fatal cases of pulmonary embolism reported annually since 1969.

It is hoped that the recent introduction of compounds containing only 30 microgrammes of oestrogen will produce a further reduction in both the morbidity and the mortality from thrombo-embolism, but no evidence of this result is yet available.

Post-operative thrombosis in women using oral contraceptives

The problem of thrombotic disease following surgery on patients using oral contraceptives was also elucidated in 1970 (Vessey *et al.*). The diagnostic indices of nineteen large general hospitals were searched to identify married women aged 16 to 40 years who had suffered post-operative deep venous thrombosis or pulmonary embolism. Patients in whom other causes could be identified, such as a recent pregnancy or chronic disease, were excluded. The remainder were compared with two controls each, matched for age, parity, and year of admission.

Forty per cent of women with post-operative thrombo-embolism had used oral contraceptives during the previous month, whereas only fifteen per cent of the controls had used them. Once again the risk was greater in preparations containing the higher dosage of oestrogen.

Stroke in young women taking the Pill

As already detailed, evidence for the association of the use of oral contraceptives and cerebral catastrophes had been found in the reports from the United Kingdom in 1968 and 1970.

Further evidence came with a report in 1973 from neurologists working in twelve major cities in the United States. During the two years beginning September 1969 (and so including a period when higher doses of oestrogen were in common use) 28.7 per cent of 429 non-pregnant women aged 15-44 years had been taking oral contraceptives shortly before admission because of a stroke, as opposed to only 13.5 per cent of controls.

Coronary occlusion in young women taking the Pill

Although in retrospective studies an association has been shown to exist between myocardial infarction and the use of oral contraceptives, an association has also been shown between Pill-usage and both an increase in blood lipids and cigarette smoking, known to be contributing causes as far as myocardial infarction is concerned. Opinion at the moment tends to the view that myocardial infarction is likely to follow use of oral contraceptives only in women with pre-existing hyperlipidaemia, in women who smoke excessively, or in women who develop severe hypertension on the Pill or, of course, where these three factors coexist.

Geographical variation

All the data quoted so far comes from developed countries. Naturally-occurring thrombo-embolic disease is rare in undeveloped countries, and it is unwise to assume that the situation with regard to this disease and oral contraceptives will apply equally in all parts of the world.

The dissentient voice

Lest it be assumed that universal agreement exists as to the role of oestrogens in the production of thrombosis, the views of Victor Drill (1972) should be mentioned. He has pointed out that retrospective studies can provide the hypothesis that an association exists between, in this case, thrombo-embolism and the Pill. Only prospective studies can show that the association has a cause-and-effect relationship. As regards the dose of oestrogen, he claims that if the figures obtained in retrospective studies are adjusted to compensate for the differing potencies of the two oestrogens used in the Pill, then the significance of the findings disappears.

Most clinicians would prefer to give their patients the benefit of the doubt, and act on the hypothesis. The long-term prospective study of the Royal College of General Practitioners may settle the question.

Alterations in blood-clotting mechanisms

The mechanism of normal blood coagulation is complex. Alterations in the mechanism have been investigated by many haematologists throughout the world, and in the United Kingdom Dr Leon Poller (1972) has reported the changes found in women taking oral contraceptives in Manchester.

The use of the combined type of oral contraceptive containing oestrogen has been found to be associated with a significant rise in the levels of Factor VII and Factor X. Many other abnormal measurements, including accelerated cephalin times, accelerated platelet aggregation times, increased platelet adhesion, a rise in fibrinogen level, and a fall in antithrombin III level have also been reported.

These changes reach significant levels from the third cycle of combined oral contraception onwards and continue for up to three months after stopping the medication.

The presumption is that these changes are in some way causally related to the occurrence of thrombo-embolism in women using combined oral contraceptives. However, some of the changes can be demonstrated in women not taking the Pill, some can be demonstrated during pregnancy, and some women with proven deep vein thrombosis after operation do not demonstrate some of the changes.

The presumption thus remains unproven. Certainly none of the measurements can be used to predict which women are likely to develop thrombosis, nor whether thrombosis is likely in any particular woman at any particular time.

The blood of patients taking progestogen-only preparations does not show these changes: indeed Poller reports a tendency to reduced coagulation in these patients. Switching from a combined preparation to one containing no oestrogen resulted in a return of the clotting mechanism to normal although this process was not complete in some cases until the sixth cycle with the progestogen-only preparation. Even progestogens which are thought to be broken down to oestrogens in the body do not seem to affect the clotting mechanisms adversely.

Clinical applications

The practitioner advising a patient who is considering starting an oral contraceptive can assure her that the risk of death from clotting is considerably less than many of the risks she runs in ordinary life, and certainly very much less than the risk of death from pregnancy, especially from unwanted pregnancy.

Assuming that the mortality from thrombo-embolism is reduced by about fifty per cent because of the lowering of the dosage of oestrogen, then the risks can be indicated as in Table VII.

Table VII. Approximate figures to illustrate the ratio of risks run by women taking combined oral contraceptives containing less than 75 microgrammes of oestrogen, and risks run from motor accidents and pregnancies.

	Aged 20-34	Aged 35-44
Annual mortality from thrombo-embolism per 100,000 users of combined oral contraceptives.	1	2
Annual mortality per 100,000 total female population from motor accidents.	5	4
Annual mortality per 100,000 maternities from all causes in pregnancy, delivery and the puerperium.	20	50

However, these are certain groups of women in whom factors which influence the risk of thrombo-embolism can be identified, and evaluation of these factors should be included in the assessment of the patient's suitability for combined oral contraception.

1. Women aged over 35, whose fertility may be declining anyway, especially if they have successfully used some other method of contraception in the past.
2. Women whose blood group is A, AB, or B.
3. Patients with severe varicose veins. There is in fact little statistical evidence as to the risk of thrombo-embolism in these patients but, in view of the tendency for this to occur even without oral contraceptives, it would seem sensible to advise that varicosities should be treated before starting to take the Pill.
4. A history of previous thrombo-embolism, other than in subsequently treated varicose veins.
5. A strong family history of cardiac infarction or cerebral or pulmonary embolism, other than as terminal events in old age.
6. Those with a cardiovascular abnormality known to be associated with emboli.
7. Those suffering from a major haemoglobinopathy (see p. 128).

These are all relative, not absolute contra-indications and as always the patient's need for efficient contraception must be assessed against the risk for each particular patient.

Indications for withdrawing combined oral contraceptives

1. Before any planned surgery. If time permits, three months before is ideal.
2. Localized pain and tenderness in the muscles of the leg may indicate the onset of thrombosis in a vein. Although the diagnosis may be uncertain, it is safer in such patients to stop the Pill immediately.
3. Oedema of a limb, especially if unilateral.
4. The sudden onset of severe chest pain. To prove that such pain is NOT due to a pulmonary embolism is almost impossible, although it may be possible to prove another cause.
5. Sudden severe headache or sudden severe migraine, especially in patients not usually suffering from these symptoms, may indicate a cerebral vascular lesion.
6. Weakness or paraesthesiae of one or more limbs, or any other indication of a stroke.

A complaint that her face 'felt funny' was made by a housewife of 42 who had been taking the Pill for three years. Examination showed a left hemiparesis which recovered completely within one month.

7. Visual disturbances.

A girl aged 23 who had taken an oral contraceptive for two years complained of 'a black worm' in front of one eye. Investigation showed thrombosis of a peripheral branch of a retinal artery.

8. Any unusual symptoms for which the clinician can find no cause.

A 29-year-old woman, who had used oral contraception for five years, complained that she could no longer play her usual round of golf because her legs started to ache halfway round the course and grew progressively worse as she continued. Partial thrombotic obliteration of the lumen at the bifurcation of the abdominal aorta was found at operation.

Conclusion

The three cases quoted above are among those occurring in my own practice. Happily none of them died, and only one will appear in any hospital statistics. They demonstrate, in my view, the fact that any doctor should prescribe any drug - including the Pill - only after considering the possible benefits to his patient in relation to the possible dangers. This trite statement is made in view of the suggestion from some quarters that oral contraceptives should be available in the United Kingdom without prescription. Every patient should have the right to be refused oral contraceptives by her family doctor.

A mother of four children, aged 43, asked to go on the Pill. She had used a cap for twelve years since her last pregnancy, but had suddenly been overcome by the thought that she might become pregnant again. Her NHS record revealed that she had a 'white-leg' after her last confinement and she was Group AB. She was advised to continue to use her cap.

Gynaecological Effects of Oral Contraceptives

VAGINITIS AND THE PILL

The complaints of vaginal discharge, and vaginal or vulval irritation, are common in general practice. Trichomonas vaginitis and gonorrhoea occur just as frequently - and no more - in women using oral contraceptives as in their sexually active sisters who do not. Because of considerable recent publicity concerning venereal disease, women with vaginitis now often express the fear that they may have VD, and it is therefore necessary for the family doctor to investigate these women carefully. To this end a swab soaked in discharge, or a drop of discharge on a platinum loop, should be mixed with normal saline and examined immediately under the microscope. Trichomonads may be seen, as may the spores and mycelia of Candida albicans if there is gross infection. Culture is often needed to demonstrate Candida in mild infection. Swabs from the cervix and urethra should also be placed in Stewart's medium for onward transmission to the laboratory for examination for gonococci. In general practice, the result is almost always negative, probably because the girl with good reason to suspect the gonococcus takes herself directly to a VD clinic, which, unlike all other consultant clinics, does not inform the patient's GP of the findings.

Just as candidal vaginitis is more common and more difficult to treat during pregnancy, so it is during treatment with oral contraceptives. Treatment of the woman with pessaries of nystatin or pimafucin will relieve an attack rapidly, but recurrences are common. Sometimes questioning will reveal that the male has suffered soreness and irritation of the penis: the application of nystatin cream to the penis twice daily is then indicated. Intercourse with pessaries and creams in place makes a satisfying form of treatment for both sexes.

Despite full courses of treatment, including oral tablets which had a vogue at one time, and after apparent bacteriological cure, relapses still occur and must be assumed to be due to re-infection. The most useful practical approach is to explain to the patient with recurrent infection that she has the choice between the Pill and candidal vaginitis, and possible pregnancy and candidal vaginitis. As a rule she will choose the variety accompanying the Pill. She should then be told to use the pessaries at the first sign of trouble until a day or two after disappearance of symptoms, and to this end should be given a small store of pessaries.

Using this method, which undoubtedly offends against all medical precepts, almost all women can avoid more than the occasional day of discomfort every few months, and happily continue with the Pill. However it must be admitted that, very rarely, the frequency and severity of candidal re-infections is such that the only advice the GP can give is to change to another method. If women on the Pill are given a course of a broad spectrum antibiotic, candidal vaginitis is likely to result. Because of this prophylaxis should accompany antibiotic therapy, either by providing vaginal pessaries to insert, or by prescribing oral tablets active against Candida as well as the antibiotic. The proprietary compound 'Mysteclin' contains both tetracycline and nystatin.

Naturally, on the Pill or not, any women suffering recurrent candidiasis should have her urine tested for sugar, since this infection is a common accompaniment of diabetes mellitus.

THE PILL AND UTERINE FIBROIDS

It is said that uterine fibroids may grow rapidly in size under the influence of the Pill. Bearing in mind the enormous variations in the estimates of the size of a fibroid uterus by different observers in the same patient that I have encountered in my practice over the years, together with the fact that fibroids are uncommon in the age and parity groups who form the bulk of Pill-users, I have doubts as to whether oral contraceptives have any effect on the size of fibroids. Red degeneration has been reported to occur during oral contraception.

The discovery of irregular enlargement of the uterus of a woman proposing to take the Pill should indicate referral to a gynaecologist for suitable investigation and treatment. If hysterectomy is advised, the contraceptive problem is solved. The presence of small fibroids is not a contra-indication to oral contraception if no other method is acceptable. If it is, then it would seem wise to avoid the Pill.

THE PILL AND CERVICAL EROSIONS

Erosions of the cervix are a common finding in women using oral contraceptives. Discharge may be profuse and a cause of considerable distress.

Admission to hospital for properly performed deep cauterization while continuing to take the Pill results in cure. Superficial out-patient cauterization does not.

Symptomless cervical erosions found on routine speculum examination should be ignored. Where symptoms are troublesome, the patient should be offered the choice between in-patient cauterization and stopping the Pill. Her estimate of her need for the method as opposed to her dislike of hospitals will dictate her choice.

Most women decide either to undergo cauterization or to ignore the symptoms. Few decide to give up the Pill.

FERTILITY AFTER THE PILL

During its short lifetime a wealth of myth and legend have grown up concerning the Pill, and nothing demonstrates this more than the question of the alleged changes in fertility of women who have used this method of contraception.

Myth 1. Women are infertile after using the Pill

This fear worries many women, and even some doctors. As always, we must point out that the effect of taking the Pill for twenty or thirty years is as yet unknown, but today we can say that after ten years we know of only three groups of women who are infertile following oral contraception.

(i) Those who have reached the menopause while taking the Pill.
(ii) Those who suffer prolonged amenorrhoea and suppression of ovulation after the Pill. This is a tiny group, considered in detail elsewhere. At best, the fertility of most of them was suspect before starting oral contraception.
(iii) Ten per cent of couples in the United Kingdom are unable to have children. Taking the Pill does not alter this percentage. As many couples use the Pill to delay the first conception, the fact that they belong to this ten per cent will not be apparent until they cease using the Pill. From this it follows that any method of contraception is unnecessary for one couple in ten of unproven fertility. A birth control method that carries a risk of mortality or morbidity used in such a patient, protecting from no danger of pregnancy, can only be bad medicine. Unfortunately, since fertile couples cannot, as yet, be identified other than by the occurrence of pregnancy, the ten per cent must run the same risks as the ninety per cent.

As the years pass, the family doctor will retrospectively be able to allocate his patients to this ten per cent. The story of one such couple may be read elsewhere (Oldershaw and Brudenell, 1972). The conclusion is that for the vast majority of the couples who use oral contraception, their fertility after its use is unchanged.

Myth 2. Women are more fertile after using the Pill

Belief in the 'rebound phenomenon' was widespread in the late nineteen-sixties. Inhibition of ovulation by the Pill was shown to be followed by an exaggerated release of gonadotrophins. Failure of ovulation was treated with oral contraception for two or three cycles, and on cessation of treatment, this exaggerated release or 'rebound' was thought to be likely to produce ovulation.

Today this idea is completely discredited, and there are various versions of its origin. My favourite, told me by Pincus, is as follows. When the initial studies of the contraceptive Pill in women were planned, he feared that if the Pill failed and pregnancy resulted, harm might come to the pregnancy because of the medication. Because of this, he chose a number of women attending an infertility clinic from whom to select volunteers. Following completion of the study, ten per cent of the women became pregnant. Despite his protestations that any method of treatment of infertility will result in a ten per cent success rate, these pregnancies became the source, first in the lay press and later in the medical, of the 'rebound phenomenon'.

Other evidence seemed at first sight to confirm the increase in fertility following oral contraception. Two groups of women of equal numbers were studied of whom one had used the Pill and the other some different method of contraception. During the three months after stopping contraception, more of those who had used the Pill became pregnant than those who had used other methods.

It was some years before anyone thought to look at the fertility record of these women before starting contraception of any sort. When they did, it became obvious that the women who were more fertile than the others after the Pill had also been more fertile than the others before the Pill. To use a phrase beloved of my patients, those women who could say 'My husband has only to take his hat off and I am pregnant' chose the safety of the Pill: they were in fact a self-selected group.

The conclusion remains, that for the vast majority of couples who use oral contraception, their fertility after its use is unchanged, and this has recently been confirmed in the interim report from the oral contraception study of the Royal College of General Practitioners (1974). This is a convenient place to examine two other myths.

Myth 3. Twins are more common after oral contraception

One hundred pregnancies after the Pill were shown to include two sets of twins. Accepting the normal incidence of twin pregnancy as one in ninety-nine, the incidence was doubled. Statistically this is obviously rubbish, yet was widely reported in the lay press and relayed to me by my patients.

Myth 4. More boys (or more girls) are likely after using the Pill
These mistaken sexual ideas have now been abandoned. Interestingly enough the suggestion reappeared in 1973, this time applied to premature babies with hyaline membrane disease. Statistically the suggestion was shown to have no significance.

FOETAL ABNORMALITY FOLLOWING ORAL CONTRACEPTION

It has been estimated that in the early 1970s about twenty million women throughout the world were using the Pill. During the decade in which it has been widely used, literally millions of women have used the Pill to delay pregnancy, and have then stopped their contraception to have their baby. No evidence of any increase or decrease in the incidence of foetal abnormality has followed these millions of women-years of usage.

Were foetal abnormality likely, it would be expected to follow in those women who, having missed Pills but unaware that pregnancy had already occurred, continued to take the Pill during the early weeks of pregnancy. This is not an uncommon situation, but even here no evidence of an increased incidence of foetal abnormality has been forthcoming.

The administration of synthetic ovarian steroids in large doses for long periods has been shown to have an effect on the foetus. The administration of progestogens in the treatment of threatened or habitual abortion may result in masculinization of the female foetus. In this condition there is fusion of the labia and hypertrophy of the clitoris, which may necessitate a plastic operation.

Stilboestrol has also been used in treatment of unwanted abortion, again in large doses and for long periods. Adenocarcinoma of the vagina has developed in children born to such patients, although instances seem rare elsewhere than in certain localities in the USA.

The use of stilboestrol in relatively large doses as a post-coital contraceptive has fallen into disrepute because of this. But, used in the low dosage contained in modern conventional oral contraceptives, there is little evidence that either oestrogen or progestogen produce any adverse foetal effects.

Suspicions that genetic abnormalities, or 'small for dates' babies may follow oral contraception have not so far progressed beyond the realm of suggestion. By contrast, it has been suggested that the respiratory distress syndrome may be less likely in premature babies born to mothers recently using oral contraceptives.

The interim report from the oral contraception study of the Royal College of General Practitioners (1974) found no difference in the incidence of abnormal babies born to 2,583 mothers who had used oral contraception and the incidence among 7,405 mothers who had not.

Thus it may be concluded that any untoward effects on the foetus following the use of oral contraceptives either do not exist, or are so infrequent that their association with the Pill has not yet been demonstrable.

Two recent papers give grounds for suspecting that the second of these conclusions may yet prove to be correct. Nora and Nora (1973) report 224 patients with congenital heart disease, twenty of whom had been exposed *in utero* to progestogen or oestrogen, as opposed to only four of 262 controls. Their findings were retrospective, and therefore subject to the disadvantages of all retrospective studies, but they report that prospective studies are proceeding. Janerick *et. al.* (1973) have suggested an association between congenital absence of a limb or part of a limb in newborn babies and the administration of synthetic sex hormones, including oral contraceptives, to the mother during the pregnancy.

Although these suggestions are as yet merely suspicions, it would seem wise to advise women to await the resumption of normal menstruation after stopping the Pill before embarking on a pregnancy. Where synthetic sex hormones, either as contraceptives or pregnancy tests, have been administered to a woman during pregnancy, then the fact of their administration would seem to reinforce any request by the mother for termination of the pregnancy.

Danger to children who eat contraceptive Pills

About twice a year I am telephoned by an anxious mother whose toddler has eaten some of her Pills. She may be reassured that no harm will result; female toddlers do not become 'early developers' nor is the opposite effect seen in males.

TIMING OF ORAL CONTRACEPTION FOLLOWING PREGNANCY

1. After confinement at term

It has long been known that women may become pregnant before the re-appearance of the menses after confinement. Lactation usually delays the appearance of ovulation, but cannot be guaranteed to do so for as long as lactation continues. Pregnancy may be followed by anovular menstruation for the first few cycles. Hence neither the periods nor lactation may be used as indicators for the timing of the administration of the Pill to recently pregnant mothers.

Sharman (1968) carried out endometrial biopsies on 285 women after birth or abortion, and came to the conclusion that ovulation had not occurred in any of them earlier than 42 days after the end of pregnancy. Correspondence in the *Lancet* in 1973 indicated that exceptions do occur, and women may become pregnant much earlier than the sixth week after delivery. My own practice is to initiate oral contraception before the twentyeighth day after confinement, and no pregnancies have resulted in ten years of adherence to this rule. The recent vogue for starting the patient on the Pill within a day or two of normal delivery seems to me undesirable. Involution of the genital tract may be delayed, breakthrough bleeding is difficult to differentiate from bleeding due to retained products, and the choice of contraceptive method or oral contraceptive preparation is transferred from the family doctor to the hospital staff. Most women today have no interest in intercourse during the first few weeks after delivery, and the fact that so many of them have had episiotomies reinforces their lack of interest. To send women home clutching packets of Pills, 48 hours after delivery, to be looked after by their family doctor seems to me quite unnecessary.

Oral contraception should be commenced not earlier than two and not later than four weeks after confinement. Each hospital should have a list of family doctors known to be desirous of supervising the contraception of their patients, and these doctors should be rapidly and fully informed of their patient's discharge from hospital, and the management of the patient left to them. Only where the family doctor does not wish to be involved should the hospital initiate contraception.

2. **After abortion**

A different situation exists when a pregnancy has been terminated, or has spontaneously aborted during the first six months. Boyd and Holmstrom (1972) demonstrated ovulation occuring ten days after abortion, although the average day of ovulation was the twenty-second. Ratten (1972) produced similar results, the earliest ovulation occurring twelve days after abortion in the first trimester, and ten days after abortion in the second trimester.

If oral contraception is to be used after therapeutic abortion (and there is a great deal to be said for the immediate insertion of an intrauterine device in such cases), it is thus imperative that it be commenced within a very few days of the operation, which will also be the time at which the patient's motivation for contraception will be at its zenith. Unless the family doctor is already involved in the care of the patient, the hospital should regard initiation of contraception as part of their duty to the patient with an unwanted pregnancy. Even where the family doctor has been involved, he may well feel it in his patient's best interests to leave choice of method and initiation to the hospital, and regard supervision and stimulation of continued motivation of use of the method by his patient as the area in which he can be most useful.

THE PILL AND LACTATION

Many studies have been made of the effect of the contraceptive Pill on lactation. Conflicting results have been obtained, probably due to the many variable factors which must be considered. Oestrogens are generally agreed to have the effect of diminishing the amount of breast milk: progestogens given by mouth in small dosage do not, but some progestogens in large doses have been shown to diminish lactation, possibly because of the production of oestrogen during the metabolism of the progestogen. The overall effect of a combined Pill on the production of milk will depend therefore on the dosage of both components and also on the weight of the mother, and whether lactation is established or not. There is no convincing evidence that the milk produced by mothers taking the Pill is in any way harmful to the baby.

In developing countries, without breast milk a baby may die. On the other hand, a new baby arriving may mean that the earlier baby may starve. Fortunately, in this country we are not faced with this type of problem, early failure of lactation usually meaning no more than disappointment for the mother.

From a practical point of view, there is usually no difficulty about prescribing oral contraceptives to recently delivered women. Many of them do not wish to breast-feed at all. Most of those who wish to breast-feed for six or nine months will not take the combined Pill in case it 'spoils' their milk, and it would be a foolhardy doctor who tried to make them do otherwise. The vast majority of women who do breast-feed intend to stop, despite what they say while in hospital, after about four weeks, and can certainly be given the combined Pill then.

Recently delivered women may be given the progestogen-only Pill without fear of suppression of lactation. My own experience with the relatively few nursing mothers who wish to take the Pill is that, providing lactation is established, the modern low-dosage combined oral contraceptives produce little discernible effect on the amount of milk produced. Lactation may not be established for several weeks after delivery, and I never advise lactating mothers to start the Pill until the baby is four weeks old. In these days of frequent episiotomies, this advice is usually welcomed by the mother.

In any event, the question is of largely academic interest in the United Kingdom. An effective contraceptive method other than the combined Pill can always be suggested while the mother feeds her baby, and the switch to oral contraception, if desired, made at the time the baby is weaned.

Recently marketed Pills containing only 30 microgrammes of oestrogen are said not to inhibit lactation, even when given early in in the puerperium.

Of one thing the doctor can be certain: if a mother's milk fails while she is taking the Pill, the Pill and the doctor who prescribed it will be blamed.

THE PILL AND THE MENOPAUSE

Fears have been expressed that the use of oral contraceptives may make the menopause appear earlier, or later. There is no evidence for either fear. There is certainly no evidence that the timing of the menopause is different in a woman who has borne no children, and a woman who has borne ten children. In the latter ovulation has been suppressed for a total of many years, a situation analogous to prolonged Pill-usage.

The use of oral contraception in women nearing menopausal age demands a balancing of the factors for and against. Beneficial factors include the certainty with which pregnancy can be avoided and the relief of the symptoms of the climacteric. Against this must be put the increased risk of thrombo-embolism at this age with oestrogen-conteining preparations and the probable diminished fertility of the woman. Each case must be decided on its merits, and the willingness of the patient to use another method, and the effectiveness of that method, are obviously of great importance in making the decision.

Women using cyclical combined oral contraceptives may continue to bleed after the menopause. Withdrawal of the oral contraceptive and substitution of an alternative method for a few cycles will indicate whether spontaneous menstruation is still occurring. On reaching the age of fifty women may be advised that taking the Pill is no longer necessary. Some prefer to continue, stating they feel better when taking it. Recent promotion of 'hormone replacement therapy' in womens' magazines has encouraged many women to ask to continue the Pill. Such senile changes as osteoporosis have been shown to be prevented by the administration of oestrogens, but this is hardly a problem of women at the beginning of the sixth decade.

The dangers of oestrogens at this age should be explained to the patient, but if she decides she still wishes to continue, then one should prescribe the Pill with the smallest dose of oestrogen that gives her the sought-after feeling of well-being.

Naturally, any abnormal bleeding pattern that develops in a woman of this age must not be attributed to the oral contraceptive unless other causes, notably carcinoma of the uterine body or cervix, have been eliminated.

THE PILL AND GROWTH

Fusion of the epiphyses of the long bones is accelerated by oestrogens. In theory, therefore, giving a Pill containing oestrogens to young girls in whom growth is not complete could result in their failure to reach their full stature. In practice it does not seem to happen. I remember being told by an eminent endocrinologist at a medical meeting that his attempts to stop promising ballet dancers growing too tall by using oestrogens had had little success. In any event, family doctors are unlikely to be asked for the Pill by girls in whom growth and development are not already well advanced.

Metabolic Effects of Oral Contraceptives

There is a great deal of evidence that women taking the Pill show alterations in the normal metabolic processes. The alterations seem to be related to oestrogen dosage, being most marked with combined Pills, less with sequential, and least with progestogen-only preparations.

For the clinician, the importance of the metabolic changes is twofold. Firstly, the effect that may be produced by the combination of metabolic disorder, latent or developed, and oral contraceptives will influence the doctor's choice of contraceptive method and his supervision of the patient. Secondly, the knowledge that abnormal metabolic test results do occur in women using oral contraception will enable the doctor to interpret such results correctly.

EFFECT ON THE LIVER

I. Hydroxylation of steroids takes place in the liver. Both the oestrogens and progestogens used in the Pill may alter the microhistology of the liver.

Certain liver function tests are regularly found to be abnormal in women using combined oral contraceptives. For example, impairment of bromsulphthalein excretion is a frequent finding.

Frank liver damage, as evidenced by the appearance of cholestatic jaundice is a very rare complication following use of the Pill. It is far more commonly reported from certain parts of the world, notably Scandinavia and South America, especially Chile, possibly indicating an ethnic or dietary difference.

In the United Kingdom the appearance of frank liver damage and jaundice following oral contraceptive use is extremely rare, and appears to have become even rarer since oestrogen dosages were decreased. One-third of the women who develop jaundice give a history of past episodes of ideopathic recurrent cholestatic jaundice of pregnancy, or of ideopathic recurrent pruritus of pregnancy. A history of either of these conditions, or of the two very rare congenital disorders of liver function, the Roter Syndrome, and the Dubin-Johnson-Sprinz syndrome, constitutes a contraindication to oral contraception using the oestrogen-containing Pill, and probably to the use of the progestogen-only Pill as well, although the evidence for this is less clear.

Stopping the administration of the Pill results in a return to normal of the liver function tests, and disappearance of the jaundice.

The Budd-Chiari syndrome, caused by hepatic vein thrombosis, has been reported in women using the Pill.

Infective hepatitis and the Pill

By far the commonest liver disease seen in general practice is infective hepatitis. Women developing this illness should stop taking the Pill, and should not return to it until three months after their liver function tests have returned to normal.

A past history of infective hepatitis followed by normal liver function tests obtained more than three months previously is not a contraindication to the use of combined oral contraception.

Other liver disease and the Pill

Given the fact that one test of liver function (BSP excretion) is frequently affected, and abnormalities of other tests sometimes occur, it would be a foolhardy family doctor who advised combined oral contraception for a women with pre-existing hepatic disease, *e.g.* cirrhosis, unless there were unusually strong reasons for avoiding all other methods - a situation difficult to imagine today.

II. Oestrogens promote the enzyme synthesis of the plasma proteins in the liver, especially the ß-globulins. These are the proteins which transport hormones and other substances, bound to them. Because there is a raised level of these transporting proteins in the plasma, there is a consequent rise in the level of the substances bound to them. This has particular application in the consideration of thyroid function and adrenocortical function.

EFFECT ON THYROID FUNCTION

Both protein-bound iodine and thyroxine levels may be raised in women using combined Pills, and the levels may reach those normally found in thyrotoxicosis. Similarly, there may be a diminished resin uptake of tri-iodothyronine. These changes take several weeks to return to normal. Two practical considerations ensue.

1. Do not attempt to assess thyroid function in women taking oral contraceptives by measurements which are affected by oral contraceptives. Either wait until six weeks after stopping the Pill to perform such tests, or make use of tests which are not affected by the Pill. The laboratory will advise what tests are available. For example, radio-iodine uptake or excretion are suitable tests to use.
2. Beware the chance finding of an abnormal test result in an oral contraceptive user.

> A patient referred to a surgeon because of persistent diarrhoea was found to have a raised PBI. A full range of tests of thyroid function was suggested, but a reminder that the patient was taking the Pill avoided unnecessary investigation.

There is no evidence that thyroid disease is either more or less likely to develop in Pill-users. Women suffering from either hyper- or hypothyroidism, often associated with low fertility, need treatment for their disease as the priority. It would seem unwise to use combined oral contraceptives until the thyroid disorder has been controlled. Afterwards, the usual considerations would apply to the choice of contraceptive method.

EFFECT ON ADRENOCORTICAL FUNCTION

Another result of the increase in the plasma protein level, is that the level of transcortin, the corticosteroid binding globulin, is also increased, with a consequent increase in the plasma corticosteroid level. Some authorities maintain that this is the explanation of the alterations in carbohydrate metabolism that may be noted in patients taking combined Pills. Others maintain that because the corticosteroid is all in bound form, this cannot be so. Whatever the outcome of this argument, there is no doubt that changes in carbohydrate metabolism do occur in patients using combined contraceptives.

EFFECT ON CARBOHYDRATE METABOLISM

Impaired glucose tolerance, a raised fasting blood sugar, and sugar tolerance curves very like diabetic curves can be shown in women taking the combined Pill. The insulin requirements of diabetic patients may alter when they start oral contraception. Usually less insulin is required, but sometimes the dosage needs to be increased, or insulin becomes necessary where diet alone previously sufficed.

Glycosuria present in a previous pregnancy may return when a patient takes the Pill. In fact the combined Pill, like pregnancy, seems to be diabetogenic. Since the general reduction of oestrogen dosage in combined Pills, the frequency with which these effects are seen seems to have diminished. No effect on glucose tolerance has been noted in patients taking progestogen-only preparations.

Pregnancy, of course, constitutes a very considerable hazard for a diabetic woman, and this the combined Pill can be guaranteed to avoid. The higher pregnancy rate with the progestogen-only Pill is a disadvantage.

How then should the GP advise his diabetic patient who seeks his advice on using the Pill? In spite of the lack of evidence that to take oral contraceptives is harmful to such women - and evidence of a slight acceleration of the diabetic disease process must be almost impossible to obtain anyway - I would advise their use only if all other methods seemed unsuitable in her particular case. And today, with the multitude of other methods available, such cases must be rare.

EFFECT ON LIPID METABOLISM

Plasma concentrations of both cholesterol and triglycerides are raised in patients taking combined oral contraceptives. The most marked cholesterol changes are reported to be found in those taking the more progestational compounds, and the most marked changes in triglycerides in those taking the more oestrogenic Pills. Women taking progestogen-only Pills have been reported to show no change, or even significantly lowered levels of both cholesterol and triglycerides. The altered plasma concentrations rapidly return to normal after stopping the Pill.

Anxiety has been expressed that increased plasma levels of these substances in women taking the Pill over long periods of time may increase the possibility of atheroma and consequent vascular disease. Although this theory remains unproven, it would seem wise to avoid combined oral contraceptives in women with primary hyperlipidaemia or with a family history of this condition.

Now that biochemical laboratories are automated, many patients taking the Pill, attending hospital for reasons quite unconnected with contraception, may be found by the autoanalyser to have high cholesterol readings. The information that a patient is on the Pill should accompany requests for biochemical tests; in any event the GP should stand ready to protect his patient from over-investigation.

Clearly abnormal values for cholesterol or triglycerides developing in a patient taking the Pill should be an indication for careful consideration of whether to continue with the method, but not for panic action.

> A girl of 29 arrived from the Continent requesting an abortion. Oral contraception had been suddenly stopped four months before because of a single serum cholesterol reading of 220 mg/100 ml, a value which would not be considered abnormal for her age in this country.

Cholesterol levels rise with age, so a small progressive increase over many years of oral contraception is not a cause for alarm.

Raised fasting and post-glucose blood pyruvate levels have also been found in women using combined oral contraceptives.

Oral contraceptives and disease

THE PILL AND CANCER

Since the introduction of the Pill there have been those who maintained that it was probably carcinogenic: there have been others who asserted that there was no evidence for this view, and what evidence there was indicated that the Pill protected against cancer. The argument continues to this day, despite enormous research efforts.

The complexity of the problem may be indicated by considering the following factors:

1. Our knowledge of the causes of cancer is small. We do not really know where to look for our answers.
2. The incidence of the different types of cancer found in the age groups likely to take the Pill is small. Because the alterations in the incidence may also be small, huge numbers of patients would need to be studied in detail before one could be quite sure that small changes were not occurring.
3. Allowance must be made in any study for a multitude of variables, among which may be listed the possible differences resulting from the differing types and dosages of oestrogens; varying types and dosages of progestogens; the length of time for which they are administered, and whether administration is continuous or intermittent, oral or parenteral; the possibility that different organs will show different effects, or even that the same organ will show different effects depending on the strength or method of administration of the same substance; there may be ethnic or geographical or dietary factors to take into account; and finally even the vehicle, or colouring matter used in the Pill may influence the outcome of an investigation.
4. Evidence from experimental animals must be viewed with suspicion, since the physiological action of a drug on an animal may not be the same as its action in a human, and because an effect shown to develop in an animal may not develop in human beings. In addition it must be remembered that

animals are sometimes chosen for research because of their propensity to develop particular tumours.

5. The 'incubation period' of cancer is thought to be of the order of ten to twenty years. In practice few women will take the Pill continuously for that length of time.

The fact that indisputable proof to implicate or exonerate the Pill has not so far appeared is therefore not surprising, but some general indications exist.

Synthetic steroids have been used in treatment for many years before the Pill appeared, and no increased incidence of malignant disease has been noted.

A review was published in 1962 of reports of 304 women treated with oestrogens for periods varying from 14 months to 27 years (average 7.8 years) with no cases of neoplasm of breast or genital tract developing.

Defares (1971) reviewed reports of 2,552 women treated with oestrogens for up to 17 years, in whom only seven cases of neoplasm developed.

In both these reviews the number of cases of cancer observed was fewer than the expected number.

It seems reasonable to assume that the uterus and vagina, the breast, the ovary and the liver are the organs most likely to provide evidence of any carcinogenic effects of the Pill.

(i) **Uterus**

(a) *Cervix*

A diminished progression from negative to positive Papanicolou smears has been reported in populations using the Pill, but the effects of removal of patients with abnormal smears from the study, and the general improvement of the economic conditions of the population during the study prevent reliance on these reports. There is evidence that some women taking the Pill develop dyskaryosis, a condition also seen during pregnancy or infection with trichomonas. Removal of the infection, the pregnancy or the Pill results in disappearance of dyskaryosis, a condition which has not been proved to be pre-cancerous anyway. One study (Melamed *et al.,* 1969) did demonstrate that women using oral contraceptives were more likely to develop abnormal Papanicolou smears than women using the diaphragm, but this could be due to the protection afforded by barrier methods against the male secretions. Nor did this study make adequate allowance for the social class differences known to exist between cap-users and Pill-users.

(b) *Endometrium*

The condition of endometrial hyperplasia is followed by the development of endometrial carcinoma in 7–10 per cent of cases. Treatment with progestogens has resulted in the disappearance of neoplastic change as a complication of the condition. In view of the hypoplastic endometrium found in long-term users of oral contraceptives, it is believed that the Pill protects against both endometrial hyperplasia and endometrial carcinoma.

(c) *Breast*

There is no evidence that malignant disease of the breast is more likely in women using the Pill. Pre-existing hormone-dependant tumours could theoretically become either better or worse. An increased incidence of breast tumours in beagle dogs given large doses of progestogen was reported some years ago. Further work has failed to show that this has any relevance to humans taking progestogen-only Pills.

There is some evidence (Vessey *et al.*, 1972) that benign tumours of the breast are less common in women using oral contraception, and the interim report from the Royal College of General Practitioners (1974) confirmed this.

(d) *Ovary*

Ovarian function is depressed during oral contraception, the ovary shrinking and follicles becoming atretic, a situation hardly likely to lead to neoplasia, and no increased incidence of malignant ovarian neoplasms has been reported.

As with the breast there is some evidence that benign tumours are less common in women using oral contraceptives, Ory (1974) reporting a tenfold reduction in functional ovarian cysts among users when compared with non-users.

(e) *Liver*

In 1966 it was suggested that mestranol might cause primary neoplastic disease of the liver. Further work has not substantiated this suggestion.

Benign tumours of the liver, in some cases causing death from haemorrhage, have recently been reported in women using oral contraceptives, but no cause and effect relationship between this exceedingly rare tumour and pill-usage has been established.

(f) *Vagina*

There have recently been reports of adenocarcinoma of the vagina in the children of mothers who had been treated during the pregnancy with massive doses of oestrogen. If this association is proved - and at the moment it is not - it may be of significance if pregnancy follows an attempt at post-coital contraception with oestrogens. There is no suggestion that this hazard exists in users of conventional low oestrogen-dosage pills.

To summarize, there is so far no evidence that women taking oestrogens or progestogens, either as treatment or for contraceptive purposes, have an increased liability to cancer of any organ, other than of the cervix. Here there is conflicting evidence.

There is some evidence that users of the Pill may enjoy some protection against certain types of tumours, both malignant and benign.

Meanwhile large scale prospective studies, such as that of the Royal College of General Practitioners, may in time give clearer answers.

Clinical implications

Because of the possibility of unfavourably influencing the growth of a hormone-dependant carcinoma of the breast, every effort should be made to exclude breast cancer before starting oral contraception. To this end, the breasts should be palpated before starting oral contraceptives, and at intervals thereafter. If the methods now being used for screening are shown to be of value, they should be applied to women using oral contraceptives.

The question of giving the Pill to a woman known to have a carcinoma of the breast is really of academic interest only. Theoretically oral contraception may be a suitable method, but practically another method would be chosen. Ovariectomy may be found necessary anyway.

Any woman starting any method of contraception should have a full pelvic examination and cervical cytology performed beforehand, and women starting oral contraception are no exception. To repeat these examinations at intervals is good medicine, but to repeat Papanicolou smears every year, without regard to the age or parity of the patient - as has been the much publicised practice of the FPA - is a waste of valuable medical and laboratory resources.

Whatever interval between smears is advised, it will be too short for some, and too long for others. The GP will find that repeating a smear not less than every two years, and not more than every three will keep the majority of his patients content, will hopefully allow very few abnormals time to develop, and will certainly keep the family doctor and his staff fully occupied.

THE PILL AND HYPERTENSION

Hypertension occurring in women taking the Pill was first reported by Woods, a British general practitioner, in 1967, and further reports came from the United States in the same year.

Changes in the renin-angiotensin-aldosterone system have been reported by several workers. The angiotensin and aldosterone concentration in the plasma is increased significantly and rapidly - within the first week of taking combined oral contraceptives, according to Beckerhoff *et al.* (1973) - while the concentration of renin in the plasma falls, due to the negative feed-back action of the increased angiotensin. The raised level of aldosterone is probably due to stimulation of the adrenal cortex by the renin-angiotensin system, and the increased aldosterone activity, causing sodium and water retention, may be the cause of the increased weight noticed by some women taking oral contraceptives.

Retention of sodium may result from the administration of progestogens alone, and water retention and oedema from administered oestrogens.

These changes are similar to those taking place in pregnancy due to increasing hormone levels.

Studies from various parts of the world have indicated that a slight increase in systolic blood pressure, of the order of 10 mm mercury, may be expected in all women using combined oral contraceptives. Rises in diastolic blood pressure have been less regularly reported.

Weir *et al.* (1974) reported their findings in a controlled prospective study of women using combined oral contraception, and suggested that both systolic and diastolic blood pressures are significantly raised after three years of therapy, and even higher figures may be recorded after four years.

The mean systolic blood pressure in 83 women showed a rise of 9.2 mmHg after three years, and in 10 women followed for four years, a rise of 14.2 mm Hg. The mean diastolic blood pressure in the same women rose 5.0 mmHg after three years, and 8.5 mmHg after four years.

Blood pressure changes in this study were not shown to be related to changes in weight, a past history of renal disease, a family history of hypertension, parity, social class or cigarette smoking. Nor did there seem to be any changes in sodium, potassium or water balance which correlated with changes in blood pressure.

However, several other investigators have shown that women developing *severe* hypertension on combined oral contraception do tend to be older, more obese, and of higher parity, and are likely to give a history of previous toxaemia of pregnancy. Mason *et al.* (1973) showed a correlation between changes in blood pressure and metabolic functions, and suggested that combined oral contraception may produce a primary biochemical effect leading to the development of hypertension in patients showing other predisposing factors.

That the risk increases the longer the Pill is taken was confirmed in the interim report of the Royal College of General Practitioners in 1974. During the first year the risk was very small, but increased until in the fifth year of contraceptive use it was two-and-a-half times as great as in the first year. Only approximate estimates of the incidence of hypertension among Pill-users were possible, but it was suggested that fewer than 1 per cent of women would develop hypertension during the first year of use, and not more than 5 per cent after five years. The dosage of oestrogen did not seem to be significant.

There have been no reports of significant changes in blood pressure in patients taking progestogen-only contraceptives. Varying amounts of progestogen in the combined oral contraceptives studied by Weir *et al.* (1974) seemed to bear no relation to the level of blood pressure changes. In my own practice substitution of progestogen-only contraception in those patients developing hypertension while using combined oral contraceptives has resulted in a return of the blood pressure to normal levels. Stopping combined therapy altogether also results in a lowering of the raised blood pressure within a few weeks.

It is well known that women will tolerate levels of hypertension which would be associated with pathological changes and decreased life expectancy in men, so the rises of blood pressure recorded do not seem to constitute any danger to the vast majority of women taking the Pill.

In a small minority, probably one patient in two hundred, combined oral contraception is associated with a severe degree of hypertension and it is most important that this minority should be identified and, where necessary, treated. For the clinician, the tabulation below seems a sensible one in the light of our present knowledge.

1. Essential hypertension occurring in patients taking combined oral contraceptives

As stated, some reports have shown that the woman most likely to develop hypertension is the older, heavier woman, who gives a history of a raised blood pressure during pregnancy or a family history of hypertension. These are in fact the patients who might be expected to be more liable to develop hypertension in any case, and to detect them it is most important that the blood pressure should be measured before starting contraceptive therapy. An initial high reading need not be a contra-indication to the Pill, but is an indication for a full investigation of the cause. Readings from both arms should be taken if hypertension is found, to detect the rare case of coarctation. Obviously regular measurements of blood pressure should continue while the patient continues to take the Pill. Once every six months would seem sensible as a routine, once every three months for those in the

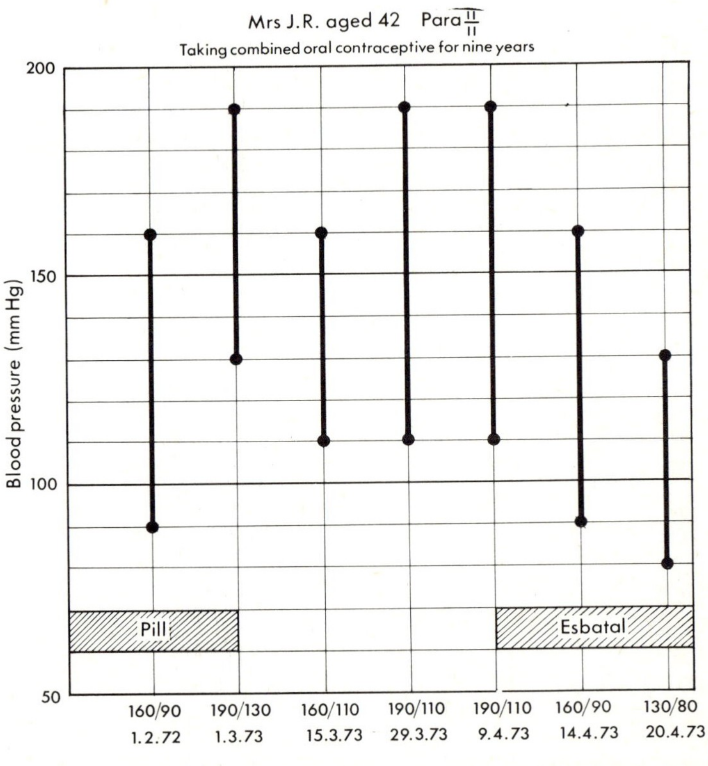

Fig. 16. Essential hypertension developing in a woman of 42 who had been taking combined oral contraceptives for nine years. Stopping the Pill made no difference to the blood pressure level. Anti-hypertensive therapy necessary.

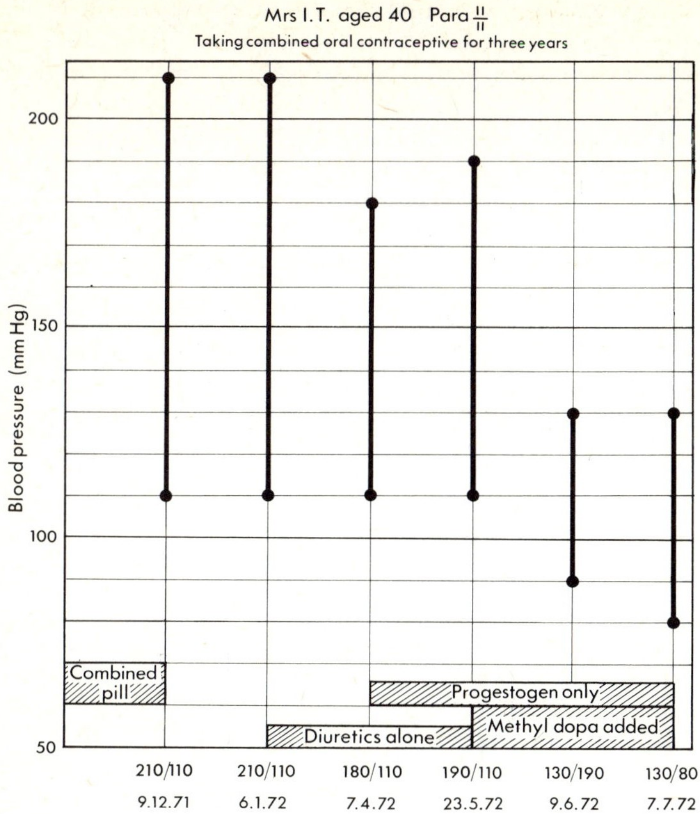

Fig. 17. Essential hypertension developing in a woman of 40 who wished to continue using oral contraception. Satisfactory control of the blood pressure resulted from treatment with methyldopa coincident with progestogen-only contraception.

group most likely to develop hypertension, and more often, according to clinical findings, in those found to be hypertensive before starting the Pill.

The blood pressure will not alter in these cases if the oral contraceptive is stopped, and the usual treatment of essential hypertension is necessary (Fig. 16).

At the moment it is not clear whether the taking of oral contraceptives causes essential hypertension to appear earlier than it otherwise would, so although finding a raised blood pressure need not be an absolute contra-indication, it would seem wise to avoid this method in such patients if alternative methods would be equally suitable and acceptable.

Patients for whom all methods other than oral contraception are unacceptable may be switched to progestogen-only contraception, and the hypertension treated in the usual way (Fig. 17).

2. **Hypertension caused by combined oral contraceptives**
This is a rare phenomenon, but cases do occur. The type of patient affected need not be the older, heavier woman. Woods, in 1967, reported that this type of hypertension did not respond to anti-hypertensive drugs, but there is little further information available on this point.

Stopping the oral contraceptive will result in a return of the blood pressure to normal within a few weeks.

Substitution of a Pill containing a progestogen alone will also result in the blood pressure returning to normal, which would suggest the oestrogen as the causative factor (Fig. 18).

It would seem therefore that the occurrence of this type of hypertension is an indication to stop combined oral contraception, but in patients for whom other methods are unacceptable, and who will accept the increased pregnancy rate, oral contraception with a progestogen alone is a reasonable alternative.

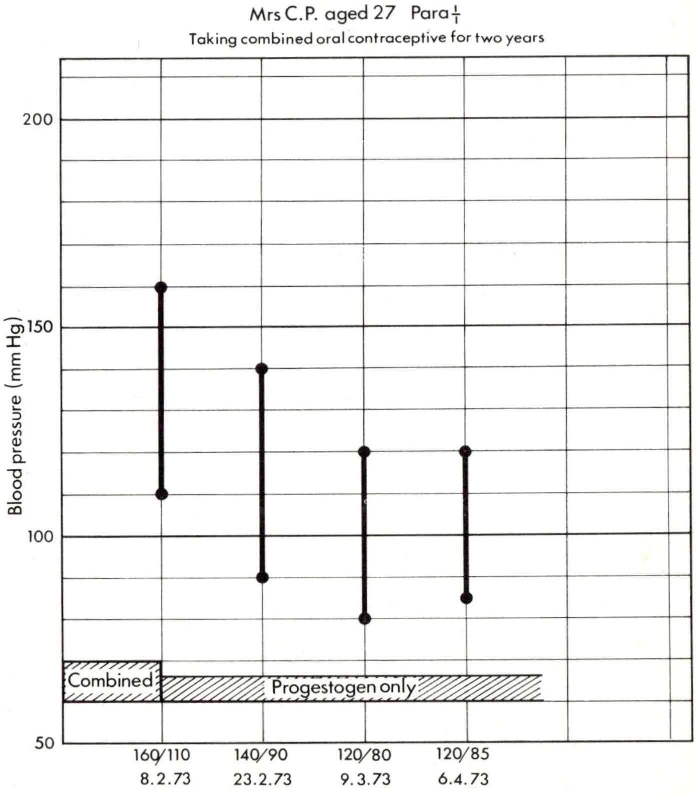

Fig. 24. Oestrogen-induced hypertension occurring in a young woman of 27 who had taken the Pill for two years. Substituting a progestogen-only Pill resulted in a return of the blood pressure to normal.

3. **Malignant hypertension occurring in oral contraceptive users**

There have been a very few reports of malignant hypertension developing in patients taking oral contraceptives. There is at the moment no evidence that the association of this condition with oral contraception is anything other than coincidental.

THE PILL AND SICKLE-CELL ANAEMIA

Most general practitioners in the nineteen-seventies look after negroid patients, some of whom have come directly from Africa, and some, by courtesy of the slave traders, from the West Indies. In their original African environment few babies with sickle-cell disease reached adult life; in the West Indies many do, and with the higher standards of medical care available in the United Kingdom, still more women with sickling disease may be expected to become adult. About 10 per cent of the coloured population of African origin in the United Kingdom have the sickle-cell trait, that is, some of their haemoglobin is haemoglobin-S. Only about one in four hundred possess haemoglobin-S alone and show the full sickling syndrome.

De-oxygenation results in crystallization of the abnormal haemoglobin within the red cell, with sickling, the development of thrombotic infarcts, and a haemolytic anaemia. If an increased tendency to thrombosis is accepted as a hazard for women using the combined Pill, then to give the Pill to a woman with sickle-cell disease, in which thrombosis is also a hazard, must be to increase the danger.

However, once more the contra-indication is only relative; pregnancy and labour are especially dangerous in a woman with the full sickling syndrome. Possibly one in fifty will die. The combined Pill will guarantee she does not run this great danger, and will ensure no offspring to inherit the sickling trait. Hence it is reasonable to say that where no other efficient method of contraception is acceptable, the combined oral contraceptive may be given to a woman with sickle-cell disease due to haemoglobin-S or one of the other abnormal haemoglobins. Each case must be decided on its merits.

Patients exhibiting only the sickling trait run no special risk of haemolysis or infarction except in exceptional circumstances of severe oxygen lack, and oral contraception poses no special problems.

THE PILL AND GALL BLADDER DISEASE

Two retrospective studies from America have indicated a definite association between the administration of oestrogens and the occurrence of gall-bladder disease.

The Boston Collaborative Drug Surveillance Programme assessed the risk of this disease developing in women aged 45-69 and calculated that whereas in women not using oestrogen it was 87 per 100,000 women per year, the risk was increased in women taking oestrogen to 218 per 100,000 women per year, a highly significant difference. Although women in this age group are beyond the need for the Pill, nevertheless of 200 women with gall-bladder disease, 31 per cent of them had been taking oestrogen-containing contraceptive pills, whereas only 20 per cent of healthy controls had done so.

This survey related to patients taking oral contraceptives containing higher doses of oestrogen than commonly used today, and of course, far higher doses than the new generation Pills containing only 30 microgrammes of oestrogen. But, because of the apparent association between oestrogens and disease of the gall-bladder, the combined Pill should be avoided where possible in women with suspected gall-bladder disease, and probably avoided in the classical 'fair, fat, fertile, flatulent woman of forty' (or thereabouts).

The interim report of the Royal College of General Practitioners in 1974 drew the interesting conclusion that the longer a woman uses the Pill, the more likely she is to develop gallstones—but not cholecystitis.

THE PILL AND OTHER DISEASES

1. Chorea

The appearance of an illness resembling Sydenham's chorea in women taking combined oral contraceptives has been reported by several observers, notably Riddoch *et al.* (1971). The hypothesis that the cause of this condition is similar to that of chorea gravidarum is obviously attractive. Pills containing only 50 microgrammes of oestrogen have been associated with the appearance of chorea.

Withdrawal of the oral contraceptive results in abatement of the disease, but opinions differ as to the advisability of following up with long-term penicillin therapy, as absence of a rheumatic element may be difficult to prove.

Where other methods are acceptable, combined oral contraceptives are best avoided in patients giving a history of chorea gravidarum.

2. Epilepsy (grand mal)

This disease has been reported as making its first appearance in women taking combined oral contraceptives, and women known to be epileptic have sometimes suffered more frequent and severe attacks after starting on the Pill. Changes in the electroencephalogram found in 60 per cent of women taking oral contraceptives studied in Cairo (Elwan *et al.*, 1973) seemed to indicate a more pathological pattern developing with higher oestrogen dosage.

Many women with epilepsy exhibit no adverse effects when given oral contraception and certainly many need the effective birth control this method offers. Hence the combined Pill should not be withheld from patients with major epilepsy, although it would seem sensible to give the lowest possible dosage of oestrogen, and supervise their progress closely. (See also 'Drugs antagonizing oral contraception, p. 131).

3. Otosclerosis

This condition occasionally shows a dramatic deterioration in pregnancy, and a similar effect may result from administering the combined Pill. Consultation with the aural surgeon caring for the patient should precede a prescription for oral contraceptives.

4. **Multiple Sclerosis**

The course of this condition is so unpredictable that it is not surprising that both improvement and deterioration have been described as following the commencement of oral contraception. There is so far no evidence that any type of Pill has any effect on multiple sclerosis.

5. **Asthma**

Exacerbation of asthmatic symptoms has been claimed to follow the ingestion of combined oral contraceptives by asthmatic patients. This must be extremely rare: asthma is a common entity in general practice, and I have never seen an asthmatic patient suffer from the addition of oral contraception. Should a GP meet such a rarity, then discontinuation of the Pill would be an obvious course of action.

6. **Porphyria**

Porphyrin metabolism is affected by the administration of both oestrogens and progestogens. Patients with porphyria of hepatic type should not be given oral contraceptives. Such patients are of course rare, but as porphyria has a genetic component it is wise to investigate the relatives of those having overt porphyria, lest administration of oral contraceptives may provoke a latent porphyria into activity (*British Medical Journal,* 1972).

The rare porphyria cutanea tarda may appear as a result of liver damage due to oestrogen administration.

GPs who have a patient suffering from porphyria on their list (as there is on mine) must ensure that oral contraceptives are included in the list of drugs such patients are warned to avoid.

7. **The Pill and urinary symptoms**

The prospective study of the Royal College of General Practitioners established that urinary tract infections were more common in women taking the Pill than in those who did not. However, it must be remembered that pyelonephritis is extremely common in women during pregnancy, and the Pill certainly avoids this category of infection. Whether women on the Pill suffer urinary infections more often because of the Pill, or because of their greater sexual activity when compared to women not taking the Pill, is not certain.

The urethral syndrome, associated with dysuria and frequency but without identifiable urinary infection, is believed by some urologists to be a consequence of oral contraception. Here again the relative increase in sexual activity in Pill-users may be causative.

8. **The Pill and neuritis**

Pain in the arm, labelled brachial neuritis, and the carpal tunnel syndrome occur both in pregnancy and in women on oral contraceptives. The presumed cause in both is pressure on nerves or nerve roots due to fluid retention.

The prospective study of the Royal College of General Practitioners detected an increased incidence of sciatica in women who had formerly taken the Pill. No evidence of such an increase has been detected in my own practice.

Other changes accompanying oral contraception

Many other changes of little or doubtful importance have been reported among women taking the Pill. Improvement of hearing, fewer complaints of wax in the ears, damage to Eustachian tubes, and alterations in the serum copper and iron level are among these. A raised ESR or alkaline phosphatase level may be associated with ingestion of oral contraceptives without any disease being present, facts which should be born in mind when interpreting laboratory results. Eczema seems to follow administration of oral contraceptives on rare occasions.

Drugs antagonizing oral contraceptives

An important recent suggestion is that the administration of Rifampicin to tuberculous women using the Pill may accelerate the breakdown of oestrogen and make the contraception less effective as a result. Hydantoin and barbiturates may have the same effect. Care must be taken if it is proposed to administer any of these drugs for long periods to women using oral contraceptives.

Miscellaneous effects of oral contraceptives

VEINS AND THE PILL

Women often complain that since starting to take the Pill the veins in their lower legs, especially varicose veins, ache more and enlarge. The increase in size is sometimes marked, and obvious to the family doctor on inspection. The patients often compare the situation to that existing during a previous pregnancy, and presumably the cause in both instances is similar, being due to increased progesterone or progestogen. Stopping the Pill results in relief of the discomfort and the veins subside. Groups of small venules in the skin may enlarge, causing a cosmetic rather than a medical problem.

Because of the possible association of varicose veins, stasis and thrombo-embolism, before starting the Pill women with varicose veins should be advised to have them treated. Women whose veins become varicose while taking the Pill should be similarly advised. Whether sclerotherapy or operation is chosen, the patient should cease oral contraception for at least two months beforehand. Following successful treatment of the veins, the patient may take the Pill again.

Occasionally a patient complains of pain and throbbing in veins which are not varicose. If these symptoms continue to worry her despite reassurance that the veins are not varicose and do not need treatment, then a change to a non-hormonal method of contraception is indicated.

The interim report of the oral contraception study of the Royal College of General Practitioners (1974) assessed the risk of superficial thrombosis of leg veins as being 50 per cent greater in women using the combined Pill than in controls. The risk attributable to the Pill was estimated at 30 per 100,000 users annually.

EFFECT ON THE EYES

Marked alterations in refraction may occur when a woman starts taking the Pill. The changes are temporary only, but an unwary optician may advise several unnecessary changes of glasses if the patient does not inform him that she is taking the Pill.

Oral contraceptives may make previously comfortable contact lenses no longer bearable. Suggested causes are alteration of the curvature of the globe of the eye, corneal oedema, swelling of the eyelids and decreased secretion of tears. Whatever the cause, women proposing to use the Pill who already wear contact lenses should be warned that there is a very small chance, possibly one in thirty, that difficulty may ensue. If it does, women usually choose to abandon oral contraception and, remembering the cost of contact lenses, who would blame them?

In the fundus, papilloedema may occur in women taking combined oral contraceptives (MacFaul, 1973), and any retinal change due to thrombo-embolism may be seen.

THE PILL AND THE HAIR

Most women do not realize that hair follicles undergo cyclic activity. Each scalp hair grows steadily for about five years and then growth ceases, the follicle entering a resting stage during which the hair is shed. About 100 hairs are shed daily, but the rate varies with age and with the season of the year. November is said to be associated with maximum shedding in the United Kingdom. After a resting stage of about four months, the hair follicle again becomes active, a new hair replacing the shed one (Rook, 1973).

An increase in the rate of shedding may follow childbirth. A diffuse hair loss, noticed by the patient on brushing or combing the hair, but without bald patches, results. Cormia (1967) described a similar hair loss in patients who had recently stopped oral contraceptives, and suggested that both types of alopecia had a similar hormonal cause. He also described male pattern alopecia developing in women taking oral contraceptives.

Figures from St. John's Hospital for Diseases of the Skin (Griffiths, 1973) indicated that despite the enormous increase in the number of women taking the Pill between 1952 and 1971 there had been no increase in the number of patients attending the hospital complaining of diffuse alopecia.

Studies of the hair follicles in women taking oral contraceptives have been made by Zaun (1972). In about half these women it was shown that a temporary increase in the number of resting follicles (and therefore shedding of the hair) followed commencement of oral contraception, but the pre-treatment status was regained after about six months. In about half of the remaining women, the number of resting follicles actually decreased.

Overall, it does not seem that oral contraceptives are likely to be associated with hair loss other than of a temporary reversible nature. Clinically, the tabulation below has been found helpful in practice.

1. **Hair loss after starting oral contraception**

(i) *Following pregnancy*

Many women start to take the Pill shortly after childbirth, and it is likely that any falling of the hair they notice is as much due to the pregnancy as to the Pill. Certainly a complaint that their 'hair is coming out in handfuls' is not uncommonly made to the family doctor looking after such women. They may be strongly reassured that such hair loss is a normal finding after pregnancy, they will not go bald, their hair will regain its full vigour within six months, and they may continue to take the Pill without a qualm.

(ii) *Not following pregnancy*

Diffuse hair loss, especially in the autumn, is a common complaint among women in general practice, and some will be taking the Pill. Provided there is no evidence of seborrhoea, excessive oiliness of the skin or associated hirsutism - conditions that might be due to excessive progestational potency - the patient may be strongly reassured that the hair loss is temporary only and probably not due to the Pill.

If evidence of excessive progestational activity exists, or if the alopecia is of the male type rather than a diffuse loss, a more oestrogenic Pill should be substituted or oral contraception stopped altogether. Such situations rarely arise in practice, possibly because highly progestogenic Pills are rarely prescribed today.

2. **Hair loss after ceasing oral contraception**

Again this is a rare complaint, when compared with the complaint of hair loss after pregnancy and starting the Pill. The patient may be reassured that it is temporary only.

3. **Alopecia areata developing in users of oral contraceptives**

Alopecia areata is a condition seen not uncommonly in general practice, and will occasionally be seen in women on oral contraception. It occurs in such women neither more nor less commonly than in their sisters who do not take the Pill, and the doctor may reassure the patient to this effect. Whether the patient will accept the reassurance if the patches of alopecia enlarge or multiply is another matter altogether and she may stop taking the Pill despite medical advice, laying herself open to the possibility of an unwanted pregnancy. Where this danger exists, it may be wiser to switch to another method of contraception.

THE PILL AND FACIAL PIGMENTATION (CHLOASMA)

Chloasma is the term applied to the appearance on the face of patches of yellowish-brown or bronze pigmentation. Situated mainly on the upper lip, cheeks, nose or forehead, the distribution may be irregular or symmetrical. Common during pregnancy (chloasma gravidarum), it also occurs in patients using combined oral contraceptives.

Fair-skinned women are less likely to develop chloasma than their dark-skinned sisters. It has been shown to be more common in countries blessed with large quantities of sunshine, and also in those cursed with endemic malnutrition, the administration of Vitamin B complex relieving chloasma in such countries (Rice-Wray, 1962). Once again the oestrogen component of the combined Pill has been incriminated as the causative agent, and both length of medication and dosage seem to be significant (Pincus and Garcia, 1964). Chloasma usually disappears completely after therapy is withdrawn.

In the United Kingdom, as one would expect from the high level of nutrition, the abysmal level of sunshine, and the low dosages of oestrogen now employed in contraception, chloasma in Pill-users is not a problem. I have noted severe facial pigmentation during oral contraception in only two patients since 1964, and Wiseman (1964) reported the same number of sufferers out of a total of 1,200 women attending the Slough Family Planning Clinic.

Treatment

Moynahan (1965) suggested that the patches of pigmentation could be bleached by the application of a simple ointment containing 5 per cent monobenzyl-ether of hydroquinone, and that the bleaching effect could be enhanced by applying 20 per cent sodium chloride in emulsifying ointment overnight beforehand. If the bleach preparation proved irritant to the skin, good results could still be obtained with lower concentrations of the hydroquinone compound.

Such treatment is worth trying if no other method of contraception is acceptable, and the patient has not completed her family. Rather than taking Pills and messing about with ointments the patient who has completed her family will probably prefer vasectomy for her husband or tubal ligation for herself.

> A woman of 35 who had been taking a combined preparation for eight years following the birth of her third child complained in 1973 of patches of brown pigmentation on her upper lip that 'looked like a moustache'. My offer of ointment was received with distaste, and my further offer of an intrauterine device was countered with the suggestion that she might be sterilized. To regain the initiative, I suggested vasectomy for her husband, but he vetoed this idea. Accordingly she was referred to a gynaecologist and tubal ligation performed. The chloasma faded

gradually, and when last seen, six months after operation, abnormal pigmentation was very difficult to detect.

The Pill and vitamin levels

A significant increase in circulating Vitamin A levels has been found in 20 young women taking combined oral contraceptives, according to a report by Gal *et al.* (1971). A 30 per cent decrease in Vitamin C levels in six young women taking combined Pills was reported by Harris *et al.* (1973). As yet there seem no clinical implications from either of these observations.

Progestogen-only contraception

Pincus in 1956, and Ishikawa in 1959, reported that large doses of progestogen alone prevented conception in women, even though inhibition of ovulation did not occur in all cases.

The following decade saw a progressive reduction in the dose of progestogen contained in the combined Pill, and investigation of the contraceptive effect of varying dosages and time schedules of both oestrogen and progestogen given alone. Oestrogen alone was found to be unreliable at low dosage as an ovulation inhibitor, and the side-effects of high dosage were unpleasant. Progestogen alone, presumably because of its effect on cervical mucus, was found to be effective in low dosage.

Between 1964 and 1967, Rudel and Martinez-Manatou in Mexico investigated the contraceptive possibilities of a progestogen, chlormadinone acetate; in varying dosage. High doses given daily throughout the cycle suppressed ovulation, altered the endometrium and made the cervical mucus hostile to invasion by spermatozoa. Low doses had little effect on ovulation or the endometrium, but the effect on cervical mucus remained.

In 1967 Martinez-Manatou reported the result of a clinical trial involving 945 women treated with 0.5 mg chlormadinone acetate for more than eight thousand calendar months. Tablets were taken by mouth, daily throughout the cycle. Only one pregnancy occurred in women who had taken tablets regularly, but a further thirteen women who had missed some tablets became pregnant. The failure rate of the method overall was calculated as 2.1 pregnancies per 100 women-years.

Considerable anxiety was widespread, both among patients and their doctors, concerning the dangerous complications of oestrogen in the combined oral contraceptives at this time. The possibility that a Pill with no oestrogen, if taken regularly, could produce a degree of protection against pregnancy approximating to that of combined Pills resulted in clinical trials of various progestogens in other parts of the world.

Unfortunately two reports doused the enthusiasm during the next few years. Mears in 1969 evaluated the contraceptive effect of four different progestogens used as daily contraception by women attending a clinic in Yugoslavia. Pregnancy rates of between 4 and 12 per hundred women-years were reported. Even more disappointing was the fact that whereas Martinez-Manatou had reported that only 2 per cent of the women had withdrawn from the trial for medical reasons, usually irregular bleeding, Mears found very much higher discontinuation rates for medical reasons. For 0.5 mg chlormadinone acetate itself the rate was 46 per cent.

The final straw was a report from the United States that administration of progestogen alone to beagle bitches had resulted in the appearance of breast tumours, and following this the only Pill containing progestogen alone marketed in the United Kingdom was withdrawn.

This report was later shown to be of little significance in human subjects taking relatively very much smaller doses of progestogen, and the concept of a Pill containing no oestrogen continued to be attractive, especially as the guilt of oestrogen as a cause of thrombo-embolism and death came to be accepted as proven, by the public if not by the medical profession.

Further work has shown that the dosage of progestogen on its own is critical. Whereas in a combined Pill the presence of oestrogen allows relatively large variation in the dose of progestogen without much alteration in the pregnancy rate, the rate will vary considerably if the progestogen dosage is changed without oestrogen to back it up. Furthermore, it has become obvious that at the optimum dosage for avoiding pregnancy, ovulation may well be suppressed as well.

A recent trial by Eckstein and others (1972) using the progestogen norgestrol illustrates that at a dosage of 0.075 mg daily a pregnancy rate for the method of 2.1 per hundred women-years may be expected, as compared with the trial in Yugoslavia, using 0.05 mg of the same substance, with a pregnancy rate of 9 per hundred women-years of use. Other factors relating to acceptability were remarkably similar in this trial to those recorded by Mears. Forty per cent of women withdrew from the trial for medical reasons connected with the method, and more than half of these were because of menstrual irregularity. One-fifth of all cycles recorded during the thirty months of the study lasted less than seventeen days.

One question remains to be answered concerning the trials in Mexico and in Yugoslavia. How could two experienced investigators, using the same daily dosage of the same progestogen, produce such widely differing results? Similar disparities were noted among reports of trials of other progestogens, and although racial or geographical difference could be the explanation in some trials, they could not explain the differences between investigations which had been carried out in neighbouring cities of the same country. Consideration of the possibilities provides an insight into the complexities resulting when doses are reduced to such critical levels.

All tablets contain inert substances used to bind the tablet together: a crumbling Pill is a powder, not a Pill. Dissolution tests in the laboratory may not exactly imitate what happens in the stomach, and the suspicion exists that in at least one preparation, the Pill was so firmly stuck together that little of it was absorbed. One answer to this difficulty may be to abandon the Pill form and use a gelatin capsule containing a solution, suspension or fine powder designed to be released in the appropriate portion of the gastro-intestinal tract.

Assuming that all the chemical ingested is available for absorption, the possibility exists that the blood level may rise rapidly and fall again equally rapidly, resulting in an adequate contraceptive effect on the target organs for only a short time each day. In order to combat this, experiments have been conducted where the dose was administered in two halves, at twelve-hourly intervals. Little alteration in pregnancy rates was observed, in fact, but the interesting finding was the willingness of many women to take twice-daily medication over long periods of time.

There are today three preparations sold in the United Kingdom for contraception which contain progestogen only.

Because of the small dose of progestogen they are sometimes called 'Mini-pills', or sometimes 'POP' pills.

Femulen	G. D. Searle (Pack of 28 Pills)	Ethynodiol diacetate	0.5 mg
Micronor	Ortho (Pack of 42 Pills)	Norethisterone'	0.35 mg
Noriday	Syntex (Pack of 28 Pills)	Norethisterone	0.35 mg

Clinical experience dictates the following conclusions.

1. The pregnancy rate among patients taking progestogen-only Pills is approximately two per hundred women-years. This rate is therefore similar to that expected in users of the intrauterine device, and nearly ten times as great as the pregnancy rate among users of combined oral contraceptives.

An illustration of the effect on pregnancy rates obtained by removing oestrogen is provided by the two Searle products 'Demulen 50' and 'Femulen', both containing 0.5 mg ethynodiol diacetate, but 'Demulen' also containing 0.05g ethinyloestradiol. The failure rate for the method using progestogen alone is 2.1 pregnancies per 100 women-years: with added oestrogen this rate becomes 0.3.

2. Cycle control is poor, especially when compared to the clockwork regularity so often seen in women taking combined Pills. In any particular patient, bleeding may be more frequent or less frequent, and the bleeding may be heavier or lighter. Long periods of amenorrhoea may occur, as also may long periods of continuous or recurrent bleeding or spotting.

The bleeding pattern may change as time goes on. In large series of patients, those complaining of bleeding tend to drop out, and complaints thus diminish with time.

Despite this rather gloomy description of the menstrual chaos which may occur, of the number of women starting to use progestogen-only Pills about half will be satisfied with their pattern of bleeding and will continue the method.

Some indeed will bleed regularly every month, and will be highly satisfied with the method. The suspicion exists that these are women in whom ovulation is not suppressed; their contraceptive safety depends entirely on the hostility to spermatozoa produced in the cervical mucus by the progestogen. The women with menstrual chaos are probably those in whom ovulation is suppressed, and as a result they are probably likely to have intercourse less often anyway, which is hardly the type of antifertility effect intended. Irregular or intermittently regular ovulation would explain the variation in bleeding patterns encountered in patients taking progestogen-only Pills over several years.

3. The usual side-effects of oral contraception, even those normally attributed to the oestrogen, seem to be complained of by the users of progestogen-only Pills. Among complaints reported are dizziness, nausea and vomiting, headache, breast tenderness, depression, lack of libido, cramps, weight gain, 'feeling bloated' and acne. Again, as usual, complaints tend to become less frequent after the first few cycles on the Pill.

However, women complaining of a particular symptom while taking combined oral contraceptives may report reduction or disappearance of the symptoms on changing to progestogen-only Pills.

4. Two of the more serious complications of combined oral contraception, namely prolonged suppression of ovulation after the Pill and thrombo-embolic complications, have not been reported. Alterations in metabolism and effects on other organs have been noted, but the degree of alteration seems less than with oestrogen-containing contraceptives. Compared to the massive research on the adverse effects of combined Pills, very little has so far been performed on progestogen-only Pills. It must be remembered that the retrospective studies reported by Inman and Vessey showed an association between thrombo-embolism and the combined Pill, which contained progestogen as well as oestrogen. The association between oestrogen dosage and thrombo-embolism has not gone unchallenged. A final verdict on the safety of the progestogen-only Pill cannot yet be given, but the results reported by Poller *et al.* (1972) on blood-clotting factors are hopeful.

The suggestion has recently been made (Bonnar, 1974) that the progestogen-only Pill may behave in a similar manner to the intrauterine device, preventing ectopic pregnancies less efficiently than intraùterine implantations. Four ectopic tubal pregnancies were reported by this author in women taking norethisterone 0.35 mg daily. Three further tubal pregnancies in patients taking various types of progestogen-only medication were reported by Hawkins the following month. When related to the number of women using the method, the incidence of ectopic pregnancy appeared to be at least as high as that to be expected among women using no contraception at all.

Whether these were chance associations or not remains unclear. Certainly one patient of the seven admitted missing tablets. Further collection of information is obviously necessary. Meanwhile, the fact that a patient is using a progestogen-only contraceptive should not prevent the clinician considering ectopic gestation as a cause of a complaint of abdominal pain. Any cases should be notified to the Committee on Safety of Medicines.

CLINICAL APPLICATIONS

As a first choice contraceptive method, the pregnancy rate puts most women off. This is certainly true today, although at times of great adverse oestrogen publicity, in 1971 for example, many women chose low-dose progestogen-only Pills as the next best to the combined Pill. Today the exaggerated fear of oestrogen is much less common, and the newer intrauterine devices offer a comparable pregnancy rate.

If the pregnancy rate is acceptable, as it may be in women who need only to delay pregnancy rather than prevent it, then it must be explained to the patient that the progestogen-only Pill will not regulate their periods, nor reduce their quantity. In fact, it may well do the opposite. Time alone will tell: they must try it and see. Some who have accepted the pregnancy rate will be put off by the chance of menstrual disorder.

As a result, today the few patients who ask for this type of Pill as a first choice are almost invariably women who are inordinately scared of oestrogens and dislike all the other methods available, or whose consorts exhibit the fear and dislike and pass on instructions to the woman.

The method is most useful in those women who have suffered severe symptoms while taking combined oral contraceptives, but prefer the oral method to all others. Such women will sometimes put up with remarkable degrees of menstrual disorganization. It is also useful as a method that the doctor can offer to women who demonstrate relative contra-indications to oestrogen, such as mild hypertension or diabetes or a history of thrombophlebitis. The scientific basis for stating that progestogen-only contraceptives are safer in these conditions is not altogether sound, but can be justified if it is felt that no other method would be used and unwanted pregnancy might supervene.

However, in practice, many women with such relative contra-indications will have completed their families and sterilization of one partner may be the best answer to the contraceptive problem.

To sum up, the family doctor will find this type of oral contraceptive a useful method to have in reserve, but will rarely find it necessary to use it at the present time.

FOLLOW-UP

The follow-up of women using progestogen-only Pills should be exactly the same as for women using the combined type, partly because many of the follow-up procedures are screening procedures in their own right, to which the patient is entitled; and partly to allay any anxiety the patient may feel at perpetually swallowing Pills. As the long-term effects of this type of con-

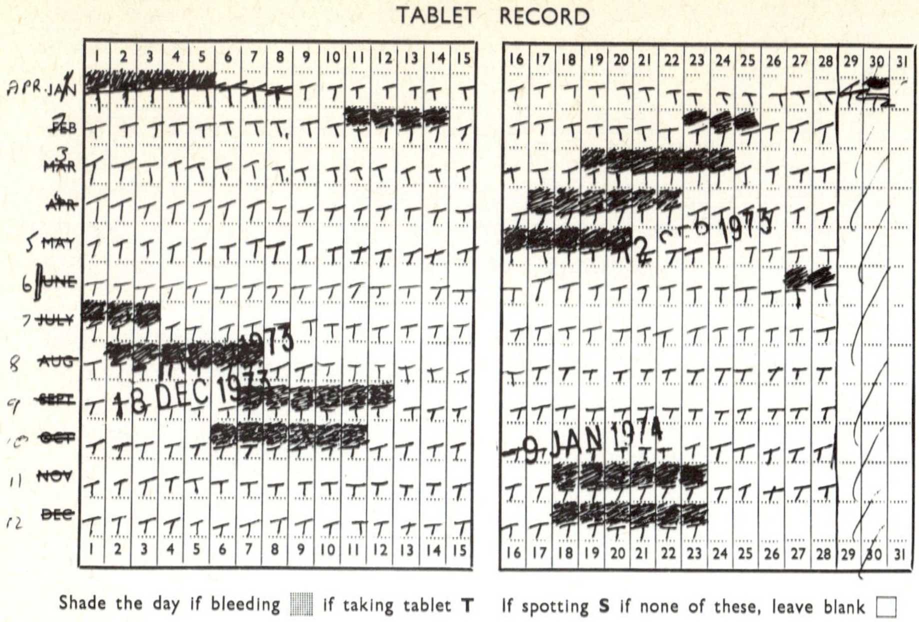

Fig. 19 Record cord illustrating one pattern of bleeding which may be seen with progestogen-only Pills. The interval between bleeds has varied from only eight days to as much as thirtyfour days. However, bleeding has never continued in this patient for more than six days at a time, and the total number of bleeds in the year was twelve.

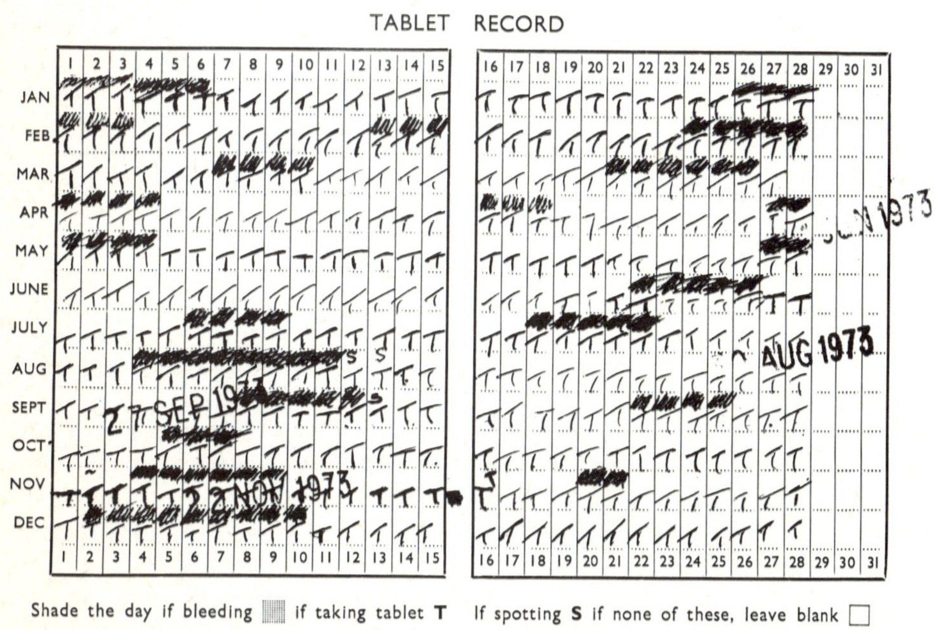

Fig. 20 'Menstrual chaos' in patient taking progestogen-only Pill. The bleeding in this case, although frequent and irregular, was not heavy. The patient wanted to use oral contraception, but feared oestrogen excessively. She chose to persevere.

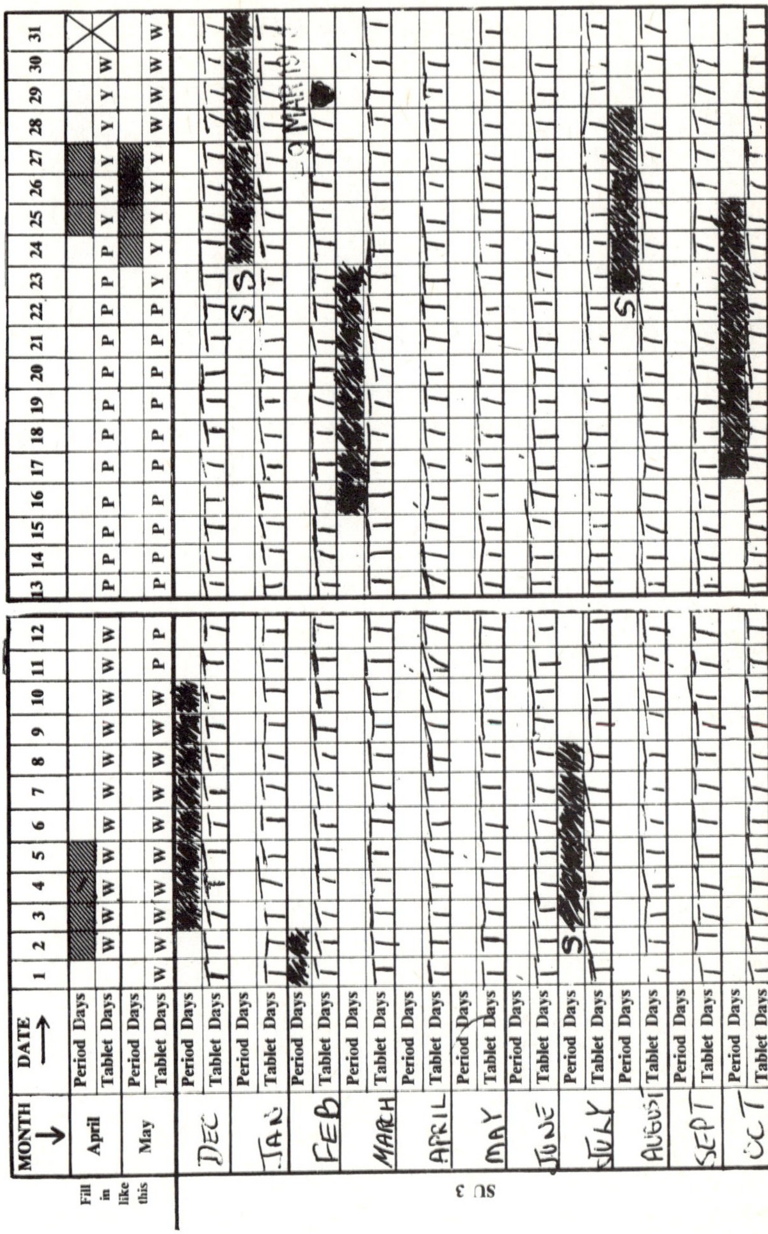

W = White tablets P = Pink tablets Y = Yellow tablets ▒ = Bleeding S = Spotting (record in "Period Days" line)

Fig. 21 Record card of patient using progestogen-only contraception. Only six bleeds appeared in one year's therapy, each lasting between six and ten days, and not heavy in character. Most women would find this a satisfactory pattern. This particular patient did not, and insisted on stopping.

traception are still unknown, only long-term follow-up will ensure that her anxiety really is misplaced.

A card on which the patient may record her bleeding is essential with this type of Pill. The mixture of frequent bleeds followed by long periods without bleeds may make it impossible for the patient to identify any pattern from memory.

But counting the bleeds on a calendar may reveal that the frequency is about twelve times a year despite the irregularity, and women are often content when this can be demonstrated.

Other Types of Hormonal Contraception

POST-COITAL CONTRACEPTION

'Look here, upon this picture, and on this' *Hamlet*

In 1963 a married woman with too many children came in tears to my surgery. During intercourse the previous night, the condom had burst. The previous night was the fourteenth of her regular 28-day cycle, and she was terrified that she might become pregnant. For two weeks she and I suffered and waited: sedatives during the day and hypnotics at night were all I could offer. The period did not arrive, and we then started waiting again, first for confirmation of pregnancy, and then to see what, if anything, could be done about it.

In 1973 a girl of seventeen told me hopelessly that her boy-friend - temporarily out of their usual condoms - had intended to withdraw, but, the ecstasy of the moment overcoming him, had ejaculated inside her. The fateful fourteenth again! She had felt that the die was cast, but the boy friend (Bless him!) had told her to consult me the next day, just in case I could do anything.

And in 1973 I could - a prescription for stilboestrol, 25 mg in the morning and 25 mg in the evening for five days. She felt slightly nauseated for two days and vomited once. Her period arrived on the twenty-seventh day, and lasted five days instead of the usual seven. And on the seventh day I inserted a copper-bearing intrauterine device.

The difference between these two tales is so marked I am sure I need elaborate no further.

Mode of Action

A great deal of research has been done with reference to post-coital agents in experimental animals, and among the ways in which such agents may be supposed to work are an increase in tubal or uterine motility, a direct toxic effect on the blastocyst, an interference with the decidual cell response or interference with enzyme systems or hormone balance.

Many substances have been investigated for their post-coital antifertility action in animals, but in the human the only compounds suitable for use at the present time are the oestrogens and progestogens. The final decision as to the mode of action of compounds used in humans has yet to be made.

Morris and Von Wagenen in 1966 used large doses of oestrogen to prevent pregnancies in volunteers, and in women who had been raped. Kuchera in 1971 published a report of 1,000 women who had been given oestrogens within 72 hours of unprotected intercourse. NO pregnancies followed - a remarkable result, since Tietze (1960) has reckoned the probability of conception resulting from a single unprotected act of intercourse as being between one in fifty and one in twenty-five.

In Kuchera's series, the unprotected coitus had taken place within three days of the date of expected ovulation in 71 per cent of the women.

Forty-five per cent of the patients suffered no side-effects, other than hardly noticeable nausea. Nausea and vomiting for one day only was noticed by 13 per cent, but another 2½ per cent vomited for between two and five days. Vaginal spotting, either during the treatment or on withdrawal of oestrogen, occurred in 1 per cent of patients. Other symptoms, similar to those complained of by women taking the usual type of contraceptive Pill, were reported by 10 per cent.

The dose of oestrogen given was large when compared with the dose in oral contraceptives in common use in the U.K. today. Diethyl stilboestrol (commonly called simply stilboestrol by general practitioners) was given in doses of 25 mg twice daily for five days.

The character of the period following this large dose of oestrogen did not vary from the normal as much as might have been expected. Forty per cent of the women reported the period as normal, both in quantity and timing. Another 10 per cent saw their period at the expected time, but in 7 per cent it was lighter, in the remainder it was heavier. Another 5 per cent came on a few days early; about the same number were a few days late. In only 6 per cent was the period delayed for more than one week.

It would appear, therefore, that the use of stilboestrol, or the equivalent dose of ethinyloestradiol, results in highly efficient post-coital contraception, without much in the way of side-effects, either as symptoms during therapy or upset of the periods afterwards, in the majority of women. As evidence of this, 117 patients returned for a second course, 65 for a third, and one patient had six courses. And herein lies the danger.

To give this large dose of oestrogens as an emergency measure, to be followed by the use of a conventional contraceptive method as a routine, is acceptable. The danger of unwanted pregnancy outweighs the dangers of the oestrogen.

As a regular method of birth control, however, there are grave objections. Even if taken only once a month, a large dose of oestrogens would be taken every year, and women with irregular cycles who could not be sure when ovulation was likely might take extra courses. If oestrogens were used after every coitus, without reference to the time of ovulation, they could be taken almost continuously.

Because of this, the Food and Drug Administration of the United States, where oestrogens are now marketed as post-coital therapy, insists on a warning of possible dangers being printed on every pack.

Progestogens alone do not seem to carry the same dangers as oestrogens, and Newton (1973) reports that in high doses they have been found to be as effective as oestrogens.

Perhaps one of the greatest difficulties associated with post-coital contraception is education. How does one tell the patients about it?

It is difficult to compose a notice to display in the family doctor's waiting room which imparts the message, emphasizes the timing, warns of the dangers, can be understood by the average patient, and yet avoids offence to the more conservative members of the practice population.

THE PRE-COITAL PILL

The action of progestogens on cervical mucus, already described, has been shown to follow oral ingestion within a few hours, and to last for 12-18 hours. If intercourse is restricted to this 'safe period', say not earlier than four hours after taking the progestogen, and no later than 15 hours, fertility control is reported to be good. Thus the method will suit those who can forecast the time of intercourse, which leaves many unsuited. In addition relatively large doses of progestogen are required, which result in irregular bleeding if taken frequently.

New progestogens whose action is more rapid in onset and of longer duration are being investigated.

ONCE-A-MONTH INJECTIONS

For those who dislike swallowing Pills, and for those who habitually forget Pills, the idea of an injection at monthly or even less frequent intervals is attractive. Trials of several different progestogens, sometimes with oestrogen added, have been conducted, especially in the United States. Administration has been by injection or by implantation of slow-release capsules.

Although the antifertility effect has been satisfactory in many of these trials, unpleasantly heavy and irregular bleeding, combined with an unpredictable delay in the return of ovulation after therapy precludes their clinical use. In one study the incidence of abnormal Papanicolou smears among women receiving long-acting progestogen injections seemed to be greater than in the general population.

PROSTAGLANDINS

The possibility that these substances could be used as 'once-a-month contraceptives' was excitedly reported in the early 1970s. Suggestions that administration could be by oral tablets, vaginal pessaries, or even through the skin (worn under a wristwatch strap) were made. It appeared that these 'new discoveries', the prostaglandins, would soon usurp the place of all other methods of contraception.

To date a great deal of investigation of the prostaglandins has taken place, and so far, all predictions with regard to contraception have remained unfulfilled.

First described in 1935 by von Euler in Sweden and Goldblatt in England, the name prostaglandins derives from the fact that they were thought to be produced by the prostate gland. Further work has shown there are several different types of prostaglandin, and they are found in a variety of different human tissues and even in other animals. Synthesis in the laboratory is now possible, and a synthetic prostaglandin E_2 is available commercially.

The action of the drug is to stimulate uterine smooth muscle, especially in the pregnant uterus, and to inhibit the contraction of smooth muscle in the cervix. Unfortunately this effect is produced in very early pregnancy only by very large doses, and the side-effects at this dosage are considerable.

After switching tablets, if changing from a high-dose to a low-dose preparation, all would agree with this advice.

Clinical Care of Patients Using Oral Contraception

INITIAL INTERVIEW AND EXAMINATION

Before prescribing an oestrogen-containing contraceptive the doctor must, by history and examination, attempt to exclude any medical contra-indications. If such contra-indications are present, then an attempt must be made to compare the risk to the life or health of the woman if she takes the Pill, with the risk which she will run if she does not take it. In this assessment of risk, it is reasonable to include consideration of the effect of a further pregnancy on both the health of the woman, and that of her existing family. If another method of contraception is acceptable to her, then this should be advised in place of the Pill.

If no other method is acceptable, and the patient needs completely effective contraception, prescription of an oestrogen-containing oral contraceptive would be justifiable even in the presence of a contra-indication, provided the risk had been explained to the patient and every effort made to induce her to use a safer method. In such women the Pill would still be safer than pregnancy.

However, in my experience a decision to prescribe the Pill under such circumstances is never necessary today. Women are only too aware of the possible dangers, and willingly accept medical advice to avoid the Pill. Doctors also have a greater choice of other contraceptive methods of almost equal reliability, and are not under the same pressure to give the Pill as the only reasonably reliable method.

The complications of oestrogen-containing contraceptives and their effects on metabolism, together with their effects on co-existing disease are discussed in detail elsewhere in this book. Their relative importance as contra-indications to starting oral contraception are summarized below.

1. **Patients to whom the oestrogen-containing Pill should not be given except under the most unusual circumstances.**

(i) Patients suffering from oestrogen-dependant neoplastic disease of the breast, or of the genital tract.
(ii) Patients who have certain disturbances of liver function.
(iii) Patients who give a past history or who have a strong family history of thrombo-embolic disease, or who suffer from a condition especially likely to be complicated by thrombo-embolism.
(iv) Nulliparous women with a history of scanty, irregular periods.

2. **Conditions where the oestrogen-containing Pill is best avoided, but may be given provided there is especially careful and frequent supervision of the patient.**

(i) Essential hypertension, cardiac or renal disease.
(ii) Diabetes mellitus.
(iii) Epilepsy.
(iv) A past history of severe depression or puerperal psychosis.
(v) A past history of severe migraine.
(vi) A past history of severe asthma.

3. **Patients for whom a prescription for a Pill containing oestrogen should be accompanied by a warning that exacerbation of the condition may ensue.**

(i) Patients with hay fever or mild asthma.
(ii) Patients wearing contact lenses.

4. **Patients for whom a prescription for a Pill containing oestrogen should be delayed until after treatment.**

(i) Those with uterine fibroids.
(ii) Those awaiting injection treatment for varicose veins.
(iii) Those awaiting surgery for any reason.

A personal and family history is taken from the patient with special reference to the identification of these contra-indications.

Assuming no contra-indications to the use of oral contraception are discovered, the next step is to take a menstrual history. The duration of the menstrual flow and its quantity are important factors when deciding the type of Pill to administer. Similarly a history of severe dysmenorrhoea would indicate that regular suppression of ovulation would be a desirable feature of any Pill prescribed. A history of acne, worse at the time of the period, or during a previous pregnancy, may be useful when it comes to the choice of the type of Pill to be used.

Finally, an obstetric history is taken including terminations, and with special reference to conditions such as hypertension and depression during pregnancy. The number of pregnancies may indicate the type of Pill needed.

EXAMINATION OF THE PATIENT

Were there no other demands on time and money, there would need to be no restriction on the complexity of the medical examination which could be performed on each new Pill applicant. A full physical examination could be followed by a battery of haematological, biochemical and X-ray investigations in every case. However, both money and time are limited, and examinations should also be limited to those aimed at eliminating reasonably common conditions known to be adversely affected by oral contraceptive usage. In addition certain base-line measurements should be taken for comparison with future findings.

It is suggested that the following procedures should precede any prescription for oral contraceptives. Any abnormalities discovered might merit further, more detailed investigation.

1. The patient should be weighed.
2. The blood pressure should be recorded, either sitting or lying.
3. The urine should be tested for sugar and albumen (Uristix).
4. The colour of the mucous membranes should be noted, and measurement of the haemoglobin performed if anaemia is suspected.
5. The breasts should be palpated.
6. Auscultation of the heart should be performed to exclude gross abnormality.
7. The abdomen should be palpated.
8. The legs should be inspected, with special attention to any varicose veins present.
9. Examination of the vulva should be followed by the passage of a speculum (without the application of an antiseptic cream) and examination of the vagina and cervix, followed by the taking of a cervical smear using an Ayre's spatula.
10. Bimanual pelvic examination should be performed.

Such physical examination, even if no abnormalities are discovered entailing further investigation, will occupy at least 10-15 minutes of the general practitioner's time. If the intention of the patient to ask for the Pill is known in advance, arrangements can be made to see her at a special time. During a quiet surgery it may be possible to carry out the examination, but during a hectic winter session it may be quite impossible, and the patient should be given an appointment to come back at a more suitable time. The temptation to omit the examination should be resisted.

However, occasions do arise where the patient appears at a time when the choice has to be made between giving the Pill without full examination or delaying the start of oral contraception for a month. The doctor may feel that the risk of pregnancy outweighs the risk of delaying the examination for a few days. The pressure under which the general practitioner may be working is difficult to appreciate for those who have never worked in a busy general practice.

INSTRUCTIONS FOR PATIENTS

Most doctors have prescribed the Pill so often that they tend to imagine that all women know how to take it, or that any gaps in their knowledge will easily be made good from the instructions enclosed with, or printed on, the packet of Pills. This may be true of women from the higher social classes, but may well not be so for the others. Some patients may not be able to read, and some who can may not have the time, patience, or intelligence to study the instructions carefully. Immigrant women may be able to hold a conversation with the doctor, yet be quite unable to understand the written word.

Because mistakes in taking the Pill may be followed by unwanted pregnancy, it is vital that the family doctor devotes adequate time to explaining how to use the method, and ensures that the woman understands him. Ideally, even though the patient is to obtain the supplies from the chemist, a specimen pack of each type of Pill habitually prescribed should be held in the surgery for demonstration to the patient during instruction.

Tablet-taking regimens vary with the type of Pill used, but the family doctor should eventually develop a mini-lecture, that he can reel off almost without thought, for each type of Pill he uses. The mini-lecture will vary for each type, but certain essential peices of information must be included:

1. The starting day

This must be identified as closely as possible, either by naming the day, if the patient's period has already started, or by giving clear instructions, as:

'You are to take the first Pill on the fifth day of your next period. For example, if your period starts on a Tuesday, then that is the first day, so Saturday would be the fifth day and you take your first Pill then'.

The fact that the human hand has five digits is useful to emphasize the timing when using preparations started on the fifth day. Whether the first Pill is to be taken on Day 5 or Day 1 of the cycle, it should be pointed out to the patient that provided she takes them correctly, the starting day will remain the same for subsequent packets.

2. The pattern of Pill-taking

That is, whether the patient is to take them for three weeks and then have a week off ('Seven days when you don't take them, and start again on the eighth'), or whether she is to take them continuously, starting the next pack immediately she finishes the first, or whether - as with Minilyn - she has six days off, taking the first tablet of the next pack on the same day of the week as she took the last tablet of the previous pack. Preparations such as Minilyn or Minovlar ED need demonstration of the pack to clarify the instructions.

3. **The timing of Pill-taking**

Patients should be told they can take the Pill at any time of day they find suitable, providing it is the same time every day. To avoid forgetting them, they should 'tie' taking the Pill to some act that they perform daily anyway, such as cleaning their teeth at night (if they clean their teeth every night) or putting on their nightie (if they ever wear a nightie).

4. **When the patient may start to rely on the Pills**

If the first tablet of the first course of a combined Pill is taken on Day 5 there is a theoretical possibility that pregnancy may occur if the patient ovulates early in the cycle. To avoid this danger, most manufacturers advise that the Pills should not be relied upon until a certain number of tablets of the first course have been taken. The number advised may be fourteen, ten or seven, although for some of the more recently marketed preparations, the manufacturers suggest that the Pill is effective from the first day. However, the suggestion is also made that if the possibility of short cycles exist, then the patient should start the tablets on Day 1.

Certainly all combined Pills may be taken on Day 1, when a slightly shorter first cycle may result, but with greater protection against unexpected early ovulation. However, an unintended pregnancy is of more immediate significance to the patient and the family doctor than to the manufacturer, and I would suggest that all patients starting oral contraception should be advised to assume that full protection against pregnancy begins only after two weeks' tablets have been taken.

After switching tablets, especially if changing from a high-dose to a low-dose preparation, all would agree with this advice.

5. **The procedure to adopt if Pills are missed**

Warning should be given against occurrences known to be frequently associated with missed Pills, e.g. going on holiday. ('Your Pills should be the first item packed in your suitcase'). If vomiting should occur within two hours of swallowing a Pill, then it should be assumed to have been lost, and another taken in its stead.

Taking a low-dose Pill up to twelve hours late is safe: taking it twentyfour hours late is not, and the patient should be warned of this and told that no reliance should be placed on the Pill until a further fourteen have been taken.

Providing the doctor's mini-lecture covers these five points there should be no mistakes in taking the Pills. However, experience shows that one common mistake should be pointed out to the patient using a 'three weeks on, one week off' Pill. Women sometimes assume that because they start their first pack on the fifth day, they should start subsequent packs on the fifth day of the period, with dire consequences if the period does not appear.

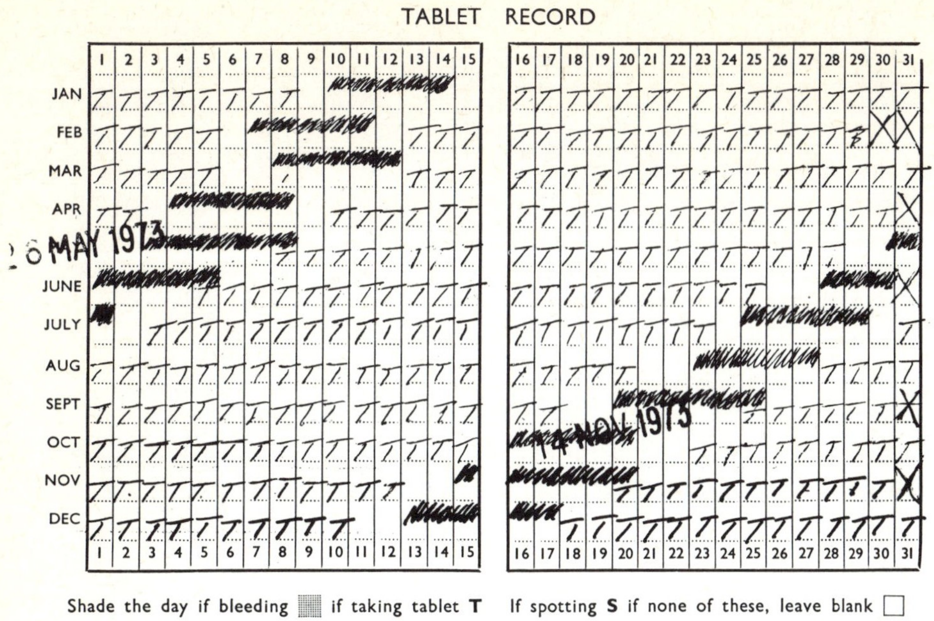

Fig. 22 A regular taker with a regular bleeding pattern.

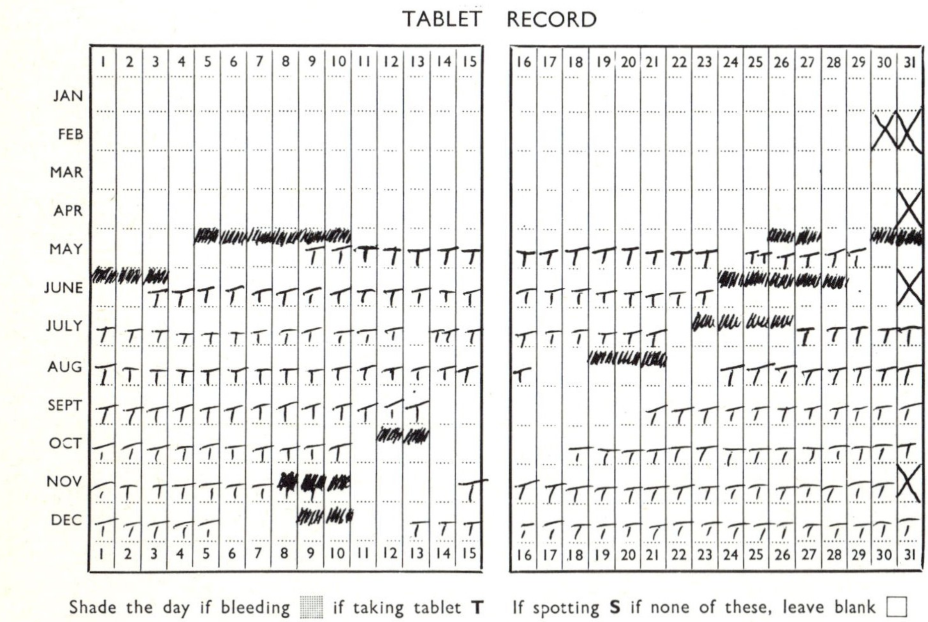

Fig. 23 Irregular bleeding pattern. Note breakthrough bleeding due to missed Pills, one episode of absent withdrawal bleed between courses, and varying number of 'days off' between courses. A somewhat vague young lady, who nevertheless successfully avoided pregnancy for three years.

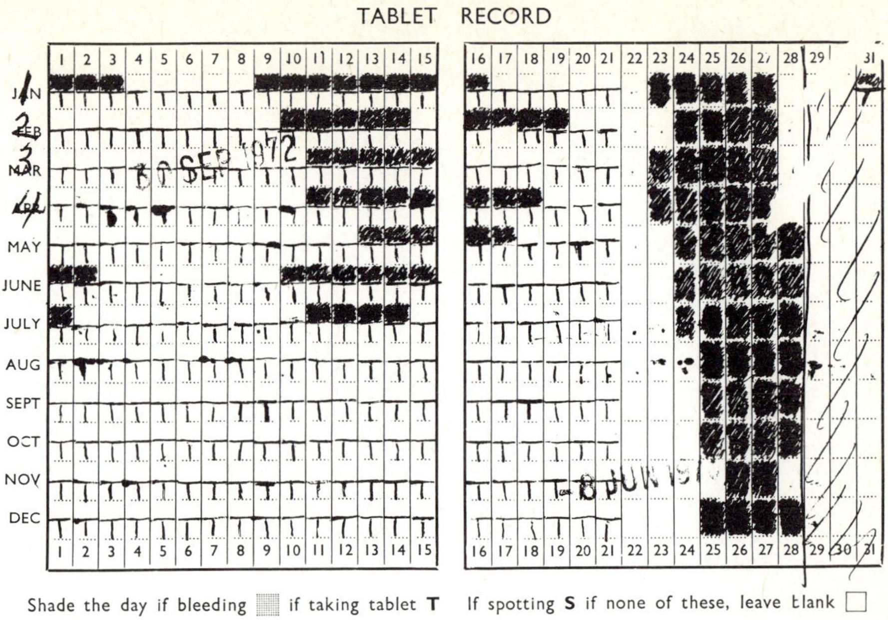

Fig. 24 Breakthrough bleeding despite regular Pill-taking for seven months. After the second month the amount of loss became very scanty, and the patient wished to persevere as she otherwise felt so well on this particular low-progestogen Pill. However, after seven months she decided enough was enough and changed to a variant containing twice the dose of progestogen. The breakthrough ceased, and happily she continued to feel extremely well.

It should be emphasized that the fifth day instruction applies only to the first pack, and thereafter it is simply seven days off, period or no period.

It is helpful to ask the patient starting oral contraception for the first time to keep a record of her bleeding pattern, and to bring it with her each time she consults the doctor. Patients seem to like doing this, and inspection of the card can save much surgery time, a glance sufficing to identify a correct pattern of Pill-taking and a regular bleeding pattern. Once the patient is established on oral contraception the card may be abandoned, the patient being told to report anything unusual (Figs. 22–24).

The doctor's telephone number should appear on the back of the card, and the patient should be told that if she has any worries, questions, or doubts, she is NOT to ask the woman at work who knows so much about the Pill, but she is to telephone the doctor and ask him. Alternatively, she may make an appointment at any surgery time.

Finally, she is wished 'Happy Pill-taking' and ushered out of the surgery to make her next appointment with the receptionist.

'EMERGENCY' ORAL CONTRACEPTION

On occasions the family doctor is confronted with a girl who is already running the risk of pregnancy, who is known to be an irregular attender for medical care and who is, at the time of seeking advice, in mid-cycle. Under these conditions, to advise her to wait for the next period and start the Pill at the proper time may be tantamount to advising her to become pregnant.

This type of patient should be given the Pill and told to take it immediately, irrespective of the date in the cycle. She should be instructed to ignore any bleeding that may happen while the Pill is being taken and, provided she does so, her period will eventually conform to the rhythm dictated by the Pill.

By this means she will receive protection against pregnancy at the earliest possible moment, and experience shows that menstrual upset is usually surprisingly small.

FOLLOW-UP OF PATIENTS ON ORAL CONTRACEPTION

The new patient should be seen after two weeks, when any early side-effects may be reported, discussed with the doctor and - as a rule - treated with explanation and reassurance. Opportunity is also given to the patient to ask any questions, or air any worries - the new Pill-user is considered fair game to all her friends and acquaintances, who will rapidly feed her all the frightening information they incorrectly remember from articles in the popular press. She may also be uncertain of the instructions given as to how to take the Pill, and the initial instructions can be reinforced. Examination is necessary only if symptoms indicate it.

One month later, after the next period and midway through the second packet of Pills, the patient should be seen again. With the exception of measurement of the weight and the blood pressure, examination is again unnecessary unless indicated by symptoms.

A further attendance follows three months later, at which the weight and blood pressure should be recorded, the urine tested, and the breasts examined.

On the anniversary of starting the Pill, and on each anniversary following, a full check-up similar to the initial examination, including a pelvic examination, should be carried out. Cervical smears should be repeated in Pill-users as often as in women not taking the Pill.

This routine is ideal for women without troubles. Those with troubles, real or imaginary, may require to be seen more often. All women should be told that they make an appointment to see the doctor at any surgery if they are at all worried.

How valuable are such follow-up examinations? From the point of view of preventive medicine they are of as much value as any other regular screening procedures: with the exception of the identification of changes in weight, urine or blood pressure they are of no value in the early detection of threatened catastrophe in women found to be normal at the initial interview.

Nevertheless, they are of considerable importance in providing opportunities for her to present her symptoms and anxieties, and for the doctor to provide reassurance and encouragement to stimulate her motivation to continue to use contraception.

The routine described is one which I have found most satisfactory. Measurements of blood pressure, weight and urinalysis may be performed by the practice nurse, and need not delay the doctor. Four doctor-patient contacts during the first year, followed by one or two during each subsequent year do not seem to me an excessive load. However, some family doctors will prefer a smaller number of planned attendances, and provided every patient feels she has immediate right of access at any time she is worried, this will be perfectly satisfactory.

What is not satisfactory is a situation where the patient continues collecting prescriptions for Pills for years at a time without any sort of check-up at all. Although it can be argued that the likelihood of adverse effects developing undetected is small, the major adverse effect is on the reputation of the general practitioner, for such patients are liable to present at clinics or at the surgeries of other doctors with the complaint that their care has been inadequate and neglectful, and with a request for a 'proper check-up'!

Conversely, some patients will object to examination, particularly pelvic examination and cervical smears. Such reluctance need not entail argument between doctor and patient, and certainly need not prevent the continuing supply of oral contraceptives. It is worthwhile recording that the proferred examination was declined, both for medico-legal reasons and to avoid inadvertently pestering the patient each time she appears.

USAGE OF ORAL CONTRACEPTION

Of the women of child-bearing age in the United Kingdom about two million, or one woman in five, use the Pill. In other countries even higher proportions of the female population at risk use it, examples being Sweden, where one in four takes the Pill, and New Zealand where one in three takes it.

Women attending FPA clinics in 1973 showed a marked preference for the Pill, 59.5 per cent of new patients choosing this method. The popularity of any method will be influenced by adverse publicity, and it is a tribute to the effectiveness and acceptability of the Pill that its usage in 1973 was so great, bearing in mind the furore caused by the suspected dangers of thromboembolism in 1970 and 1971.

However, the appearance on the scene of other methods offering a similar degree of reliability will also affect the popularity of any form of contraception, and where the newer IUDs, vasectomy and female sterilization are readily available (as they are in my practice area) an increasing number of couples are deserting the Pill. The FPA practice of holding separate clinic sessions for the IUD has probably influenced the choice of patients randomly attending a session for the first time. Unless they happen to choose an IUD session in the first place, a second visit will be required. A study of the timetables of clinics in London show that IUD sessions are outnumbered several times by general sessions at which the Pill is offered.

Evidence from general practice has been produced by Barley (1973) working in a family planning clinic in a group practice of five doctors. Here both IUD and Pill were equally available, and 48.4 per cent of patients choose the Pill, 41.7 per cent chose the IUD and only 9.9 per cent chose other methods.

The Second Hull Family Survey (Peel, 1972) described the social profile of couples using oral contraception. A proportionately higher usage was found amongst semi-skilled and unskilled manual workers. Pill-users were more likely than the rest of the sample to have had two children, and more likely to have changed to the Pill after failure of another method. The average age of couples using the Pill was less than that of the sample as a whole.

That young people seeking advice from the family doctor usually ask for the Pill is undoubted. Barnard-Jones (1973) compared patients requesting oral contraception with those requesting the IUD, and confirmed that the younger patients asked for the Pill, the older for the IUD. A group made up entirely of young people, students at Aberdeen University, were investigated by McCance and Hall (1972). The most frequently used method of contraception for those who had had intercourse during the previous six weeks had been the Pill for 30 per cent of students. For students who had already been pregnant, 60 per cent had used the Pill as their method of contraception during the past six weeks.

At the moment we can say that women requesting the Pill will probably show one or more of the following characteristics.

1. They will belong to the lower social classes rather than the higher.

   One reason for this may be that other methods are too expensive, both IUD and sterilization having required a relatively large capital outlay in most areas of the country until recently. Such women also tend to be more fearful of a further pregnancy than of any harmful effects of the Pill.
2. They will be young nulliparous women, either unmarried or in the early years of marriage.

   For these women the convenience and reliability of the Pill are the attractions.
3. They will be women who have had two or more pregnancies and may be changing to the Pill from another method because of its greater reliability.
4. They will be the women who have used the Pill as nulliparae and are now using it to space their families.
5. They have had at least one termination of pregnancy.
6. They will be using the Pill as much for its therapeutic results (relief of dysmenorrhoea, regulation of periods, etc.) as for its contraceptive effect.

Excluding this last group, it is interesting to consider whether the other five groups will continue to request the Pill in the future. The preponderance of the lower social classes among Pill users will cease as the IUD , vasectomy and female sterilization become increasingly available without payment, and more of the higher social classes will use the Pill following reassuring reports as to its safety.

Couples who have had two or more children will more and more choose sterilization, possibly after a few years during which the IUD is used.

Young nulliparae and those spacing their families now have an alternative effective method in the newer types of IUD, but so far there has been little indication in my practice that such women are choosing this method in significant numbers.

More women are choosing the modern IUD as a contraceptive method after termination, fearing that as the termination fades in their memory, so will their determination to take the Pill.

My own feeling is that in the United Kingdom Pill-usage has reached its zenith, and will now decline. Time will tell whether I am right or not.

ADVANTAGES OF ORAL CONTRACEPTION

At the time of its introduction, the most commonly used contraceptive methods in the United Kingdom were coitus interruptus and the condom, both essentially under the control of the male. The only methods available to women were the cap or diaphragm and chemical contraception. Both methods had to be used at the time of intercourse, were regarded by many women as messy and troublesome, and interfering with the spontaneity of the sex act. Merely to swallow a Pill appeared by comparison far less troublesome, and was certainly not messy. In addition the method had the great advantage of divorce in time from the act of intercourse, which could therefore be as spontaneous and uninhibited as when no contraception was being used, and repeated as often as desired without replenishment of chemical or replacement of cap.

The method also found favour in the eyes of the family doctor, the prescription of oral medication being an activity to which he was well accustomed. But for both patients and doctors the greatest advantage was without doubt the reassuring efficiency of the method in preventing pregnancies.

EFFICIENCY OF ORAL CONTRACEPTION

1. Combined oral contraceptives

Extremely low pregnancy rates have been reported by many investigators. Drill (1966), quoted by Peel and Potts (1969), summarized published data on Enavid and found a pregnancy rate of 0.028 per 100 women-years. On the other hand, Peberdy (1965), working with problem families in Newcastle, reported a failure rate of 9.0 pregnancies per 100 women-years. The vast difference between these two figures illustrates that motivation and regular and correct use of the method markedly influence its efficiency.

Patients attending family planning clinics are likely to be highly motivated, as Cartwright (1970) found that many patients had to travel long distances and wait for long periods of time at clinics, and in terms of the periods for which clinics were open, had restricted access to their facilities. Most studies in the United Kingdom relating to the use effectiveness of oral contraceptives have been carried out on clinic populations.

In general practice one finds a cross-section representing all types of patient, the highly and the poorly motivated, the intelligent and the stupid and, as might be expected, reports from general practice indicate pregnancy rates midway between the two extremes reported by Drill and by Peberdy.

John (1973) found a failure rate of 0.2 per 100 women-years among patients in his practice, and eighteen general practitioners in the United Kingdom found a pregnancy rate of 0.3 per 100 women-years among 1,686 women over 22,839 cycles. Patients who had not taken Pills correctly had been excluded from both studies, so it would seem likely that the modern combined Pill, with the low dosage of oestrogen, has a failure rate, when properly used in accordance with the manufacturer's instructions, about ten times greater than that found by Drill in 1966.

In my opinion, one of the reasons for the increase in pregnancy rate is the persistence in the instructions of most manufacturers that if one Pill has been missed, provided the missing Pill is taken within the following 24 hours the contraceptive 'cover' will be unimpaired. That this was so with the early high-dose pills is undoubted; that it is not so with the present low-dose pills does not seem to be generally recognized, and I feel that patients should be warned of the possibility of pregnancy in these circumstances.

2. Sequential preparations

Comparison of failure rates between highly efficient methods is difficult. With sequential preparations it was particularly difficult since the products of different manufacturers showed variations in both the type and dosage of oestrogen and progestogen, and in the regime for taking tablets. Some regimes entailed taking oestrogen alone for the first 11 days of the cycle, whereas with other regimes the progestogen was added only after 15 days. A further complication arose where patients formerly using combined Pills were transferred to sequential tablets, when pregnancy seemed particularly liable to follow the changeover.

Working with sequential therapy in general practice most doctors had the impression that they were seeing more pregnancies than with combined Pills, although the numbers involved were too small for any one GP to be sure of their significance. However, the suggested benefits of this method - decrease in the incidence of depression, weight gain and breast tenderness - did not seem significantly obvious, and the fact that bleeding between courses of tablets approximated more to a normal menstrual loss was not considered a benefit by the majority of patients.

Eventually the Committee on Safety of Drugs announced that pregnancy following sequential preparations was being reported relatively more often than after combined Pills, and most general practitioners ceased to recommend their patients to use the method.

Today, only two sequential products are marketed in this country. The 'Ovanon' regime embodies oestrogen for seven days, with progestogen added for a further fifteen. The 'Serial 28' regime differs in that oestrogen is taken alone for sixteen days, the progestogen being added for a further five, followed by seven lactose tablets.

Failure rates with both these preparations are low, being of the order of 1.0 per 100 women years. However, the daily dose of oestrogen in both exceeds the norm of 50 microgrammes now advised, and consequently neither are very popular among prescribing doctors.

3. **Progestogen-only Pills**

The use-effectiveness of these preparations is very much a part of the story of the appearance of these Pills on the UK market, and is dealt with in some detail in the section on progestogen-only contraception (p. 135).

The failure rate of the products on the market today (Femulen, Micronor, and Noriday) is between 2 and 2.5 pregnancies per 100 women-years.

Thus sequential preparations are approximately four times, and progestogen-only preparations seven times less effective than combined oral contraceptives at preventing pregnancy.

REFERENCES

ADAMS, P. W., WYNN, V., ROSE, D. P. *et al.* (1973). *Lancet*, **i**, 897.

ARRATA, W. S. M. and DE ALVAREZ, R. R. (1972). *American Journal of Obstetrics & Gynecology*, **112**, 1025.

BARLEY, N. H. (1973). A family planning clinic in general practice. *Journal of the Royal College of General Practitioners*, **23**, 663.

BARNARD-JONES, K. (1973). A study of two forms of contraception in general practice. *Journal of the Royal College of General Practitioners*, **23**, 658.

BECKERHOFF, R., ARMBRUSTER, H., VETTER, W., LEUTSCHER, J. A. and SIEGENTHALER, W. (1973). Plasma-aldosterone during oral contraceptive therapy. *Lancet*, **i**, 1217.

BONNAR, J. (1974). *British Medical Journal*, **1**, 287.

BOSTON COLLABORATIVE DRUG SURVEILLANCE PROGRAMME (1973). Oral contraceptives and venous thrombo-embolic diseases, surgically confirmed gall-bladder disease, and breast tumours. *Lancet*, **i**, 1399.

BOYD, E. F. and HOLSTROM, E. G. (1972). *American Journal of Obstetrics & Gynecology*, **113**, 469.

BRITISH MEDICAL JOURNAL (1967). Rate of thrombo-embolic disease in women taking oral contraceptives. A preliminary communication to the Medical Research Council by a sub-committee. *British Medical Journal*, **2**, 355.

BRITISH MEDICAL JOURNAL (1972). The Pill and porphyria. Editorial. **3**, 603.

CARTWRIGHT, ANN (1970). *Parents and Family Planning Services.* Routledge & Kegan Paul, London.

CARTWRIGHT, ANN and WAITE, M. (1972). General practitioners and contraception in 1970–1. *Journal of the Royal College of General Practitioners*, **22**, Suppl. 2, 21.

CORMIA, F. E. (1967). *Journal of the American Medical Association,* **201,** 635.

DEFARES, J. G. (1971). *Lancet,* **i,** 135.

DJERASSI, C. *et al.* (1954). 19-norprogesterone, a potent progestational hormone. *Journal of the American Chemical Society,* **76,** 4092.

DRILL, W. A. (1966). *Oral Contraceptives.* McGraw-Hill, New York.

DRILL, W. A. (1972). Oral contraceptives and thrombo-embolic disease. *Journal of the American Medical Association,* **219,** 5.

ECKSTEIN, P. *et al.* (1972). Clinical and laboratory findings in a trial of Norgestrel, a low-dose progestogen-only contraceptive. *British Medical Journal,* **3,** 195.

ELWAN, O., MADKOUR, O., KAMA, I. and ABDULLAH, M. (1973). Report delivered at 10th International Congress of Neurology, Barcelona. Reported in *Pulse*, 27 October 1973.

GAL, I. *et al.* (1971). *British Medical Journal,* **2,** 436.

GOLDITCH, I. M. (1972). Postcontraceptive amenorrhea. *Obstetrics & Gynecology,* **39,** 903.

GOLDZIEHER, J. W. (1963). The use of sequential oestrogen and progestin to inhibit fertility. *Proc. Seventh IPPF Conference, Singapore.* IPPF, London.

GOLDZIEHER, J. W. *et al.* (1971). A placebo-controlled double-blind crossover investigation of the side-effects attributed to oral contraceptives. *Fertility & Sterility,* **22,** 609.

GRIFFITHS, W. A. D. (1973). *British Journal of Dermatology,* **88,** 31.

GUTTMACHER, A. F. (1965). *25 Month Club Study.* Planned Parenthood-World Population, New York.

HARRIS, A. B. *et al.* (1973). *Lancet,* **ii,** 201.

HAWKINS, D. F. (1974). *British Medical Journal,* **1,**387.

HERZBERG, B. N., DRAPER, K. C., JOHNSON, A. L. and NICOL, G. C. (1971). Oral Contraceptives, depression and libido. *British Medical Journal,* **3,** 495.

INMAN, W. H. W. and VESSEY, M. P. (1968). Investigation of deaths from pulmonary, coronary, and cerebral thrombosis and embolism in women of child-bearing age. *British Medical Journal,* **2,** 193.

INMAN, W. H. W., VESSEY, M. P., WESTERHOLM, B. and ENGELUND, A. (1970). Thromboembolic disease and the steroid content of oral contraceptives. A report to the Committee on Safety of Drugs. *British Medical Journal,* **2,** 203.

JANERICK, D. T., PIPER, J. M. and GLEBATIS, D. M. (1973). Birth defects and oral contraceptives. *Lancet,* **ii,** 96.

JOHN, A. P. K. (1973). Contraception in a practice community. *Journal of the Royal College of General Practitioners,* **23,** 665.

KUCHERA, L. K. (1971). Post-coital contraception with diethylstilboestrol. *Journal of The American Medical Association,* **218,** 4.

MACFAUL, P. (1973). The adverse effects of some drugs on the eye. *Prescriber's Journal,* **13,** No. 3.

MCCANCE, C. and HALL, D. J. (1972). Sexual behaviour and contraceptive practice of unmarried female undergraduates at Aberdeen University. *British Medical Journal,* **2,** 694.

MARTINEZ-MANATOU, J. *et al.* (1967).Daily progestogen for contraception: a clinical study. *British Medical Journal,* **2,** 730.

MASON, B., OAKLEY, N. and WYNN, V. (1973). Studies of carbohydrate and lipid metabolism in women developing hypertension and oral contraceptives. *British Medical Journal,* **3,** 317..

MEARS, E. *et al.* (1969). Preliminary evaluation of four oral contraceptives containing only progestogen. *British Medical Journal,* **2**, 730.

MELAMED, M. R., KOSS, L. G., FLEHINGER, B. J., KELISKY, R. P. and DUBROW, H. (1969). Prevalence rates of uterine cervical carcinoma in situ for women using the diaphragm or contraceptive oral steroids. *British Medical Journal,* **3,** 195.

MORRIS, J. M. and VAN WAGENEN, G. (1966). Compounds. *American Journal of Obstetrics & Gynecology,* **96,** 804.

MOYNAHAN, E. J. (1965). Correspondence. *British Medical Journal,* November 13.

NEWTON, J. (1973). Future developments in contraception. *Update,* **7,** 405.

NORA, J. J. and NORA, AUDREY , H. (1973). Birth defects and oral contraceptives. *Lancet,* **i,** 941.

OLDERSHAW, K. L. and BRUDENELL, J. M. (1972). Contraception and infertility. *British Medical Journal,* **3,** 637.

ORY, H. (1974). Functional ovarian cysts and oral contraceptives. *Journal of the American Medical Association,* **228,** 68.

PEBERDY, M. (1965). In *Biological Aspects of Social Problems.* ed. Meade, S. E. and Parks, A. S. Oliver & Boyd, Edinburgh.

PEEL, J. (1972). The Hull Family Survey II. *Journal of Biosocial Science,* **4,** 333.

PEEL, J. and POTTS, M. (1969). *Textbook of Contraceptive Practice.* Cambridge University Press.

PINCUS, G. and GARCIA, C. R. (1964). In *Proceedings of a Symposium on Recent Advances in Ovarian Steroids and the Control of Ovarian Function.*

PINCUS, G., GARCIA, C. R. and ROCK, J. (1959). *Science,* **130.**

PINCUS, G., ROCK, J. and GARCIA, C. R. (1959). Field trials with norethynodrel as an oral contraceptive. *Proc. Sixth IPPF Conference, New Delhi.* IPPF, London.

POLLER, L., THOMSON, Jean M. and THOMAS, P. W. (1972). Effects of progestogen oral contraception with norethisterone on blood clotting and platelets. *British Medical Journal,* **4,** 391.

RATTEN, G. H. (1972). *Australian & NZ Journal of Obstetrics & Gynaecology,* **12,** 217.

RICE-WRAY, E. (1957). Field study with Enavid as a contraceptive agent. *Symposium on 19-norprogestational steroids.* G. D. Searle & Co, Chicago.

RICE-WRAY, E. (1962). *Journal of the American Medical Association,* **180,** 255.

RIDDOCH, D., JEFFERSON, M. and BICKERSTAFF, E. R. (1971). Chorea and the oral contraceptive. *British Medical Journal,* **4,** 217.

ROCK, J., PINCUS, G. and GARCIA, C. R. (1956). *Science,* **124.**

ROOK, A. (1973). Disorders of the hair. *Practitioner,* **211,** 593.

ROYAL COLLEGE OF GENERAL PRACTITIONERS (1967). Oral contraception and thrombo-embolic disease. *Journal of the Royal College of General Practitioners,* **13,** 267.

ROYAL COLLEGE OF GENERAL PRACTITIONERS (1974). *Oral Contraceptives and Health. Interim report from the Oral Contraception Study of the Royal College of General Practitioners.* Pitman Medical, London.

SHARMAN, A. (1968). *Clinical Trials Journal,* **5,** 67.

STEELE, S. J., MASON, B. and BRETT, A. (1973). Amenorrhoea after discontinuing combined oestrogen-progestogen oral contraceptives. *British Medical Journal,* **4,** 343.

TIETZE, C. (1960). Problems of pregnancy resulting from a single unprotected coitus. *Fertility & Sterility,* **11,** 485.

VESSEY, M. P., DOLL, R., FAIRBAIRN, A. S. and GLOBER, G. (1970). Post-operative thrombo-embolism and the use of oral contraceptives. *British Medical Journal,* **3,** 123.

VESSEY, M. P., DOLL, R. and SUTTON, P. M. (1972). Oral contraceptives and breast neoplasia. A retrospective study. *British Medical Journal,* **3,** 719.

WEIR, R. J., BRIGGS, E., MACK, A., NAISMITH, L., TAYLOR, L., and WILSON, E. (1974). Blood-pressure in women taking oral contraceptives. *British Medical Journal,* **1,** 533.

WISEMAN, A. (1964). in *Proceedings of a Symposium on Recent Advances in Ovarian Steroids and the Control of Ovarian Function.*

WOODS, J. W. (1967). Oral contraceptives and hypertension. *Lancet,* **ii,** 653.

ZAUN, H. (1973). Quoted in Hair loss and oral contraceptives. *British Medical Journal,* **2,** 499.

SUGGESTED FURTHER READING

COMMITTEE ON SAFETY OF MEDICINES (1972). *Carcinogenicity Tests of Oral Contraceptives.* HMSO, London.

INTERNATIONAL PLANNED PARENTHOOD FEDERATION (1970). *Comments on Steroidal Contraception.* IPPF, London.

WORLD HEALTH ORGANISATION (1966). *Clinical Aspects of Oral Gestogens. Report of a WHO Study Group.* WHO, Geneva.

SWYER, G. I. M. (1973). Advances in hormonal contraception. *Practitioner,* **211,** 535.

11

THE INTRAUTERINE DEVICE

The idea of inserting a foreign body into the uterus in order to prevent pregnancy is not new. Many centuries ago small stones were put inside the uteri of camels before long journeys across the desert in order to achieve this effect. During the nineteenth century 'wish-bone' and 'collar-stud' pessaries were in use. Peel and Potts (1969) describe these as being gold-plated, and it is interesting to speculate whether their effect was wholly mechanical, or partly chemical due to ionization of the gold.

The Grafenberg ring is usually described as being of silver, but in fact contained copper, and certainly may have had a chemical action. In 1973 a silver Grafenberg ring, thought to date from the early 1920's, was discovered at the Marie Stopes Clinic. A small portion had been broken off, and this portion was sent by Dr J. S. Templeton on behalf of A. H. Robins Co Ltd to the Analytical Research and Development Unit at Harwell. The 'silver' was found to be a silver-copper alloy containing about 12 per cent copper. Grafenberg started using this device, made of coiled silver wire, in the 1920s and reported very good results. Despite this, the medical profession in this country disapproved of the idea of inserting a foreign body into the uterus: it was thought that infection was bound to occur, and any contraceptive effect must be due to the infection. During the two decades following 1930, any medical innovations from the Continent were looked at with disfavour, although a few independent spirits continued to fit Grafenberg rings in the United Kingdom.

After World War II, Japan legalized abortion which came to be used as a method of contraception, and stimulated workers there to re-examine all methods of preventing pregnancy, including intrauterine methods. By this time man-made fibres and various types of polythene were available, which were inert when placed inside the human body. Surgeons were using these materials for a variety of purposes, and it was not surprising that trials of intrauterine devices made from the same substances followed. In view of the American occupation of Japan, and the close association of medical schools in these two countries after the war, it was to be expected that further work along these lines would be carried out in the United States, and the early reports by Ishihama from Japan in 1959 were followed by reports from

Oppenheimer from the U.S.A. in the same year, and then by Jack Lippes in 1962. The device that bears his name, the Lippes loop, became the most widely used in the United Kingdom in the late 1960s.

The major advantage of the many varieties of intrauterine device which appeared during the 1960s was the fact that polythene has a memory. Whatever shape was used, it could be crushed flat or stretched out straight for introduction through the undilated cervix, but would recoil into its original shape when inside the uterus. Once inserted, it could be removed simply by pulling it out, when its pliability allowed it to negotiate the undilated cervix with the minimum of discomfort to the patient. To facilitate removal, most devices had a tail or thread which traversed the cervical canal and protruded into the vagina.

The ease with which these devices could be inserted and removed compared favourably with the original Grafenberg ring which in most cases needed dilatation of the cervix under anaesthesia as a prelude to either.

The wheel turned full circle, when Zipper (1969), working in Chile which boasted both a formidable population problem and abundant supplies of copper, reported the use of a device bearing copper wire which added a chemical contraceptive effect to the easily inserted inert polythene, with consequent increase in contraceptive efficiency.

Investigation is presently proceeding of a device made of a special plastic which contains progesterone, which is released into the uterine cavity over a period of one year. Hormonal intrauterine contraception thus becomes a possibility for the future.

TYPES OF INTRAUTERINE DEVICE

For those who care for such things, a complete list of devices, with illustrations, provides a surfeit of bizarre shapes and fascinating names. About sixtyfive different designs have been patented. The average doctor will meet few of them in practice, and the list below includes all that it is necessary to consider.

Intra-uterine contraceptive devices

Of historical interest	Grafenberg ring
First generation devices	Antigon Birnberg bow Lippes loop Margulies spiral Saf-T-Coil
New generation devices	Dalkon shield Gravigard (the copper seven)

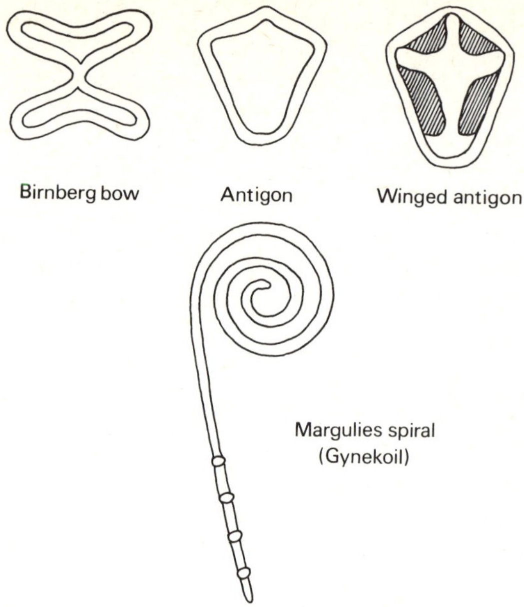

Fig. 25. Three intrauterine devices.

The Margulies spiral possesses a plastic tail, with plastic beads at intervals along it. After inserting the device, the doctor cuts off the superfluous tail in the vagina, leaving a fairly rigid stem protruding the length of the cervical canal with a bead at the external os. The enthusiastic lover is liable to impale his eager glans on this beaded stem, resulting in a sudden loss of enthusiasm. If the GP wishes to remain friends with his patients, this device is not recommended.

For practical purposes only four devices need be considered at the present time, the Lippes loop, the Saf-T-Coil, the Gravigard, and the Dalkon shield.

DESIGN OF IUDs: GENERAL CONSIDERATIONS

In general the larger the device, the greater the surface area and the stiffer the material of which it is made, then the less likely is the patient to become pregnant, or the device to fall out. Unfortunately, associated with these low rates are higher rates for bleeding and pain, and for removals because of these symptoms (Table VIII).

The larger and stiffer the device and the greater the size of the introducer, the more difficult is insertion through the nulliparous cervix. Paradoxically, therefore, the only type of conventional device suitable for insertion in nulliparous women is the smaller one with a higher pregnancy rate. Yet such women often require the most effective contraception.

The position of an IUD within the uterine cavity is also important, the

Table VIII. Pregnancies, expulsions, and removals for bleeding or pain per 100 users of Lippes loops over 2 years.

	Lippes loop size			
	A *Smallest*	*B*	*C*	*D* *Largest*
Pregnancies	11.8	8.2	5.8	5.1
Expulsions	31.2	29.3	28.3	18.3
Removals for bleeding/pain	15.9	20.8	18.8	19.5

Adapted and reprinted with the permission of the Population Council from 'Evaluation of intrauterine devices: ninth progress report of the Co-operative Statistical Programme'. Tietze, C. and Lewitt, S. Studies in Family Planning: Vol. 1, No 55, July 1970, Page 11, Table 9.

contraceptive effect being maximal when the device is placed, and remains, at the fundus.

The newer devices illustrate attempts to avoid these difficulties.

The size of the uterine cavity was measured by various workers, using silicone moulds and hysterographic methods, and great efforts followed to ensure that IUDs conformed to the average size and shape of the female uterus.

Davis, in 1970, reported his results using a Dalkon shield. This device embodied a large area of soft pliable plastic, with protrusions at the edge pointing outwards towards the lateral walls of the uterine cavity, and also slanting downwards towards the internal os. Contractions of the uterus would tend, by squeezing these lateral projections, to force the device upwards within the uterus, thus minimizing the chances of expulsion. A smaller device, tailored to fit the average size and shape of the nulliparous uterus, was also produced. Being of soft plastic, and carried on, rather than within, an introducer which could therefore be very thin, it was hoped that it could pass easily even through a nulliparous cervix. The method of insertion, correctly performed, entails pushing the device and inserter up to the fundus, and then withdrawing the inserter, leaving the device in the best position for most efficient contraception.

The Gravigard was developed on the basis that if an anti-fertility agent were to be carried on the device, then the device could be made smaller and less stiff. Trials carried out by Dr Jaime Zipper showed that wire made of copper or zinc, placed in one horn of a rat's uterus, prevented pregnancies in that horn, but not in the other. None of the many other metals tried produced as satisfactory an effect as copper. Silver, gold and platinum thankfully were among these less satisfactory metals.

Later, in clinical experiments on the human female, Zipper showed that the pregnancy rate of about 20 per cent associated with the use of a small T-shaped device could be reduced to about 1 per cent by winding copper wire around it. The pregnancy rate was inversely proportional to the surface area of the copper wire.

Folding the 'T' to insert into the introducer meant that three thicknesses - that of the stem and those of the two arms of the 'T' - had to be accommodated. By changing to a '7' shape, two arms resulted, and the diameter of the introducer could be cut to only 3 mm, which meant that insertion through a nulliparous cervix was possible. The '7' shape accords nicely with the shape of the uterine cavity in the transverse plane, the arm of the seven lying in the fundus between the cornua, and the curve of the stem lying in the long axis of the uterus. Contractions of the myometrium exert a minimal effect on the shape and position of the device which, being made of soft polypropylene, affords minimal resistance to contractions.

As with the shield device, the correct method of insertion entails pushing the inserter to the fundus, and then withdrawing the inserter to leave the device, with the copper wire wound around its upper part, in the upper part of the uterine cavity.

The Antigon and the Birnberg bow are examples of closed-loop devices. When loaded onto their introducer, the external diameter is such that few cervical canals are large enough to allow them passage. Because of the absence of strings they cannot be simply pulled out, a hook being required to effect removal. Although they are unlikely to be expelled into the vagina, and the absence of strings makes it impossible for dissatisfied husbands to remove them, the closed-loop devices have one great disadvantage. If one escapes into the peritoneal cavity the intestine is liable to become strangulated within its polythene coils. Because of this, the Birnberg bow should today never be used.

Revised versions of the Antigon are now being evaluated. The Antigon-F has a plastic membrane filling the central hiatus of the device, thus increasing the area in contact with the uterus and avoiding the possibility of intestinal strangulation. The 'Winged' Antigon has projections from the plastic into the central open area. Both these versions have strings attached facilitating removal. Pregnancy and expulsion rates with these versions are said to be very low, but as they are not as yet available for use in the surgery they will not be considered further.

MODE OF ACTION OF IUDs

At the moment this is not clear. Tubal motility has been shown to be affected in monkeys, and it has been postulated that the ovum, normally fertilized in the tube, may be hurried through the genital tract too fast for proper implantation to occur. Distortion or stretching of the uterus by the device may have a similar effect, but since most of the newer devices have been designed to avoid distortion or stretching and are associated with a lower pregnancy rate, this suggestion may be discounted.

The presence of a device results in a mobilization of polymorphonuclear leucocytes into the cavity of the uterus and, to a lesser extent, into the endometrium and myometrium. The possibility has been considered that this leucocytic infiltration represents a low-grade infection which interferes with implantation. However, although the degree of leucocytic infiltration correlates well with the antifertility effect of the device, reaching a maximum at about the third month after insertion when protection against pregnancy also reaches a maximum, there is no correlation with the presence or absence of infection. The leucocytosis probably does not indicate infection, but a specific reaction to the presence of a foreign body in the uterus.

It is unlikely that any effect is produced on spermatozoa. Were there to be such an effect, one would expect both intrauterine and tubal pregnancy to be affected equally, whereas tubal pregnancies are not prevented by intrauterine devices as efficiently as are intrauterine pregnancies. Devices carrying copper do produce an increase in the amount of copper in cervical mucus, but although *in vitro* experiments have shown that copper does possess a spermicidal action, the occasional occurrence of accidental pregnancy with a device *in situ* shows that any spermicidal effect is not infallible. The suggestion has been made that sperm capacitation may be impaired by the copper in the mucus, but this is unlikely since partial extrusion, where the copper lies entirely in the mucus of the cervical canal, is associated with an increase in the pregnancy rate.

As well as an increase in the amount of copper in the cervical mucus, there is also an increase in copper in the cells of the endometrium, and it is here that the major antifertility effect of copper-bearing devices is thought to exist. It is postulated that interference with enzyme systems in the endometrium, in particular with the carbonic anhidrase reaction in which the copper competes with zinc, results in the prevention of implantation.

Ovulation seems to be unimpaired in the presence of an intrauterine device. Because at the present time the action of all types of IUD is thought to be on the endometrium, the fact that the endometrium is shed every month is regarded as a guarantee that no harmful effects will ensue with long-term use.

DANGERS OF COPPER USED AS A CONTRACEPTIVE

The Dalkon shield contains copper, but it is not released from the device. The slow release of copper from the Gravigard is an integral part of its action, and fears have reasonably been expressed regarding the action of this ionic copper on the human body.

1. Effects on the patient

The copper-bearing device at present in use carries 200 mg copper wire, although trials are taking place of devices carrying larger quantities. About 50 microgrammes of copper are released daily from 200 mg and this is released locally inside the uterus. The usual dietary intake of copper is about three milligrammes daily, and, as a normal trace element, mechanisms exist for the regulation of copper in the human body. No alterations in copper levels can be detected in the serum of women using the device (Hagenfeldt, 1972; Elstein and Daunter, 1973)

Increased copper levels are found in the cells of the myometrium and the endometrium, and also in the menstrual discharge and cervical secretion. The fact that the endometrium is renewed every month and the copper-bearing cells and secretions are discharged from the body is regarded as a guarantee that harm will not ensue from the local accumulation of copper.

Eczema occurring shortly after the insertion of a copper-bearing device has been blamed on sensitization to copper. However, eczema is a very common skin condition, and the association has not yet been proven to be more than coincidental.

To summarize, there is no evidence that the purely local release of copper is associated with any adverse effects in humans. Indeed, it has been believed by the lay public for generations that copper worn as rings, necklaces or bracelets has a beneficial effect on rheumatic disorder. Perhaps a copper-bearing IUD will have similar antirheumatic properties.

2. **Effects on the foetus**

The possible effect of intrauterine copper on the developing ovum, in cases where the contraceptive effect has failed to prevent pregnancy, has also been a cause of anxiety.

Chang *et al.* (1970), transferring blastocysts from normal rats to rats wearing copper wire in one horn of the uterus, have shown that the effect of the copper seems to be on the endometrium to prevent implantation, and there is no interference with development of the fertilized ovum. Teratological studies have shown no evidence, in animals or humans, of any increased tumour development. No chromosome abnormalities have been observed in cells of human tissue cultures in contact with copper-bearing contraceptives (Jones *et al.*, 1973).

Among children born to mothers wearing a copper-bearing device there has so far been no evidence of an increased incidence of abnormality. However, in view of the small number of accidental pregnancies occurring in women using such devices, and the fact that many of these women will request that the pregnancy be terminated, it will be a long time before sufficient data is available to be quite certain that there is no deleterious effect at all.

3. **Effect of diathermy treatment**

Short-wave diathermy should not be applied to the abdomen of a patient wearing a copper-bearing device because of the danger of burns to the endometrium, although an experiment in 1973 by Sandler seemed to indicate that this is not a serious hazard. However the same investigator has shown that distortion and loss of flexibility of any polythene device may result from the application of short-wave diathermy.

INSERTION OF AN IUD

Before inserting an IUD it is most important that the doctor allows adequate time to interview the patient. Many women saying, 'I want the coil fitted, doctor', have very little information on the subject. They tend to imagine that the efficiency of the IUD is identical to that of the combined Pill, but without the side-effects of that method, or indeed any side-effects of its own. Usually their introduction to intrauterine contraception has been a glowing account given by a friend or neighbour who has found the IUD an ideal method. Those whose friends give adverse reports do not ask for a coil.

The patient must be willing to accept a pregnancy rate of two or three pregnancies per hundred women per year. She must be told an IUD will not regulate her periods, indeed may make them heavier, so that it is unsuitable for the woman who already bleeds heavily or frequently. If fear of oestrogen has brought her to request an IUD, the correct figures of the risks involved with the combined Pill should be given her, as many of these patients have exaggerated ideas of both the risks of oral contraception, and the lack of side-effects from the IUD.

Having made sure that the patient's request is based on a sound knowledge of the expectations of the method, consideration can be given to the choice of device to be inserted.

At the time of writing, neither patient nor family doctor have a free choice in this matter, since only the Lippes loop and the Saf-T-Coil are available on National Health Service prescription, and if such prescription is used no fee may be claimed by the GP for insertion or subsequent care of the patient. Hopefully this unsatisfactory state of affairs will soon be altered.

Contra-indications to the insertion of an IUD

All are relative. The needs of the patient and the history of previous methods attempted may make it advisable in a particular case to override any of these contra-indications.

1. Genital neoplasms.

(NOT carcinoma-in-situ of the cervix).

2. Uterine abnormality.

The desirability or even possibility of inserting a device will depend on the degree of abnormality present.

3. Pelvic inflammatory disease.

An IUD should not be inserted in the presence of acute salpingitis, cervicitis, or vaginitis, which should be treated. A past history of infection need not prevent insertion, but a past history of recurrent infection may make it unwise if any other method is possible.

4. A history of heavy or prolonged periods, which have caused the patient to seek medical advice.

5. Uterine scars.

The presence of a Caesarean section scar, especially a classical scar or the scar of hysterotomy or myomectomy, should indicate careful consideration before selection of this method, and great care during insertion if this method is chosen.

6. Reluctance of the patient to accept the known risk of pregnancy for the device.

7. Severe dysmenorrhoea.

The patient who already complains of severe dysmenorrhoea is likely to complain even more after insertion of an IUD. In most cases other methods are to be preferred.

8. Nulliparous patients.

Dilatation of the nulliparous cervix is not a surgery procedure, and in any event may be associated with cervical damage, so that rigid forms of IUD were not suitable in women who had not borne children. First generation devices could be inserted without dilatation, but many nulliparous women found insertion painful, and suffered severe cramps afterwards. The smaller devices were more satisfactory in these respects, but had higher pregnancy rates.

In addition, the possibility that infection might follow insertion, with subsequent tubal blockage and sterility, made the use of the IUD as a method of contraception unpopular among both nulliparous women and their medical attendants.

Gamma irradiation of packaged devices has reduced the dangers of infection and the problems of size and insertion of the device have been overcome by the development of the small Dalkon shield, the Saf-T-Coil 25S, and the Gravigard, which seem eminently suitable for many nulliparous patients.

Once patient and doctor have agreed that an IUD should be fitted, the place and time should be considered. An adequately equipped surgery (i.e. one containing at least a handbasin and a sterilizer) is perfectly suitable for this procedure. The single-handed family doctor can manage quite successfully: those working in purpose-built premises with nursing staff to assist are that much more fortunate. The ideal time to fit the device in the patient not recently pregnant is at the end of menstruation, preferably during the last day of bleeding. One can then be quite certain that the patient is not already pregnant, and the cervical os is already slightly dilated. The ideal arrangement is to ask the patient to telephone on the first day of the period. An appointment can then be made for the last day with reasonable accuracy.

This is much easier to arrange if devices are inserted at a set time on any working day, rather than on a particular day of the week. The numbers to be inserted in any one practice are small, and it is quite feasible to insert them at the end of morning surgery, for example. If it is arranged as the last procedure of the morning, then there need be no fear of having to hurry. One of the many reasons patients give for their dislike of clinics is the feeling of being on a production line (non-production line?). If only one or two devices are fitted each day then there is no feeling of pressure from a waiting queue, for either doctor or patient.

Insertion after pregnancy or abortion

Immediate insertion after delivery is possible, but about a quarter of IUDs inserted then will fall out again. Devices inserted during the first few weeks after delivery are associated with a greater risk of perforating the uterus, and since pregnancy is most unlikely to occur during the first four weeks of the puerperium, insertion is best left until four to six weeks after the baby is born.

Insertion immediately after termination of pregnancy by the vaginal route is possible, and often desirable, as subsequent attendance of such patients cannot be guaranteed.

Equipment required

Small cervical dilator or uterine sound.
Swab-holding forceps.
Cusko's vaginal speculum.
Tenaculum forceps.
Scissors.
Sterile dressing pack with bowls for antiseptic solution and cream.
Sterile gloves.
Face-mask.
Intrauterine device and introducer.

Procedure (The description which follows refers to a doctor working with no assistance.)

The instruments, ready sterilized and covered, are laid up before the patient enters. She should empty her bladder and, after removing her lower clothing, place herself on the examination couch. A cervical smear, if not performed in the recent past, is taken before any antiseptics are introduced into the vagina. At the same time any infection of the cervix or vagina may be noted. A simple erosion is not a contra-indication to insertion of an IUD. Gross cervical or vaginal infection is, and swabs should be taken and the insertion postponed.

Bimanual examination, wearing an ordinary disposable non-sterile glove. is carried out and any pelvic abnormalities noted. The uterus is then carefully palpated noting its size and position (whether anteverted or retroverted). The glove can then be removed and the patient placed in the desired position for insertion. This may be the lateral position, with the thighs fully flexed on the abdomen or, better, the lithotomy position. This latter position may be obtained easily and efficiently by the use of a webbing sling as shown in Fig.

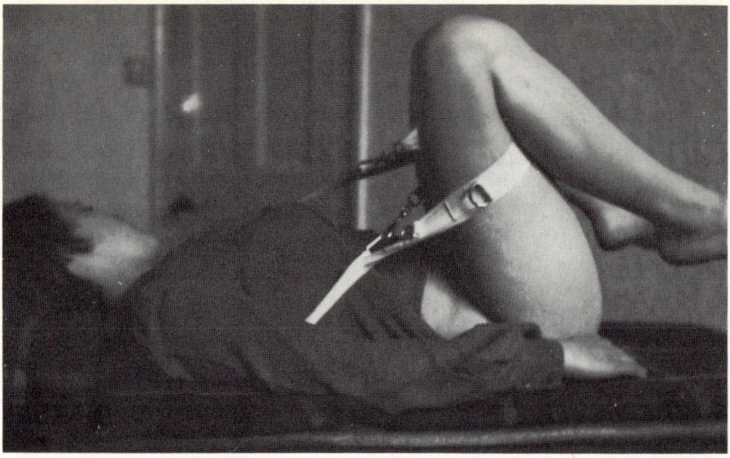

Fig. 26. Webbing sling used to obtain lithotomy position.

26 and is quite comfortable for the short time needed to insert an IUD. In both the lateral or the lithotomy position the long axes of the cervical canal and the vagina tend to come into alignment, and so these positions are preferable to any other. To have the couch at the correct height and to have a good light to work by are obvious essentials.

The doctor then removes the IUD and its introducer from its sterile pack,

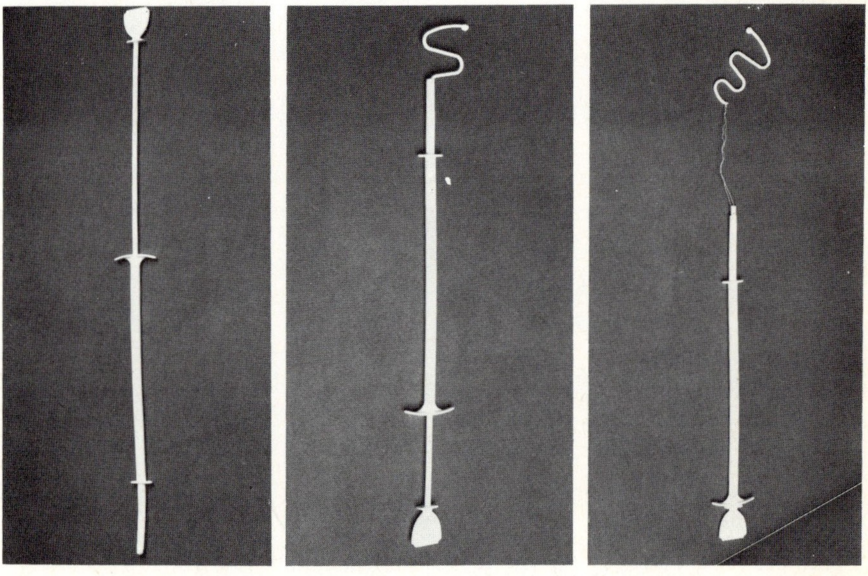

Fig. 27. Lippes loop. Loaded, half-extruded, extruded.

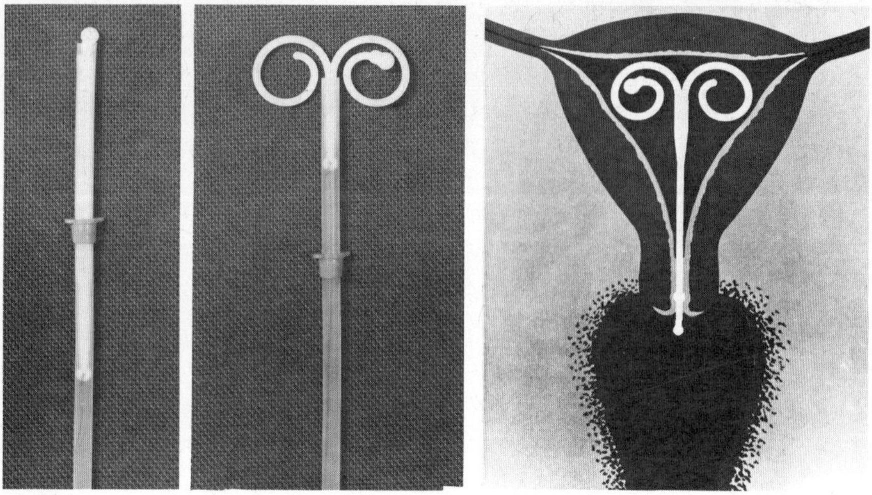

Fig. 28. Saf-T-Coil. Loaded, half-extruded, in situ.

and uncovering the instruments, drops it among them. He puts on the mask, scrubs up and dons sterile gloves. The device is then loaded into the introducer. Both the Lippes loop (Fig. 27) and Saf-T-Coil (Fig. 28) are loaded by pulling back the plunger of the introducer which, fastened by a thread to the base of the device, pulls it into the tube of the introducer. The

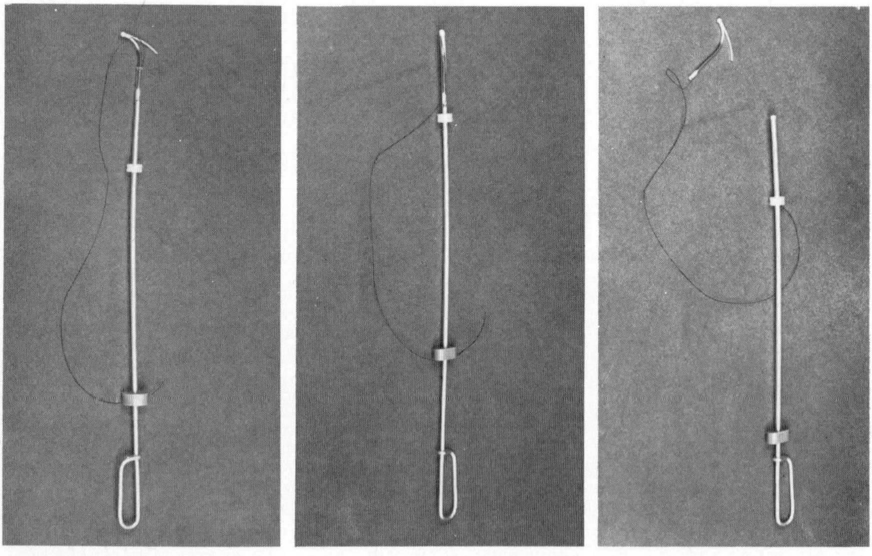

Fig. 29. Gravigard. As packed, loaded, extruded.

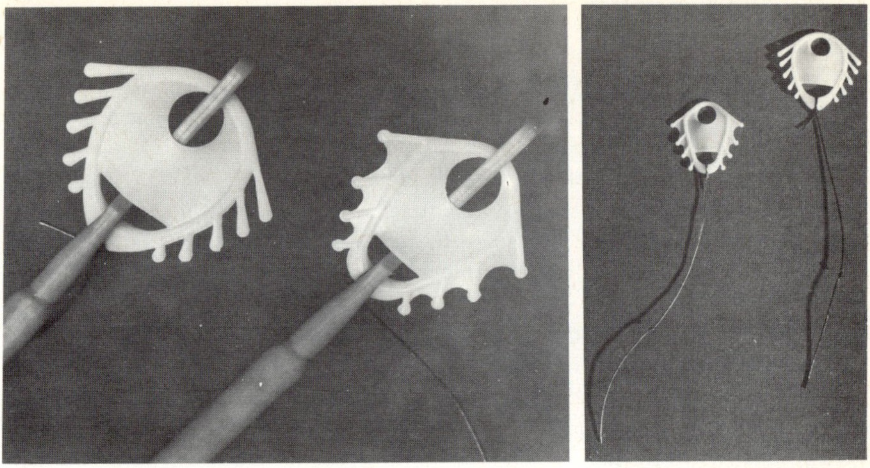

Fig. 30. Large and small Dalkon Shields. As packed; extruded.

Gravigard (Fig. 29) needs to be inserted manually into its tube, and can be rather 'fiddly'. It is best to hold the device at the junction of the two arms, insert the stem of the '7' into the tube, and then bend it laterally, bringing the arm of the '7' into apposition with the stem, when it can be pushed into the tube relatively easily. The doctor is advised to practice this loading procedure in advance.

The loading of the device into the introducer must be done as late as possible, since the longer it is compressed within its tube, the less likely it is to resume its original shape after expulsion from the tube.

The Dalkon shield (Fig.30) is already fitted in position on the introducer and is ready to be inserted on removal from the sterile pack.

The Cusko speculum is now inserted, the cervix visualized, and the speculum locked open. Each action of the doctor is explained in advance to the patient, who is often remarkably apprehensive. Efforts to relieve this apprehension are most important in an attempt to minimize the likelihood of shock developing.

A sterile swab is soaked in antiseptic solution (e.g. 0.1 per cent aqueous solution of acriflavine) and the cervix and upper vagina thoroughly, but gently, cleaned.

The small dilator is tipped with antiseptic cream (e.g. Hibitane) and inserted into the external os. In parous women the opening of the cervical canal may be large and bowl-shaped, and gentle probing within the area may be necessary to find the entrance to the cervical canal. This in its turn may have snags and blind alleys leading off it, and the tip of the dilator must be gently 'felt' into and along the canal. Spasm of the internal os occasionally occurs, making further progress impossible. A few minutes' light banter with the patient may result in the spasm passing. If not, then it is best to postpone the insertion. Dilatation may be achieved by injection of local anaesthetic into the cervix, but in my opinion this is not a suitable procedure for the surgery. Amyl nitrite by inhalation may result in both cervical dilatation and a splitting headache. Patients prefer postponement.

Some operators use a uterine sound. This instrument seems to me to be much more suitable for uterine perforation than the small dilator which can be used quite successfully as a sound. If sounding shows the uterus to be upright, applying a tenaculum - which in some women is a painful procedure is unnecessary. However, where more than a small degree of flexion of the uterine body in relation to the cervix exists, then traction on the cervix is necessary to align the cervical canal with the cavity of the uterus. Unless this is done, at worst the device or its inserter will be pushed through the uterine wall: at best the introducer will be impossible to insert 'round the bend' or will kink after insertion.

Once the dilator has traversed the cervical canal, it is gently pushed into the uterine cavity until the resistance of the fundus is reached. The size of the cavity, as measured by the distance the instrument can be inserted, is often surprisingly large, lengths of between three and four inches from external os to fundus being not uncommon. There is little relationship between the estimation of size on bimanual examination and the length of cavity on actual measurement. Even the height or parity of the woman cannot be used as a reliable indication of the length of the uterine cavity.

The dilator is then removed from the uterus, the mark reached at the external os having been noted, and is then measured against the introducer. This measurement varies according to the device used, as both the Lippes loop and Saf-T-Coil are pushed from the introducer into the uterus, whereas the introducers of the Gravigard and Dalkon shield are inserted to the fundus, and then withdrawn to leave the device in the uterine cavity.

Whatever type of device is used, its position in the inserter must be noted before it is hidden within the uterus in order that correct positioning in the transverse uterine plane is obtained. Detailed instructions for insertion are enclosed with each device, and should be carefully followed.

After insertion the introducer is removed. The Dalkon shield introducer is angled and notched: a turn through ninety degrees frees the device from the notch and the introducer can then be withdrawn. The thread, bearing a knot which, if the device is correctly positioned, lies at the external os, is not fastened to the introducer, as is the case with the Lippes loop and Saf-T-Coil. Care must be taken with removal of the introducer of these devices lest accidental traction on the thread pulls the device out of position.

It is usually advised that about two centimetres of thread should be left protruding from the cervix. Often the thread seems to be drawn up inside the uterus during the first weeks after insertion. It is preferable to leave more protruding, e.g. four centimetres, and trim it as necessary later.

The insertion is now complete. The vagina and vulva are swabbed dry, the sling supporting the legs removed and both legs lowered together to avoid straining the patient's back. The lower abdomen is palpated, and the patient should feel no pain nor discomfort suprapubically.

At this stage, not before, I show the patient a device similar to the one inserted. I encourage her to feel both the thread and the lower end of the device, explaining that to feel the thread in the vagina is evidence that the device is still present, but to feel the device means that it is no longer in the correct position, and its contraceptive action absent. I do not suggest to women that they explore their vagina regularly, as some find the idea distasteful. Having felt the difference between the threads and the device some women proceed to examine themselves regularly, others do not.

When first inserted, the thread in the vagina is stiff and protrudes away from the cervix. After some weeks the thread softens, and coils up against and around the cervix. I advise women to use a pad, not a tampon, for the first three periods after insertion to avoid accidental removal of the device by entanglement of the thread with the tampon. Husbands who find they can feel the thread on the penis may be advised that when the softening and coiling has occurred they will suffer no longer.

There is no doubt that warning patients that certain symptoms may appear predisposes to their appearance. Nevertheless, I think it proper that the family doctor should warn his patient, in the least worrying way possible, of common side-effects such as bleeding and pain, and simple measures the patient may take to relieve them. He should also tell her, as emphatically as possible, that he is available to advise her at any time, either by telephone or at the surgery. This knowledge will reassure her, and will help to minimize symptoms.

Difficulties during insertion of IUDs

In nine patients out of every ten the insertion of an IUD is an easy and satisfying procedure, taking between five and ten minutes. In the tenth patient some difficulty delays insertion, and in about one in five of these, insertion is found to be impossible.

Perforation of the uterus may occur, especially in the soft pregnant uterus. Insertion at the end of a period will minimize this possibility. The early puerperal uterus is also especially liable to perforation, and insertion is best avoided at this time.

The greatest danger of perforation exists where the uterus is acutely flexed and the long axes of the cervical canal and uterine cavity form an acute angle. Any attempt to force an instrument, be it sound, dilator, introducer, or the device itself, past such an angle may result in a false passage into or through the uterine wall.

THE INSERTION OF AN IUD IS NOT AN URGENT PROCEDURE. If the internal os is in spasm, and the dilator won't go through – leave it until another day. If all the passages in the cervix turn out to be blind alleys - leave it until another day. If the uterus is so acutely flexed that the introducer cannot be persuaded to enter the uterine cavity - leave it, either for another day or for someone else to perform. The consultant gynaecologist at the local hospital, working with assistants and an anaesthetic, will succeed where you have failed.

No loss of face will be involved in the referral of such a patient to a consultant. Frantic efforts to force a device into such a uterus may result in perforation, and referral of the perforated patient does mean loss of face.

Difficulty or failure to insert

Shock may develop while insertion is being performed. This is a rare condition, as indicated by the fact that it has appeared only once in my last two hundred insertions. Peel and Potts (1969) make no estimate of its incidence, and three very experienced operators writing in *Update* (March, 1973) do not mention it at all. However it is very frightening, both to the patient and the doctor, and so deserves mention. Probably the combination of a difficult insertion and a nervous patient predisposes to the appearance of shock. The patient may say she feels unwell, respiration becomes gasping, the pulse becomes weak and slow, the skin pale, cold and clammy. The blood pressure falls, being 60/40 in my one case.

Peel and Potts suggest that removal of the device is not necessary to aid recovery, but most GPs would be unwilling to test this hypothesis in the surgery. Shock may occur before insertion is completed. The patient should be kept warm, and allowed to rest, and the shock will pass off in a few minutes.

The 'kinked introducer'

The slender flexible introducer of the Gravigard may kink after insertion, the

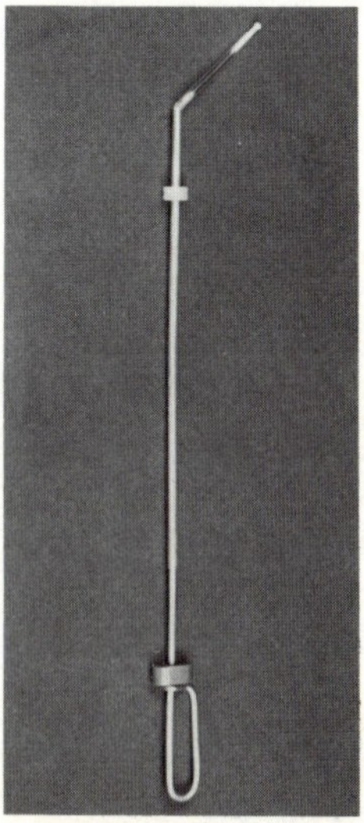

Fig. 31. 'Kinked' Gravigard introducer.

kinking of the sleeve occurring at the junction of the base of the device and the top of the plunger (Fig. 31). It is especially liable to happen in the acutely flexed uterus, but occasionally there seems to be an invisible flaw in the sleeve, allowing kinking to result after the easiest of insertions into an upright uterus.

Clinically, the result is that the operator finds that withdrawal of the sleeve along the plunger is impossible. The introducer and device must be withdrawn, and a new set substituted. On no account should one attempt forceful expulsion of the device by pushing the plunger up into the sleeve. The plunger is likely to be pushed through the kink of the sleeve into and through the uterine wall.

Insertion after oral contraception

Theoretically, oral contraceptives may result in increased tone of the myometrium and cervical os, and because of this it is sometimes advised that an IUD should not be inserted in patients taking the Pill, or in those who have been taking it recently. Apart from the risk of pregnancy in such women if insertion is delayed, experience shows that this is only a theoretical objection, and IUDs may be inserted, even in nulliparous women, during oral contraception with no more difficulty than in those not on the Pill.

As the risks of pregnancy and of excessively heavy periods are greatest in the first few months after insertion, then provided the Pill is not being stopped for medical reasons, and provided the woman is willing, it is quite helpful to ask her to continue to take the Pill for a further two or three months with the IUD *in situ*.

A delayed period after stopping the Pill may cause suspicion of pregnancy, even in the presence of an IUD, but the suspicion can be easily allayed by examination and a pregnancy test. To await a period after stopping the Pill before inserting a device may mean a wait of two or three months.

Follow-up after insertion

Every doctor will adopt the routine he thinks most suitable, and no ideal can be advised. Provided the patient knows that access for advice is available at any time—as should be the case with a GP—no routine for follow-up is any better than any other.

Personally I see my patients one week after inserting the device, partly to reassure us both it is still present and partly to enable the patient to express any anxieties or seek advice about symptoms. If all is well I see them again one month later, when they will have finished their next period. After that a further visit three months later is followed by annual checks.

The type of examination performed at each visit will be varied to suit the circumstances. The annual check, for example, offers an opportunity to carry out a variety of screening procedures, not directly related to the presence of the IUD. As a minimum, at each visit the cervix must be visualized and the continuing presence of the threads confirmed.

There is no evidence that the presence of an IUD affects the cytology of Papanicolau smears in any way, but the usual procedure is to repeat them annually.

It is wise to insert a probe into the cervical canal to feel for the stem of the Gravigard. Partial expulsion may result in this device occupying the cervical canal rather than the uterine cavity, with consequent reduction in antifertility action. The tip of the stem may be visible at the external os but, especially if a considerable amount of mucus is present, it may be extremely difficult to see. If the cervical canal is long, then the tip may not reach the external os. It is reassuring to be unable to feel the stem in the cervical canal.

'The missing threads'

If no threads can be seen in a good light, after careful swabbing - for the light-coloured threads can be very difficult to see amidst a mucoid discharge - pregnancy should be excluded, and then a sound passed through the cervix. The plastic device may often be felt indirectly by this means, rather as a piece of glass can be felt but not seen in a wound. The patient may be reassured that her contraception is still operative, and the threads in such a case sometimes reappear with the menstrual flow. The other possibilities are expulsion, rarely pregnancy, and very rarely extrusion, and are dealt with under the appropriate headings.

How long can an IUD remain in the uterus?

Many patients, after a symptomless first year of use, default later check-ups, and it is not uncommon to see patients in the surgery who have visited for reasons unconnected with contraception, and are found to be happily wearing the same IUD six or eight years after insertion.

However, with the passage of time the inert plastic devices sometimes become covered with accretions of calcium and phosphorus salts and lose their flexibility. The nylon threads lose their strength, and are liable to break when removal is attempted. For these reasons it is probably best to change Dalkon shields, Lippes loops, and Saf-T-Coils after three or four years of trouble-free use.

The copper will be exhausted from the Gravigard after some years and contraception will become inefficient. It is advised that the Gravigard at present in use, having 200 sq.mm of copper, should be changed every two years, although trials taking place at the moment seem to indicate that a longer period will eventually be advised.

Planned removal of a device

Those devices having threads attached may be simply pulled out again, in theory.

In practice, although the Lippes loop and Saf-T-Coil need little force applied, both Dalkon shield and Gravigard may need a considerable pull, particularly in nulliparous patients. The slender thread of the Gravigard may indeed snap under the strain.

Devices without threads or tails, and devices whose threads have parted company with the device, or have disappeared inside the uterus, must be fished out using either a hook (e.g. that designed by Dr Soonawala of Bombay) or a fine pair of ovum forceps. Parous women may generally be dealt with as out-patients, but nulliparous women and very nervous women may need admission and a general anaesthetic.

Unless the general practitioner is particularly experienced in removing things from the uterine cavity - and most are not - it is safer to leave this procedure to the hospital gynaecologist.

Removal by pulling on the thread may be undertaken at any time in the cycle, but is easiest when the cervix is open towards the end of a period and this time should always be chosen in nulliparous patients. Removal at this time will also ensure that pregnancy has not already occurred, or will not occur as a result of spermatozoa deposited in the vagina prior to removal.

COMPLICATIONS FOLLOWING INSERTION

1. Bleeding

A little bleeding immediately after insertion is almost inevitable. The periods are often heavier with a device in place than they were before insertion, especially for the first two or three months. After this they often settle down. Intermenstrual bleeding or spotting may occur.

As already stated, the incidence of bleeding varies with the size and type of device inserted, but tolerance of the bleeding varies greatly from woman to woman, and is reported to be less troublesome among women from the lower social classes. To some extent the doctor is dependant upon the patient's history: if she says the bleeding is excessive and asks for removal of the device, then it is wise to agree. Clinics tend to be reluctant to remove devices for this cause, and it is not uncommon for patients to present with a history of refused requests for removal. This type of patient is unhappy with the method, and her wishes should be respected.

If the patient does not demand removal, it is sometimes helpful to encourage her to keep a diary of the bleeding, which may demonstrate that the loss is not in fact as great as she had supposed. Haemoglobin estimations will show whether frank anaemia is developing. Although oral iron may correct it, if iron has to be given continuously, then other methods of contraception should be considered. The administration of ascorbic acid is advised in notifications sent to GPs by the Family Planning Association, but seems to produce little benefit.

Advice from the same source to administer oral contraceptives to patients bleeding heavily because of an IUD would seem to be completely unjustified, the patient then being liable to the dangers of both methods.

Administration of aminocaproic acid in a dosage of three grammes three times daily is alleged to lessen heavy bleeding associated with the Saf-T-Coil (MacMath, 1973).

Some patients are so anxious to succeed with the device that they will make light of the amount of bleeding they suffer, becoming progressively anaemic. Often such women are unaware that acceptable alternative methods exists, and they regard the IUD as their last chance. The GP must be on the look out for such women: timely removal of the device and sterilization will avoid much chronic ill-health.

Prolonged bleeding, even if only little in amount, may act as a bar to intercourse rather than to pregnancy, and constitute a reason for removal. It is, of course, particularly unacceptable to some religious groups, for example Jews, for whom it represents 'uncleanliness'.

2. **Pain**

Cramping pain, similar to period pains or after-pains may follow a few hours after insertion, but usually disappears in a day or two. It may recur at period times. Again the size and type of device and the pain threshold of the individual patient influence the number and degree of complaints of pain. Mild analgesics such as Anadin or Phensic should relieve it. The regular use of stronger compounds is inadvisable.

Pain occurring immediately after insertion, or at times other than period times, must raise the suspicion of perforation. More commonly, improper positioning of the device, which is not lying comfortably in the transverse plane of the uterus, is to blame. Removal and re-insertion may relieve pain of this type.

Any patient wearing an IUD who complains of pain should be examined carefully. The abdomen should be palpated, the cervix visualized and bimanual pelvic examination performed. The examination itself in many cases seems therapeutic, the patient ceasing to complain of pain afterwards, no doubt due to relief of her anxiety about the pain.

Continuing severe pain indicates removal of the device.

3. **Expulsion**

All types of IUD may be expelled through the cervix. Expulsion occurs most commonly during the first three months after insertion. Repeated expulsions may occur in the same patient. Larger devices or those of a different shape may be tried, but often the patient has become disillusioned with the method and requests another.

Expulsion may be complete, the device lying in the vagina or being found on a pad. Occasionally the patient does not notice its departure, which is worrying both because pregnancy may occur and because there is no evidence that the device is not still somewhere inside the patient.

Expulsion may be confirmed by failure to demonstrate the device on X-ray, as all devices now in use are radio-opaque. A soft tissue technique may be needed to demonstrate the thin Dalkon shield. Partial expulsion may result in the device lying in the cervical canal instead of in the uterine cavity, with consequent reduction in contraceptive efficiency.

4. **Extrusion**

In addition to perforation occurring at the time of insertion, IUDs sometimes gradually work their way through the uterine wall, coming to lie in the Pouch of Douglas or freely in the peritoneal cavity, in which case they have a tendency to migrate to a sub-hepatic position, or within the folds of the broad ligament. This process is sometimes called extrusion, or translocation, to distinguish it from traumatic perforation at the time of insertion.

In fact it is difficult to be certain that a device found outside the uterus many months after insertion was not in fact misplaced by perforation at insertion, the patient being symptomless during the interval.

The incidence of perforations varies with the type of device, the Birnberg bow being particularly notorious in this respect. Esposito (1966), in a study of 62 reported cases of perforation, found that 80 per cent were associated with this device. The bow had been inserted in three of the four cases of perforation reported by Mills (1967) in 1300 patients in Birmingham, England. Tietze (1966) suggests a rate of four perforations per 10,000 insertions of devices other than the bow.

The rigid, slender Dalkon shield introducer seems especially liable to perforate the uterus at insertion. Snowden (1974) reported five perforations occurring in two series totalling 5,000 insertions.

Closed devices, such as the Birnberg bow, may result in intestinal obstruction. This is a very rare complication, only fifteen cases being reported by more than six thousand consultant gynaecologists in the USA in response to a circulated questionnaire.

Provided insertion during the first month after delivery is avoided, open-ended devices are used rather than closed, and unhurried insertion is performed gently, especially in acutely-angled uteri, the general practitioner should never see a case of perforation of the uterus due to an IUD.

However, in the very rare case where it has occurred, it may sometimes be felt lying in the Pouch of Douglas or within the broad ligament. All devices now in use are radio-opaque and an X-ray will demonstrate its position in the abdomen, although hysterography may be necessary to decide whether it is inside or beside the uterine cavity. Ultrasound may be used in place of X-rays.

Closed devices must be removed because of the risk of obstruction: open devices made of inert material, causing no symptoms, may be allowed to remain under observation.

Devices in the Pouch of Douglas may be removed by colpotomy. Laparotomy may be needed to remove other devices, but laparoscopic removal is the method of choice in most cases.

5. **Infection**

As insertion takes place through the unsterile vagina and cervix, it is almost inevitable that infection will occur around the IUD in the uterine cavity. In addition, the presence of a thread lying along the cervical canal would seem to invite infection. Bacteriological investigation shows that although infection develops in almost all cases immediately after insertion the cilial flow along the tubes, the secretion of the endometrial and endocervical glands, and the 'flushing' effect of the menstrual flow usually results in disappearance of the infection after menstruation following insertion.

Occasionally purulent infection of one or both tubes and of the uterine cavity develops. The patient complains of severe lower abdominal pain, worse on one side if one tube is badly involved, and a foul discharge. Examination reveals fever and abdominal tenderness. Purulent discharge coming through the cervix can be seen with the speculum, and the uterus is very tender.

In such a case, the folly of attempting treatment with the device *in situ* can be demonstrated by removing it, when several millilitres of pus may cascade into the vagina. The IUD should be removed, swabs taken for culture, antibiotics started, and an alternative contraceptive method advised for when the patient feels better.

Some authorities advise that antibiotic treatment should precede removal, which may tend to spread the infection. This advice is presumably based on the analogy between treatment of infection with a device *in situ*, and treatment of an infected incomplete abortion. I do not believe the analogy stands examination. To remove a foreign body and at the same time promote drainage of pus is good surgical practice, and provided antibiotics are given at the same time, there is no need to fear that the non-pregnant uterus will behave in the same way as when pregnant.

Milder cases may be treated with the IUD in place. When unilateral tubal tenderness exists, the possibility of a tubal pregnancy should be considered. Reinsertion of an IUD is possible after the infection has subsided, but usually the patient finds the experience somewhat disillusioning, and opts for another method.

Theoretically, infertility may follow where the tubes have been damaged by infection. In practice most GPs have met patients who, despite repeated septic abortions, or attacks of salpingitis, still manage to become undesirably pregnant. The practical risk is probably smaller than the theoretical risk, and for the multipara who has completed her family, the risk of infertility does not constitute a risk at all.

However, the risk is a real one, albeit small, for the young nulliparous patient, in whom an intrauterine device should not be inserted without a careful consideration of the suitability of other methods, and a frank discussion with the patient of the risk of subsequent infertility.

A mucoid discharge, which may be quite heavy, is not uncommon in women wearing an IUD. Repeated bacteriological investigation reveals no pathogens, and the cause is presumably excessive normal secretion in response to the intrauterine foreign body. Excessive discharge may result because the device has slipped down inside the uterine cavity, its lower end lying in the upper reaches of the cervical canal, irritating the glands lining the canal. Removal and re-insertion will cure the discharge in such cases. Some women tolerate a remarkable degree of this type of discharge quite happily: others find even a small amount intensely unpleasant. One of my patients wearing a Gravigard declares she can 'smell the copper' in her discharge.

It has recently been suggested that the discharge in patients wearing copper-bearing devices may be bactericidal for some organisms, particularly the gonococcus.

6. **Pregnancy**

Unplanned pregnancy may occur despite the use of any IUD so far invented. It is more likely during the first few months after insertion and becomes progressively less so as time goes by. Because of this, it is sometimes advised that a spermicidal cream should be used in addition during the first three months after fitting. Correct positioning of the device is more probable if the operator is experienced, and the pregnancy rate may be expected to vary accordingly. Pregnancy may follow expulsion of the device, but the device may be correctly positioned in the uterus and still it occurs.

If the device is not in the uterus it may have been expelled through the vagina, unknown to the patient. The expulsion may be only partial, the device lying in the cervical canal. In such a case the patient may have felt the threads in the vagina without realizing that the device was no longer fully effective.

The device may have perforated the uterine wall, and be shown on X-ray to be lying elsewhere in the abdomen. The decision whether to leave it, or to remove it, then or later, will depend on its position, the stage of pregnancy and the position of the device, and this decision is one for the consultant gynaecologist. Whether the pregnancy is wanted or unwanted, and the patient's feelings with regard to operation are factors to be considered.

It used to be thought that pregnancy with an IUD *in situ* presented no special hazards to either mother or foetus. However, a recent report (Steven and Frazer, 1974) from Edinburgh has thrown doubt on this concept.

Of 82 patients who became pregnant with an IUD in place, four had extra-uterine pregnancies, and a further 55 aborted, 31 spontaneously. Three of the remaining patients had premature labours, there were five Caesarean sections and only 14 patients had spontaneous vaginal deliveries.

Another report relating particularly to the Dalkon shield (Templeton, 1974) tells of four maternal fatalities following septic mid-trimester abortion in patients wearing this device. Christian (1974) gives details of these four deaths, adds a further similar death in a patient pregnant with a Lippes loop *in situ*, and records seven further cases of severe illness due to mid-trimester septic abortion, six of whom were wearing the shield device.

Because of these and other reports, the wisdom of allowing unplanned pregnancies to continue with any sort of IUD *in situ* is questionable. The Dalkon shield has been withdrawn from sale pending further investigation.

Removal of a device by gentle traction at the time an early pregnancy is diagnosed is advised, and failure to do so would indicate termination of the pregnancy. If, knowing the risk, the mother decides to continue with the pregnancy then especially careful observation is necessary. After delivery the device must be looked for in the membranes. If it cannot be found then the uterus must be explored to remove it, to be certain that perforation has not occurred.

Ectopic pregnancy

About five per cent of pregnancies in women with an IUD *in situ* are ectopic, as compared with about 0.3 per cent of all pregnancies. Ectopic pregnancy is thus more common in women pregnant despite the IUD. But pregnancy itself is much less common in women who wear devices, so that the incidence of ectopic pregnancy in a population using the IUD is less than in a population using no contraception.

Tietze (1966) calculated that the frequency was in fact much less than was to be expected. He reported 25,000 women-years of experience. Calculating the number of ectopic pregnancies that would have been expected in that number of women over that length of time, he estimated that there should have been between 200 and 300 ectopic pregnancies. In fact, there were only 23.

The conclusion to be drawn is that an IUD prevents both uterine and ectopic implantation, but prevents uterine more efficiently than ectopic.

USE OF THE IUD IN GREAT BRITAIN

The great advantage of the IUD is that, once in place, it continues to function without further effort by the patient. It cannot be forgotten - as can the Pill, nor be unavailable at the crucial time - as may be the cap or the sheath.

In contrast to all other methods of contraception, the patient with an IUD in place must be motivated towards action to become pregnant, rather than to continue to avoid pregnancy. She must take positive action to cease contraception, rather than to continue it.

Pregnancy rates are still approximately ten times as great for the IUD as for the combined Pill, so it is not the method of choice for most single women, nor for women who have completed their family, when sterilization of one of the partners would be preferable. Despite this, for women afraid to take the Pill, or unwilling to undergo operation, it is the most efficient alternative method available. It is particularly valuable in women of low intelligence, or of high fecklessness, as motivation is needed only for insertion, not for continuation.

After termination of pregnancy, especially after repeated terminations, and especially where pregnancy has resulted from failure of the patient to use other methods properly, the IUD is often the contraceptive method of choice.

The enormous adverse publicity associated with the Pill at the time of the Scowen report in 1969 resulted in an increase in the number of women asking for intrauterine devices. Despite this, it remains a little used method. In 1973, 11 per cent of first attenders at FPA Clinics chose intrauterine contraception. In the United Kingdom about 350,000 women are estimated to use the IUD, as opposed to, for example, the two million who use the Pill. Only 3 per cent of the families included in the Hull Family Survey (Peel, 1972) had ever used the IUD as a method of contraception, whereas more than 50 per cent had used the Pill, and 60 per cent had used the condom. These figures illustrate the fact that the IUD tends to be the method of choice for the older woman, seldom being used before the first pregnancy.

As a method of family spacing it is gaining in popularity. As a method for use after families are completed it was popular, but the newer methods of sterilization are today being chosen by more couples.

The part played by general practitioners in the provision of intrauterine contraception has so far been small. A report in 1973 (Bone) pointed out that whereas IUDs are fitted in 40 per cent of clinics, only 12 per cent of family doctors provide this service.

GPs have in general been indifferent, or even antagonistic to the IUD. The reason for their attitude lies in their virtual exclusion from existing contraceptive services. Many local authorities and hospitals supply and fit the IUD free of charge. The National Health Service did not. Certain devices, not all, became available on NHS prescription only in 1973. The GP had to look to the patient for payment, which was often simply not possible, either because the patient could not afford it, or for some other reason.

> A patient known to be far from impecunious consulted a GP colleague. A twenty-minute interview embraced a discussion of all forms of contraception, and resulted in a decision by the patient to have an IUD fitted. Arrangements were made for insertion, but the patient later telephoned to say that her husband said it was daft to have to pay for the device - and pay the GP for fitting - when the local clinic would do it free. My colleague could only agree the system was daft, and regret he had not arranged for the twenty-minute interview to take place at the clinic.

In addition, the GP has found that the clinic which fitted the IUD was likely to be closed at the time a patient needed help because of some side-effect, so the GP was called instead.

Even patients who took their side-effects back to the clinic might be sent on for the GP to treat; as a result he tended to see a larger proportion of the complications of intrauterine contraception and developed a jaundiced view of the method.

A 28-year-old multipara presented at morning surgery complaining of abdominal pain. She did not volunteer the information that she had an IUD fitted, but full pelvic examination revealed one, associated with gross infection. As the clinic was in operation that day, the GP sent her back to it, with a letter detailing his findings. He was astonished to find the patient again in his surgery that evening, still with the IUD, still infected, but with a letter from the clinic requesting that he gave treatment.

The insertion of an intrauterine device is a procedure easily performed by any GP with obstetric experience and, with a little training, by any GP who is interested. The follow-up of patients using intrauterine contraception is ideally performed by their GP. The financial inducements to persuade patients to go to clinics have been misguided, and sometimes not in the patient's best interests.

Future developments of the contraceptive services in this country should include arrangements for GPs to play a full part, on conditions of equality, with doctors working in clinics.

THE IUD IN DEVELOPING COUNTRIES

Because of the continuing contraception resulting from one insertion and the relative cheapness of the device, the IUD is a very suitable method for use in developing countries. Where medical personnel are in short supply, paramedical workers can be trained to insert IUDs. The dangers of inexpert insertion and lack of supervision, while unacceptable in a country such as the United Kingdom, may be less than the dangers of uncontrolled fertility in an undeveloped country, and so acceptable.

COMPARATIVE EFFICIENCY OF TYPES OF IUD

When assessing the performance of a particular IUD, its ability to prevent pregnancy is obviously of major importance, but the number of expulsions, and the number of removals necessitated by bleeding or pain that occur in any group of women using that device are also of importance. Expulsion, especially unnoticed or partial expulsion, may be followed by pregnancy, as may removal for medical reasons. And high rates of removal for bleeding or pain, even with a low pregnancy rate while the device is still in position, will indicate that the device is unlikely to be acceptable to large numbers of the population at risk. The continuation rate, that is the proportion of acceptors happily continuing with the device after a stated length of time, is probably the best guide as to the acceptability of any device.

There are many factors influencing the performance of IUDs.

1. Factors related to the device itself

As well as size, stiffness and surface area, factors already considered, performance may be influenced by contraceptive substances carried on the device, copper or progesterone for example, and the dosage of this substance.

2. Factors related to the patient

Age and parity are important factors here. Younger women are more fertile than older, and pregnancy rates are likely to be higher if a trial includes large numbers of young women. If large numbers of nulliparous women take part in a trial of the performance of a device, the fact that an unknown number of infertile women will of necessity be included will affect results. The smaller nulliparous uterus may react to a device placed inside it in a different manner to the larger parous uterus, and the higher parity uterus may react differently when compared with one of low parity.

As well as these purely physical factors, the enthusiasm of a patient using a new type of device must be taken into account, since in her desire to be 'one up' on her friends and neighbours she may put up with a degree of discomfort from bleeding or pain that she would otherwise not tolerate. Women will put up with a certain amount of suffering in order to be leaders of fashion, even of IUDs.

Research has demonstrated that race, religion and social class all have an influence on the performance of any pattern of IUD.

3. Factors related to the investigator

The results produced from a trial of any device may reflect the expertize of the investigator rather than the efficacy of the device. Most initial trials are performed by an expert gynaecologist (perhaps the enthusiastic inventor of the device) or particularly experienced workers in the family planning field. When the device comes to be inserted by less expert and less experienced personnel then less favourable results may appear.

Enthusiasm for a new device may affect doctors as well as patients. The 'removal threshold', the point at which a doctor will decide to remove a device because of bleeding or pain will vary from doctor to doctor. Some would be happy to leave a device in place and prescribe iron, or even oral contraceptives in addition, whereas others faced with the same patient would advise removal of the device and a change of method.

It has been shown that when a patient constantly sees a single doctor, removal for medical reasons is less likely than if more than one doctor is involved in the care of the patient. In other words, we are all more likely to agree to remove a device inserted by somebody else, and less likely to destroy the result of our own efforts.

Before passing any final opinion as to the efficacy of any device therefore, one must await results from trials involving many insertions, followed over several years, performed by doctors of varying experience on patients of all types, enthusiastic, intelligent and feckless, drawn from all social classes. Parameters to be examined should be not only the occurrence of accidental pregnancy, but also the rates for expulsion and medical removals. Because of the differing 'removal thresholds' multicentre trials involving many doctors are essential. Care must be taken to record any advice to use other contraceptive measures in addition to the IUD at any stage after insertion and to assess the effect of this advice. The influence of race, religion, social class, age and parity on the performance of any device needs separate assessment.

Few trials conforming to this pattern have taken place in the United Kingdom. Patients attending the clinics of the Family Planning Association have often been used to provide volunteers for trials, and such patients are in general of higher social class then those attending general practitioners' surgeries or hospitals. The expertize of those inserting devices has not been taken into account, follow-up of defaulters has been poor, and results have not been expressed in a standard manner, making comparisons between centres and types of device difficult. For those devices which have been in use for many years, almost all the detailed information collected has come from the United States.

However, trials now in progress in this country show improvement in design. The manufacturers of the Gravigard are conducting trials using hospitals, clinics and general practitioners as investigators. The Family Planning Research Unit at the University of Exeter collects data from twenty-two clinics, obtaining information about ten thousand new users of IUDs each year, and is now engaged in collecting and analysing data for the new devices.

It is to be hoped that in the future workers in the contraceptive field will be much better informed as to the merits and demerits of the various types of IUDs, and as a result will be able to give more accurate advice to their patients.

First generation devices

One of the most comprehensive reviews of the efficiency of intrauterine devices was provided by the Cooperative Statistical Programme set up by Christopher Tietze in the United States in 1963 and reported in 1970 (Tietze and Lewit).

Calculated according to the Life Table method, this study involving thousands of women using a variety of devices over two years has provided a base line against which the newer second generation devices may be compared (Table IX).

From this table it can be seen that devices giving a reasonably low pregnancy rate were invariably associated with unreasonably high rates of removal and expulsion. Excluding the large bow, because of the risks associated with closed devices mentioned previously, the large Lippes loop D presented the least unsatisfactory picture.

Second generation devices

Early reports of the performance of the new generation of IUDs were very optimistic. Davis (1970), using the Dalkon shield in the United States,

Table IX. Gross Cumulative Rates of Events and Closures by Type of Termination, per 100 Users: All Devices, by Type and Size, All Segments, Two Years of Use.

Events, closures, first insertions, and woman-months of use	Loops				Spirals		Bows		Steel ring	Double coil
	A	B	C	D	Small	Large	Small	Large		
Events										
Pregnancies	11.8	8.2	5.8	5.1	6.4	3.3	18.0	8.8	10.6	4.9
Expulsions										
First	25.5	24.1	19.4	12.9	37.1	26.9	5.6	2.1	20.52	20.2
Later	5.7	5.2	8.9	5.4	12.7	8.8	1.9	1.4	5.4	4.6
Removals										
Bleeding	15.9	20.8	18.8	19.5	16.2	24.7	18.6	17.9	14.0	25.0
Other medical	8.4	7.1	6.8	6.9	7.3	13.8	5.2	6.8	4.2	7.0
Planning pregnancy	4.7	1.5	3.9	3.3	5.4	3.6	5.4	2.7	5.7	3.1
Other personal	8.9	5.7	4.5	5.1	14.8	7.9	9.1	4.8	4.3	3.3
Closures										
Pregnancies	9.7	7.5	5.0	4.3	3.6	2.5	14.5	7.1	9.3	4.7
Expulsions										
First	7.7	7.8	6.1	4.1	11.0	8.4	1.4	0.9	6.0	8.8
Later	2.9	2.8	3.9	2.9	4.8	2.5	0.4	0.6	2.7	2.3
Removals										
Bleeding/pain	10.5	18.8	16.9	16.9	10.6	16.1	10.6	14.8	11.7	23.7
Other medical	3.7	5.7	5.3	5.0	5.3	7.3	4.3	5.5	3.9	6.3
Planning pregnancy	2.2	1.5	3.0	2.4	3.0	3.1	4.0	2.1	4.4	3.1
Other personal	6.9	5.6	4.0	4.4	11.8	5.9	7.8	4.0	4.1	3.0
First insertions	1,015	1,305	3,489	7,553	448	2,203	1,476	2,259	1,706	2,463
Woman-months of use	13,453	12,463	50,775	121,566	5,938	29,331	19,636	41,755	25,829	22,619

Reprinted with the permission of the Population Council from 'Evaluation of intrauterine devices: ninth progress report of the Cooperative Statistical Program . Tietze, C. and Lewit, S., Studies in Family Planning, Vol. 1. No. 55, July, 1970, Page 11, Table 9.

reported a pregnancy rate of only 1.1, expulsions of 2.3 and only 2.0 medical removals, all calculated by the life table method after one year of use. The continuation rate after one year was 94 per cent. Newton *et al.* (1972) using the Gravigard device in London, reported after nine months of use a pregnancy rate of 1.08, and a medical removal rate of only 2.95. The continuation rate after nine months was 94 per cent.

Without for one moment doubting the accuracy of these results, it must be pointed out that they do not accord with those obtained following use in the surgery, and are an example of the results obtainable by expert and enthusiastic doctors, working with a new device engendering enthusiasm among the patients.

The enthusiasm displayed for a new device may be quite extraordinary. My practice area is included in the district served by the King's College Hospital contraceptive clinic from which John Newton and his colleagues reported the figures above. I have received glowing reports of the efficiency and lack of side-effects of the 'new copper curl' from many of my patients, some of whom were attending the clinic as patients, but some of whom were nursing staff, secretaries, clerks and even cleaners. In such an atmosphere of enthusiasm, how could any method fail?

Countrywide multicentre trials of both devices have been carried out under the supervision of the Family Planning Research Unit at Exeter and I am most grateful to Dr Robert Snowden, the Project Director at this unit for allowing me to make use of the results obtained. Much of what follows is based on the findings of this Unit at Exeter.

Accidental pregnancies

The number of accidental pregnancies occurring in users of various types of device at one year of use, according to various trials, is indicated in Table X.

Table X. Accidental pregnancy rate per 100 users at one year, calculated by the life table method.

Device	*Investigator*	*Number of women*	*Pregnancy rate*
Lippes loop D	Tietze and Lewit (1970) (CSP)	7,553	2.7
Saf-T-Coil	Tietze and Lewit (1970) (CSP)	2,463	2.8
Dalkon shield	Davis (1970)	640	1.1
	Snowden and Williams (1974)	4,191	2.8
	Jones *et al.* (1973)	377	4.7*
Gravigard	Williams and Snowden (1974)	2,002	2.8
	Newton *et al.* (1974)	1,156	1.8

* This pregnancy rate, was expressed as 4.7 per HWY, but the author stated in a letter that recalculation by the life table method had shown a 'not dissimilar' rate.

Accidental pregnancy rates for the newer devices do not seem to be markedly different at one year from those obtained with the more satisfactory types of older device. However, at two years the Dalkon shield, with a cumulative rate of 3.6 (Snowden and Williams, 1974), does seem rather better than the Lippes loop D (5.1) or Saf-T-Coil (4.9). Results at two years for the Gravigard are even better, Newton *et al.* (1974) reporting a gross termination rate due to pregnancy of 2.5.

Thus although the published results of all devices show that a decrease in the number of accidental pregnancies may be expected in the second year of use, the Dalkon shield seems to excel in this respect, possibly due to the low expulsion rate, since some pregnancies will follow expulsion not noticed at the time.

Accidental pregnancy is more common with all devices during the first few months after fitting. Because of this many centres advise the use of spermicidal preparations for the months after insertion. Snowden and Williams report conflicting evidence relating to the influence of this additional method. Centres reporting that spermicides had been advised in addition to the Dalkon shield in more than half the patients, reported pregnancy rates one-third as great as those reported by centres not giving such advice. However, for the Gravigard the reverse seemed to be true. Obviously further elucidation of the effect of additional methods is needed.

Expulsion

All first generation devices have a greater risk of expulsion during the first year after insertion when compared with the risk in subsequent years. Table XI illustrates reported rates for various devices after one and two years of use.

Table XI. Net cumulative expulsion rates per 100 users per type of device at stated length of use.

Device	*Investigator*	*At one year*	*At two years*
Lippes loop D	Tietze and Lewit (1970) (CSP)	9.5	12.9
Gravigard	Williams and Snowden (1974)	7.2	?
	Newton *et al.* (1974)	8.4	9.7
Dalkon shield	Snowden and Williams (1974)	2.0	2.0
	Jones *et al.* (1973)	6.3*	?

* Rate per 100 WY.

Both the new generation devices show some improvement over the Lippes loop D as far as expulsion is concerned, but the Dalkon shield seems particularly unlikely to be expelled, and there is no increase in the risk of expulsion during the second year.

As with accidental pregnancy, expulsion seems more likely to occur in younger women, under the age of 30, and no clear relationship with parity emerges.

Medical removals

Bleeding or pain or both continue to be troublesome accompaniments to the wearing of an IUD, even with the newer devices. Table XII gives some indication of comparative rates to be expected with various types of device.

Table XII. Cumulative removal rates for bleeding/pain per 100 users at stated length of time.

Device	*Investigator*	*At one year*	*At two years*
Lippes loop D	Tietze and Lewit (1970) (CSP)	12.9	19.5
Saf-T-Coil	Tietze and Lewit (1970) (CSP)	14.7	25.0
Gravigard	Williams and Snowden (1974)	5.1	?
	Newton *et al.* (1974)	4.1	7.6
Dalkon shield	Snowden and Williams (1974)	4.2	8.8
	Jones *et al.* (1973)*	9.5	?

* Expressed as rate per 100 WY

Both second generation devices show an improvement in the rates of removal for bleeding or pain when compared with earlier devices. Parity seems the most important factor influencing removal for bleeding or pain, women having had three or more babies being particularly liable to need removal of the Gravigard for this reason, and those having had one or two babies being particularly liable to suffer bleeding or pain while wearing the Dalkon shield. Snowden and Williams postulate that the small size and linear shape of the Gravigard may enable it to move inside the bulky multiparous uterus and thus cause symptoms. That movement has taken place inside some patients has been demonstrated radiologically.

As expected, considerable variations were noted in the rates of removal for medical reasons reported from different centres.

Continuation rates

It is generally accepted that about 75 per cent of women will continue to wear a Lippes loop D after one year, the percentage steadily falling to reach about 40 per cent after six years. Continuation rates for the Saf-T-Coil are about 5 per cent lower. Although too early to give accurate figures for long-term use, the continuation rates presently being reported for the second generation devices are very encouraging. Snowden and Williams estimate 90 per cent of women are continuing with the Dalkon shield at one year, and 82 per cent at two years, and for the Gravigard their estimate is 86 per cent at one year. Newton *et al.* (1974) report a continuation rate of 68.9 per cent at two years for all patients using the Gravigard, reflecting a high discontinuation rate for planned pregnancy.

These rates should be borne in mind when comparing the efficacy of the IUD at preventing pregnancy with that of combined oral contraceptives, for which disappointingly low continuation rates of 60–70 per cent at one year have been reported.

WHICH INTRAUTERINE DEVICE FOR OUR PATIENTS?

I assume that all types of IUD will eventually be available to all women by prescription on EC10, and therefore differences in cost to the patient and availability need not be considered.

As yet no perfect intrauterine device is available. All have their advantages and disadvantages, but it would seem that the vast majority of patients seen in the GP's surgery will be suited by either the Lippes loop D, the Gravigard or the Dalkon shield. Because of its higher rates for expulsion and removal, and its lower continuation rate, without benefit of a lower pregnancy rate, I would only use a Saf-T-Coil today to replace another inserted some years previously, and known to be well tolerated by that particular uterus. I never use the smaller sizes of Lippes loop.

The preference of the patient may indicate which device to use. She may dislike the idea of copper as a contraceptive, or she may have heard good reports of a particular device. The expertize of the practitioner must be considered. The Lippes loop and Gravigard are easy to insert, whereas the Dalkon shield can be downright dangerous in inexperienced hands, but its exceedingly low expulsion rate may make it the device of choice for patients who have demonstrated their ability to expel other devices. For easy painless insertion in nulliparous women the Gravigard reigns supreme.

At some time in the future we may be able to decide by examining the patient and taking a history, which particular device will suit her best. At the moment we cannot do so, except with regard to factors such as age, parity and previous expulsions, already discussed.

POSTSCRIPT

The information relating to the Dalkon shield has been allowed to remain in this chapter despite withdrawal of the device from sale in the United Kingdom because the Food and Drug Administration in the USA has already permitted it to be distributed again there, and it is expected that the device will be made available again in the United Kingdom shortly.

Because of the suggestion that infection accompanying use of the Dalkon shield was due to pathogens 'wicking' up the inside of the polyfilamentous thread, the device when reissued will be fitted with a monofilament thread.

REFERENCES

BONE, M. (1973). *Family Planning Services in England and Wales*. HMSO, London.

CHANG, C. C., TATUM, H. S., and KINCL, F. A. (1970). The effect of intrauterine copper and other metals on implantation in rats and hamsters. In *Introduction to Copper Contraception*, G. D. Searle, Chicago.

CHRISTIAN, C. D. (1974). Septic abortion and IUDs. *American Journal of Obstetrics & Gynecology*, **119**, 441.

DAVIS, H. J. (1970). The shield interauterine device. *American Journal of Obstetrics & Gynecology,* **106,** 155.

ELSTEIN, M. and DAUNTER, B. (1973). Copper absorption from IUDs. *British Medical Journal,* **2,** 776.

ESPOSITO, J. M. (1966). *Obstetrics & Gynecology,* **28,** 799.

HAGENFELDT, K. (1972). *Acta Endocrinologica,* Supp. 169.

JONES, R. W., GREGSON, N. M. and ELSTEIN, M. (1973). Effects of copper-containing intrauterine devices on human cells in culture. *British Medical Journal,* **2,** 520.

JONES, R. W., PARKER, A. and ELSTEIN, M. (1973). Clinical experience with the Dalkon shield intrauterine device. *British Medical Journal,* **3,** 143.

McMATH, I. F. (1973) Antifibrinolytic control of menorrhagia after IUD insertion. *Practitioner,* **210,** 417.

MILLS, W. (1967). *British Medical Journal,* **1,** 428.

NEWTON, J., ELIAS, J. and McEWAN, J. (1972). Intrauterine contraception using the CU7 device. *Lancet,* **ii,** 951.

NEWTON, J., ELIAS, J., McEWAN, J. and MANN, G. (1974). Intrauterine contraception with the Copper 7: Evaluation after two years. *British Medical Journal,* **3,** 447.

PEEL, J. (1972). The Hull Family Survey II. *Journal of Biosocial Science,* **4,** 333.

PEEL, J. and POTTS, M. (1969). *Textbook of Contraceptive Practice.* Cambridge University Press.

SANDLER, B. (1973). *British Medical Journal,* **3,** 458.

SNOWDEN, R. and WILLIAMS, M. (1974). *The Dalkon Shield. Field Trial in the United Kingdom (Second Report).* Family Planning Research Unit, University of Exeter.

STEVEN, J. D. and FRAZER, I. S. (1974). Pregnancy after IUD failure. *Journal of Obstetrics & Gynaecology of the British Commonwealth,* **81,** 282.

TEMPLETON, J. S. (1974). Septic abortion and the Dalkon shield. *British Medical Journal,* **2,** 612.

TIETZE, C. (1966). *British Medical Journal,* July 30.

TIETZE, C. and LEWIT, S. (1970). Evaluation of intrauterine devices: 9th progress report of the Cooperative Statistical Program. *Studies in Family Planning,* **1,** 11.

WILLIAMS, M. and SNOWDEN, R. (1974). *The Gravigard Device. Field Trial in the United Kingdom (First Report).* Family Planning Research Unit, University of Exeter.

ZIPPER, J. *et al.* (1969). Metallic copper as an intrauterine contraceptive adjunct to the 'T' device. *American Journal of Obstetrics & Gynecology,* **105,** 1274.

12

STERILIZATION

Before the end of the nineteenth century sterilization was performed by barbarous and mutilating means, often with castration, often as retaliation or punishment. In the twentieth century the substitution of surgery for butchery has made possible the use of sterilization as an acceptable means of fertility control, although once again the Roman Catholic Church is out of step with other religious groups, the Papal Encyclical of 1968 forbidding sterilization as a means of birth control.

Compulsory sterilization for eugenic reasons, mainly for severe mental defect, has been legally possible in the United States since 1907. Infinitely preferable is voluntary sterilization, a procedure that has become more frequently practised throughout the world as this century has progressed.

In 1934 the report of the British Departmental Committee on sterilization stimulated consideration of the operation on grounds other than purely eugenic and in Aberdeen the policy of Sir Dugald Baird and his colleagues from 1935 onwards was to offer sterilization to all women who had failed to prevent recurrent pregnancies undermining their health.

In 1939 came the Second World War and the Nazi policy of forcible sterilization on eugenic, racial and 'moral' grounds had the effect of halting further liberalization of the operation in the world as a whole and caused such revulsion in countries occupied by the Nazis that even today sterilization plays a relatively small part in their fertility control programmes.

With safer, easier and more effective sterilizing operations in both the male and female, and the modern view that individuals have the right of choice of control over their own fertility, the indications for the operation have widened from eugenic reasons, or reasons connected with the preservation of health, to its use as a method of birth control both for the individual and for a population.

The use of sterilization as a means of controlling population growth has already been discussed. Like all other methods, its use in isolation has many disadvantages. As part of a planned programme of use of all available methods however, it has great value both on the personal and the community level. All the contraceptive methods in use today are relatively inefficient, and unwanted pregnancies will occur. Abortion may be a solution for the patient with unwanted pregnancy, but sterilization can avoid both abortion and pregnancy, and therefore should be available to all who are attempting permanent, completely effective contraception.

INDICATIONS FOR STERILIZATION

Sterilization may be indicated to preserve the life or health of a woman in the presence of co-existing disease, mental or physical, which might be worsened by pregnancy and delivery. Two previous deliveries by Caesarean section are usually regarded as an indication for sterilization at the third, although some gynaecologists would advise it after the second. Patients suffering from hereditary disease may seek the advice of their general practitioner as to the advisability of sterilization. The help and advice of specialist genetic counsellors should be sought in such cases. Grand-multiparity and advancing age are likely to result in maternal ill health and this in its turn to result in the mother being unable to care for her children properly, with resulting poor health in the children. The relationship between age and number of children has led to the introduction of formulae on which the decision to sterilize is made; for example, the '120 rule':

Age of woman x number of children = more than 120,
sterilization offered.
Age of woman x number of children = less than 120,
sterilization not offered.

Thus a woman of 30 who has four children and wishes for five should be offered sterilization whereas a woman of 40 who wants no more than her existing two children should not be offered it. This is obvious nonsense, as is the rule existing today in some vasectomy clinics than men aged less than X years should not be offered the operation. Why X? Why not X plus 1 or X minus 1 or any other number one cares to choose?

Granted the safety of modern sterilizing operations, there is no logical reason for restricting it to patients of any particular age or parity. A couple who have completed their family may regard sterilization as the most acceptable and efficient method of birth control open to them, and they should be allowed to make use of it - provided they understand all the implications. Infant mortality is today so low in the United Kingdom that the possibility that the existing family will be reduced by death is remote. Any morbidity or mortality from the operation must be compared with that resulting from failure to perform it, with the possible occurrence of unwanted pregnancy and abortion, or even with the risks of using oral contraceptives over several decades. The risk to the mother of an unplanned pregnancy and confinement at the end of her reproductive life is probably greater than the risk of her sterilization in her late twenties, and certainly greater than the risk of vasectomy in her husband.

I would suggest that today there are two broad headings under which one can classify the indications for sterilization.

1. *Medical,* i.e. where the medical attendant, because of his specialized knowledge, can forsee dangers inherent in any future pregnancies which are not obvious to the patient. Repeated Caesarean section, maternal disease and genetic disorders may be cited as examples.

In such cases it is the duty of the medical attendant to point out the dangers and to take the initiative in offering sterilization.

2. *Socio-economic,* i.e. where the patient wishes to avoid any further pregnancies. The reasons may include completion of family, dislike of children, a wish to conserve family finances for existing children, a wish to avoid using contraception over long periods of time or failure to use contraception effectively.

In such cases it is the duty of the medical attendant to seek contraindications, not to consider whether the patient should be 'allowed' sterilization.

If this view of sterilization as an extension of contraception is adopted, then the importance of counselling becomes obvious, and it is in the field of counselling that the family doctor has the major role. Few will have the skill to perform the operative procedures involved, but all should be able to advise their patients.

Female sterilization

OPERATIVE PROCEDURES

The operations most frequently performed are those aimed at interrupting the continuity of the Fallopian tubes.

The Madlener operation is performed by crushing the middle third of the tube and tying it with a ligature.

The Pomeroy operation consists of excizing the middle third of the tube between two ligatures.

Irving's operation requires excision of a portion of the tube, with ligation of both cut ends and their burial; the distal end within the broad ligament and the proximal within the wall of the uterus.

The more complicated the operation, the lower the failure rate due to recanalization of the tubes. The most complex, that of Irving, has virtually no failure rate.

Bilateral salpingectomy is a more serious operation, but again is extremely effective.

Hysterectomy should be used only where uterine pathology such as fibroids co-exists, and would necessitate the operation in the future.

Laparoscopic sterilization

The use of the laparoscope for sterilization was first described by Dr Hans Frangenheim on the Continent and popularized by Mr Patrick Steptoe in this country. Under general anaesthesia, carbon dioxide or nitrous oxide gas is introduced into the peritoneal cavity through a needle. The laparoscope is introduced through a small incision below the umbilicus, and the uterus, tubes and ovaries examined visually. The diathermy forceps are passed through another small incision in the abdominal wall and one tube is coagulated. By means of a rigid instrument placed transvaginally within its cavity, the uterus may then be rotated to allow access to the remaining tube.

Steptoe (1970) reported a failure rate of 0.2 per cent for this method, as opposed to a rate of 0.4 per cent for the Pomeroy operation (Peel and Potts, 1970). Its great advantage lies in the minimal upset caused to the patients, almost all of them being able to leave hospital the day after the operation.

It is, however, a procedure not without dangers. The Medical Defence Union (1973) reported accidental burning of bowel, ureter and other structures, as well as direct trauma to major blood vessels during the introduction of the trocar and cannula through which the laparoscope is inserted. Laparoscopic sterilization should not be undertaken by the 'occasional' operator.

The operation may be technically very difficult or even impossible to perform in women who are grossly obese or who have undergone previous lower abdominal surgery, when adhesions may interfere with the circulation of gas within the peritoneal cavity. Indeed, unforseeable difficulties may arise in any patient, and for this reason all women on whom it is proposed to perform laparoscopic sterilization should be warned that formal laparotomy may be found necessary, and the consent form should be appropriately worded.

Other methods

Operations designed to obliterate the tube using an approach through the vagina and uterus have been designed. To obliterate the tubes, at or near the utero-tubal junction, heat (diathermy), cold (cryosurgery) and various chemicals have been used. Although such methods would have the advantage of being possible as out-patient procedures, the high failure rate so far makes them inferior to the conventional abdominal approach.

The approach through the vagina, using either colpotomy or culdoscopy to gain access to the tubes via the Pouch of Douglas, has not found favour in this country because of the restricted surgical field available in case of unexpected emergency.

Variations in the abdominal approach to the tubes have been described, including the use of a bivalve speculum, a proctoscope or a sigmoidoscope, with either ligatures or tantalum clips to occlude the tubes and avoid the dangers of diathermy. The small incisions necessary make some of these procedures possible under local anaesthesia, with consequent reduction of the patient's length of stay in hospital.

Immunization against pregnancy, by inducing antibodies to either trophoblast or spermatozoa, is an intriguing possibility and is being investigated in various centres.

All these methods must be considered as being only at the research stage at the moment.

Reversible procedures

At this moment in time sterilization operations should be regarded as irreversible, but a simple reversible procedure would constitute a highly effective method of birth control in patients unable to use any other method. Frangenheim (1964) has described tying the tubes with a polythene thread by means of forceps attached to a laparoscope, and also the application of tantalum clips to the tubes using the same method. Thread or clips may later be removed at laparoscopy, and tubal patency and function restored.

From America come reports of the injection of silicone via the uterus to form a firm mass occluding the lumina of the tubes, capable of later removal.

Various operations of ovariopexy have been attempted, and enclosure of the ovaries in silastic bags is referred to by McEwan *et al.* (1973).

Other experimental techniques are being investigated. Meanwhile reversal of the commonly used methods is not very successful. Tubal patency may be restored at operation, but tubal function often is not.

In any event, reversal of sterilization should rarely be necessary if the patient has been adequately counselled before operation. In addition, it is doubtful whether in this country valuable gynaecological time and effort should be expended on such a task at a time when there are long waiting lists for operations for such conditions as prolapse and fibroids.

Post-partum sterilization

Sterilization after confinement is often requested by women and this is a good time to perform the operation from the point of view of avoiding further interruption of her domestic life. The risk of thrombo-embolism following operations performed in the puerperium can be largely avoided by operating during the first three days of the puerperium. Neither Irving's operation nor laparoscopic sterilization are suitable at this time, due to the possibility of excessive bleeding. The patient should remain in hospital for a week after sterilization.

Sterilization may also be performed after termination of pregnancy and the laparoscopic method then is eminently suitable. Many older women and those who have completed their families accept the offer of sterilization with alacrity at such a time. The practice of offering termination only if the patient agrees to sterilization as well is a form of blackmail which happily seems to have disappeared since the Abortion Act.

Surgical risks of sterilization

There are no operations which carry no risk of sudden death, haemorrhage or infection, and operations for sterilization are no exception. Where the operation has been performed because of pre-existing disease the risk is increased because of the disease. In healthy women the risk to life or health of modern methods of sterilization properly performed is tiny.

Peel and Potts (1970) suggest the mortality rate following female sterilization is about one in five thousand operations.

Male sterilization

Vasectomy has become an extremely popular method of sterilization over the past decade. Indeed, it has become almost a status symbol. The vasectomy tie, the vasectomy wristwatch, the vasectomy badge - all are worn with pride by the vasectomized male - and sometimes, with cunning, by the unvasectomized.

Between 1960 and 1966 the Simon Population Trust (later to become the Crediton Project) reported 1,600 vasectomies; since then the operation has become almost commonplace. The difficulties in the early years were mainly due to a shortage of genito-urinary surgeons to perform the operations and the necessity for a general anaesthetic and hence admission to hospital or similar institution. Both these factors resulted in a high cost for the operation, charges of forty to sixty pounds being made.

The use of local anaesthesia has enabled all but the most nervous of males to be operated on as out-patients, and lesser mortals, trained by the genito-urinary surgeons, have proved quite capable of performing the operation. The establishment of 'VAS', the Vasectomy Advancement Society, under its enthusiastic chairman Dr Michael Altman, has done a great deal to promote the proper instruction and training of general practitioners in the performance of vasectomy.

The National Health Service, as is usual with all advances in fertility control, has lagged well behind, but in 1972 made vasectomy available for health reasons. Such organizations as the Family Planning Association and the International Planned Parenthood Federation set up vasectomy clinics, halving the previous charges, and were almost swamped by the demand. Predictably the local authorities stepped in and some provided the service to their ratepayers free of charge (i.e. as a charge on the rates). In 1974 vasectomy, as a form of birth control and not necessarily for health reasons, became available under the NHS.

Some indication of the numbers of operations being carried out in Britain is given by a report of 1,000 cases performed in little over a year, ending in 1972, at one centre in London. In America it is estimated that more than one million vasectomies are performed annually, and by 1973 thirteen million vasectomies had been performed in India. Such figures indicate that vasectomy has a significant part to play in world population growth control, as well as in the solution of personal birth control problems.

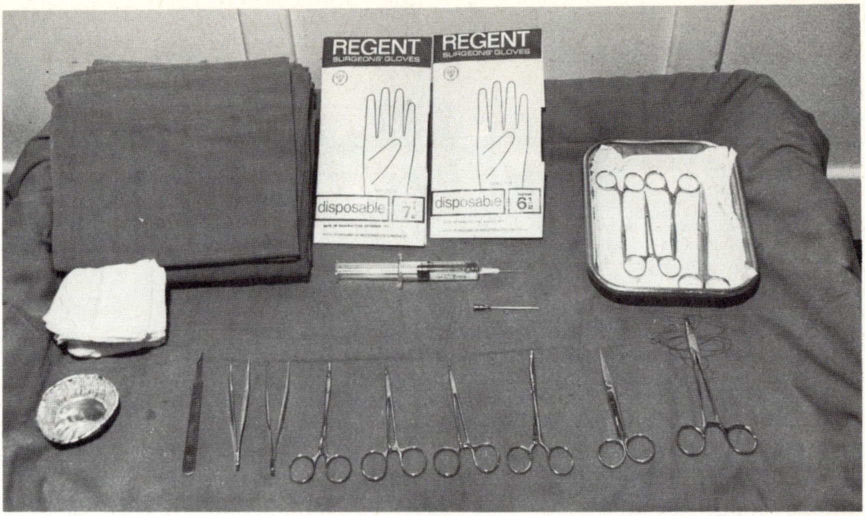

Fig. 32. Instruments required for vasectomy.

Operative methods

All methods are aimed at removal of a short portion of the vas deferens as it lies in the upper part of the scrotum. Differences in technique relate to the treatment of the cut ends, which may be ligated singly or doubly or doubled over and ligated; buried in different fascial planes, or passed across to the other side of the scrotum; occluded with tantalum clips, or plugged with silicone or plastic materials. The lumina of the cut ends may be treated with diathermy.

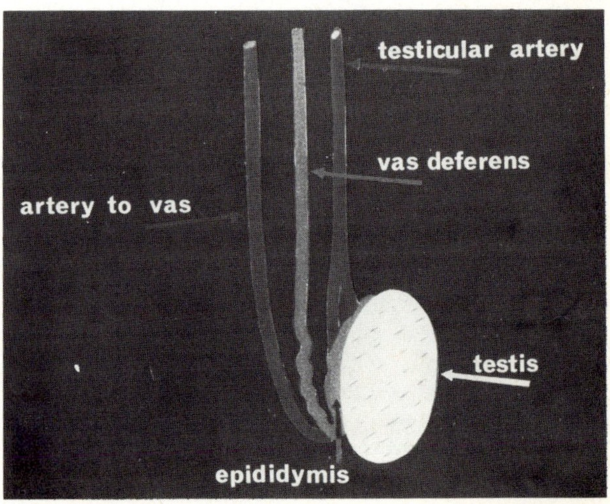

Fig. 33. Anatomy of the spermatic cord.

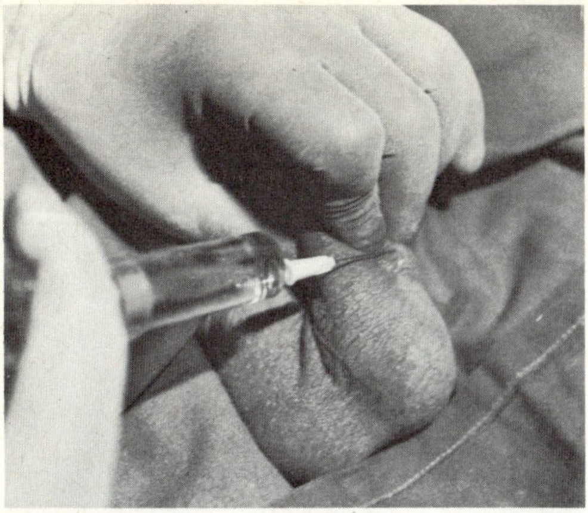

Fig. 34. Vas held beneath the skin by two fingers and local anaesthetic injected.

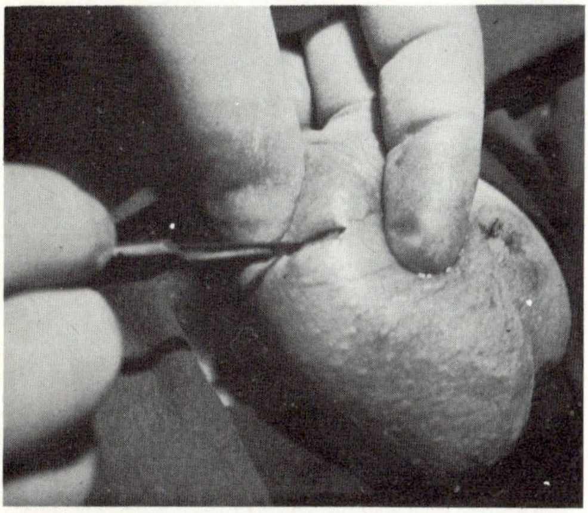

Fig. 35. Transverse incision 5 mm long across the line of vas.

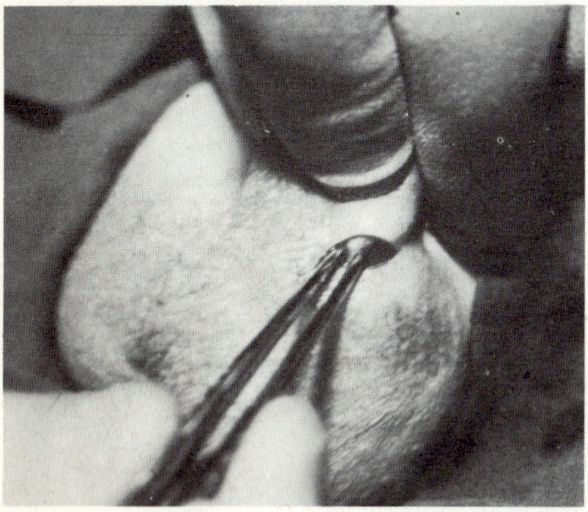

Fig. 36. Toothed forceps pulling vas out of incision.

Figs 32–40 and 42–44 are from 'Outpatient Vasectomy', a 35 mm colour filmstrip and slide set presented by Mr J. A. Newton and produced and published by Camera Talks Ltd.

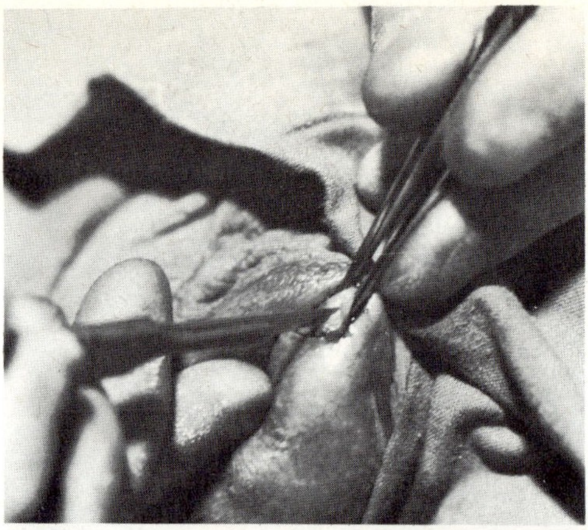

Fig. 37. Longitudinal incision 5 mm long through spermatic fascia.

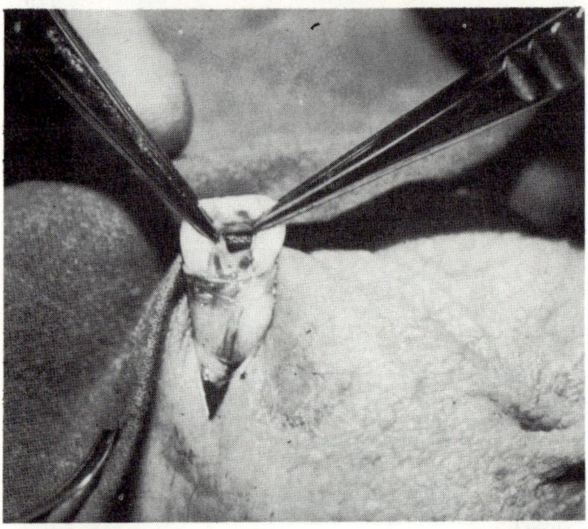

Fig. 38. Vas itself withdrawn through incisions.

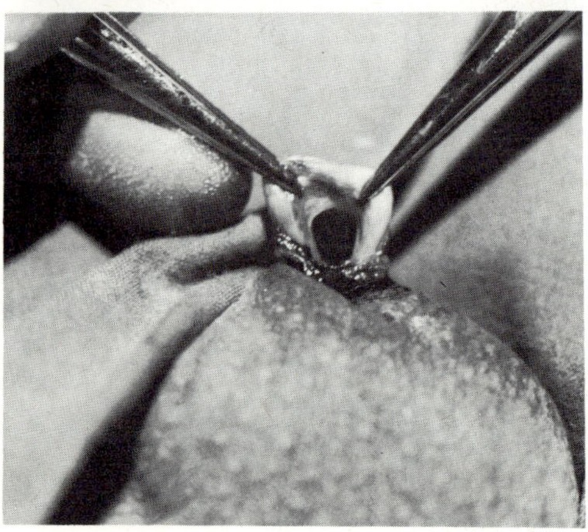

Fig. 39. Fascia cleaned from underside of vas. two artery forceps clamped at each end of loop, and loop divided near upper artery forceps.

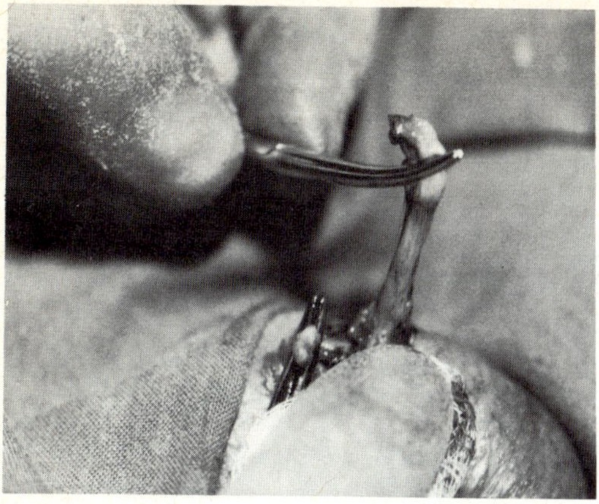

Fig. 40. Traction on lower portion of vas to display 3 cm length to be excised.

Before operation the general health of the patient should be assessed. The presence of diabetes or severe anaemia may have a bearing on the likelihood of subsequent infection. The presence of a hernia, varicocele or a large hydrocele, or previous operations in the area with possible distortion of the anatomy, must be considered. In such circumstances a local anaesthetic may not be suitable and the operation for vasectomy may be performed at the same time as the in-patient repair of the pathological condition. A history of sensitivity to local anaesthetics should be sought, and the presence of heart disease would make the addition of adrenalin to the local anaesthetic unwise.

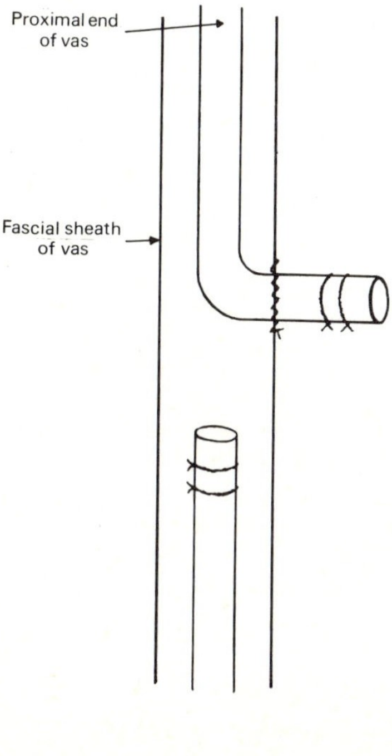

Fig. 41. Technique of burying cut ends of vas in different fascial planes.

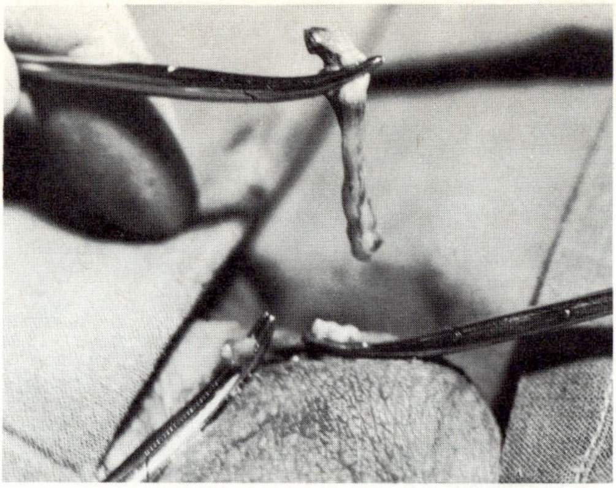

Fig. 42. Excised portion of vas, prior to placing in labelled container for histology.

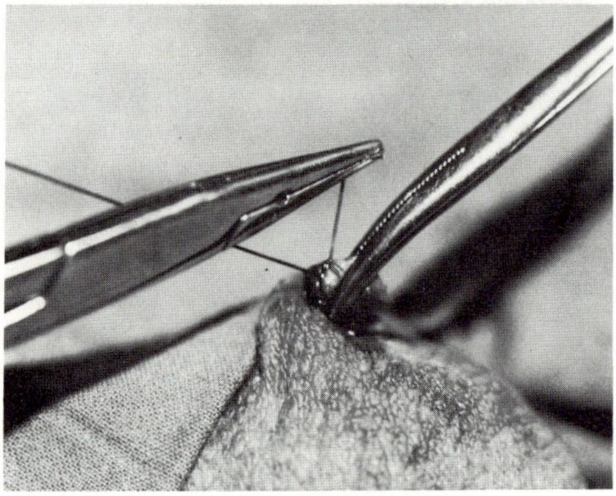

Fig. 43. Both ends of vas doubly ligatured with catgut.

The spermatic cord is palpated through the skin and a small transverse incision made over it. The sheath of the cord is incised longitudinally and the vas lifted out and dissected free of the other structures in the cord. The length of vas removed may be between one and four centimetres, some surgeons preferring to remove as little as possible to facilitate reconstruction later if required and some preferring to remove a larger amount in order to prevent the re-canalization of the vas.

Irrigation of the proximal end of the cut vas may be performed in order to accelerate the disappearance of spermatozoa from the semen. The irrigating fluid may be sterile water, euflavine or other spermicidal solution.

In order to avoid sperm granuloma formation and to facilitate reconstruction, some surgeons bury the cut end of the vas in different fascial planes. One end is doubly ligated and allowed to retract within the fascial sheath of the vas. The other end, also doubly ligated, is passed through to the outside of the fascial sheath which is then closed and stitched, the sutures fastening the vas in position with its cut end outside the fascial sheath (Fig. 41).

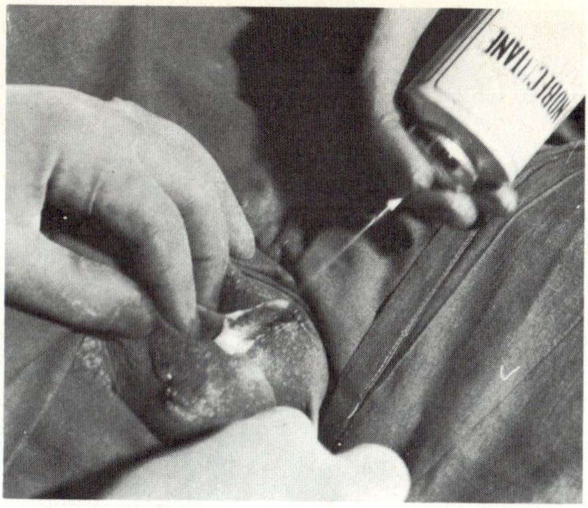

Fig. 44. Subcuticular skin sutures. Wound sprayed and plastic dressing.

The portion of vas removed must be sent for histological examination. Occasionally there is an extra vas deferens on one or both sides, and in such cases it might be legally imperative at a later stage to prove that the structure removed was indeed the vas. The testicular vein may be mistaken for the vas under certain circumstances.

The skin is then sutured, subcuticular absorbable sutures being much appreciated by the patient. Strict attention to haemostasis is most important at all stages of the operation in order to avoid subsequent haematoma formation, with possible infection. The operation is then repeated on the other side.

The patient should rest during the next day, but will be able to return to his work, other than the heaviest types of manual labour, the day after that. Clinics should be held on Friday evenings to enable men to avoid missing work. A scrotal support should be worn for two weeks after operation to avoid dragging pain which otherwise may occur.

Complications of the operation

Haemorrhage may result in the formation of a haemotoma beneath the skin. Small haematoma are common, and most absorb satisfactorily. Larger ones may cause extreme pain, and because of this, and the possibility that infection may supervene, should be evacuated. Superficial haemorrhage from the skin edges sometimes occurs, resulting in a call to the family doctor. Local pressure by the patient deals with such bleeding quite easily. About five per cent of patients develop haemorrhagic complications, but the majority of these are mild in degree.

Infection may follow the operation, either beneath the skin of the scrotum or as an epididymitis. The latter may in some cases be due to bacterial infection; in others it may represent a 'back-pressure' phenomenon due to the sudden obstruction to the outflow from the semeniferous tubules.

Sperm granuloma (Schmidt, 1966) may affect the cut end of the vas.

A series of 1000 vasectomies under local anaesthesia performed on out-patients attending the Margaret Pyke Centre in London was reported in 1973. The incidence of haematoma requiring treatment was 0.7 per cent, of sepsis 1.2 per cent and of other minor local symptoms 5.6 per cent.

Post-operative supervision

Spermatozoa do not disappear from the seminal fluid immediately after operation, appearing from the seminal vesicles, prostate, the posterior urethra and its glands for some time. The length of time during which they appear varies.

Factors which are reported to increase the speed of their disappearance include the age of the patient (in general the younger the quicker), the number of ejaculations the patient has enjoyed since operation (in general the more the better), and irrigation of the vas at operation.

Craft and McQueen (1972) used sterile water to irrigate the proximal end of the vas and reported that following this procedure, a greater proportion of men had negative seminal analyses at both 12 and 15 weeks after operation, compared with men who had not been irrigated. Urquhart-Hay (1973) used euflavine as the irrigant fluid, and reported no motile spermatozoa in any seminal specimens collected at intervals of between 10 and 158 days after operation. Irrigation is not a generally accepted procedure at most clinics, however, because of the possible risk of infection.

There is considerable debate at the moment as to the significance of the finding of non-motile spermatozoa - are they really dead or may they have been motile in the body before ejaculation? - and as to the significance of finding only occasional spermatozoa, that is, a condition of induced oligozoospermia, known to result in infertility anyway.

Dead spermatozoa take up vital dyes such as trypan blue, but some non-motile spermatozoa do not take up such dyes, and are therefore questionably dead. Frozen sperm from 'sperm banks' are non-motile but on thawing motility may return.

Finally there is argument as to whether semen should be centrifuged before microscopy or examined plain on a slide. These questions will no doubt be answered in time, and repeated seminal analysis following vasectomy will possibly be unnecessary in the future.

Meantime the procedure adopted by most clinics is that after operation the patient is presented with a clean plastic or glass jar with a secure stopper, and instructed to attend the clinic with a specimen of semen in three months time. During the waiting period he should have intercourse regularly, a minimum of twelve ejaculations being suggested. The importance of continuing contraception until his operation is pronounced successful is emphasized.

The patient should be told that the seminal specimen may be produced either by masturbation, or by withdrawal at coitus. Collection of specimens in a condom should be discouraged as the lubricant may interfere with sperm motility. The specimen should reach the laboratory as soon after collection as possible, and should be examined without delay.

Techniques for examination differ. If uncentrifuged, relatively large quantities of seminal fluid must be examined, and use of a low-power lens is more convenient. At King's College Hospital twelve high-power fields of a centrifuged specimen are examined. The presence of spermatozoa, their numbers and their motility should be recorded. Their morphology is, of course, unimportant.

Seminal examination should be performed at three months, and thereafter at monthly intervals until two consecutive negative specimens are obtained. A negative specimen is defined as one in which NO spermatozoa are found. 75 per cent of men will produce negative specimens at three and four months after operation. A further 10 per cent will be negative at four months and five months. 5 per cent more will be negative at five months and six months. The remaining 10 per cent will include those who are lost to follow-up, and those who are still producing spermatozoa six months after operation.

If the spermatozoa are motile, or if non-motile are present in large number - say ten or more - the patient must be questioned as to frequence of coitus. Assuming that he has been ejaculating with a satisfactory frequency, then the operation must be pronounced a failure and re-operation under general anaesthesia as an in-patient advised.

Persisting motile spermatozoa

There may be three explanations of the persistence of motile spermatozoa after vasectomy.

1. The structure divided was not the vas. A histological report will settle this question.
2. There was a third vas present in that particular patient which has not been divided. This is a very rare cause, occurring in about 0.1 per cent of cases.
3. Re-canalization of the properly divided vas has taken place. This is a rarity, occurring in less than one per cent of patients according to published series.

It is especially liable to result from the formation of a sperm granuloma, which may contain cavities lined with epithelial cells, communicating with each other, and eventually growing to communicate with the lumina at the ends of the divided vas. Such a situation is more likely where the cut ends have not been buried in different fascial planes, and only a short section of vas has been excized. Presumably also the length of time needed for epithelial growth to bridge the gap will depend on the length of vas removed. Examination of seminal fluid too early may not detect the reappearance of motile spermatozoa later.

Persisting non-motile spermatozoa
The presence of non-motile spermatozoa in large numbers presents no difficulty - the operation must be repeated. The difficulty arises where only one or two non-motile sperm are found in successive specimens, or where such specimens alternate with the others containing no sperm at all. From a medical point of view, the chances that pregnancy would result from a patient oligozoospermic to this degree must be exceedingly remote. However, every doctor performing this operation must bear in mind the possibility that his assessment of its success may have to be justified in a court of law, so he must tell the patient that his operation has not been demonstrated to be entirely successful.

The situation should be carefully explained to the patient, who may choose to accept his oligozoospermia as adequate. If not, a further series of monthly checks may eventually result in two consecutive negative specimens. If it does not, then admission for further operation will be necessary.

Post-operative seminal analysis
From what has been written above it would seem that post-operative seminal analysis must not be expected to reveal definite evidence of permanent sterility. The most that can be expected is either evidence of *probable* sterility - as evidenced by complete absence of spermatozoa or low counts of non-motile spermatozoa - or clear evidence of failure of the operation - as evidenced by the continuing presence of motile sperms. Hence the importance of emphasizing to the patient beforehand that no guarantee of success will be forthcoming, either before or after operation.

Reversal of vasectomy
Attempts to devise reliably reversible methods of sterilization are being undertaken but so far no such operation exists. Reconstruction of the vas is possible in cases where a minimal amount of vas has been removed and many surgeons claim a high success rate for the restoration of vasal continuity after vaso-vasostomy. But the reappearance of motile sperm in the ejaculate must not be equated with fertility and the successful restoration of fertility is not so frequent, only one quarter of apparently successful operations being followed by pregnancy in the consort. More favourable results have been reported by surgeons in India.

Testicular damage and alterations in hormonal balance have been reported to follow ligation of the vasa of rats, and sperm agglutinating and immobilizing antibodies have been found in men after vasectomy. The significance of these findings is not yet clear but they may explain cases where the apparently successful operation is not accompanied by the expected fertility.

As with female sterilization, it is doubtful whether attempts to restore fertility in adequately counselled males is justifiable in the United Kingdom at a time when surgical skills are in short supply and waiting lists for prostatectomy and other genito-urinary operations are long.

REQUESTS FOR STERILIZATION

Ten years ago most requests for vasectomy came from men in social Classes I and II. The publicity from the Simon Population Trust and other organizations, added to the appearances on television of vasectomized men extolling the virtues of the operation, resulted in a greater spread of awareness of the existence of this method of family restriction. Men from social Classes III, IV and V began to make enquiries about, and undergo, the operation. Men from social Class V, however, constituted only two per cent of the men undergoing vasectomy in the Simon Population Trust series, and also in another series at King's College Hospital, London.

Nevertheless there is still considerable reluctance to be sterilized on the part of males compared with females, although the man who steadfastly refuses to entertain vasectomy for himself will often cheerfully agree to his wife's sterilization. Women of course do the actual child-bearing, and so, especially in multiparous women, the choice is between pregnancy, labour and looking after the baby on the one hand and a simple operation on the other. To choose the simple operation from these two alternatives is possibly easier than to choose, as must the man, between a simple operation and no effort on his part at all. Laziness, and a feeling that to prevent further pregnancies is her job, not his, are in part the reasons for male unwillingness to submit to vasectomy.

Ignorance of anatomy and physiology, and therefore of the effects to be expected from the operation, are another cause. To many men, sterilization is castration and will, they believe, be followed by impotence, loss of masculinity and his image - to females, other males and himself - as the master, as he who impregnates. West Indian immigrant males belonging to the lower social classes are particularly opposed to vasectomy, probably due to the reasons enumerated above, but also because many of them originate from a culture that still venerates fertility for its own sake.

Simple cowardice, so often evident in the male's attitude to application for contraceptive advice, is possibly a cause for some male reluctance to undergo vasectomy and is certainly a cause for his failure to initiate discussion on vasectomy in many cases, the wife being deputed to raise the matter with the doctor and bring home the information for discussion between them.

Doctors should be a little careful under such circumstances. The reporting to the husband of what the doctor said may not be entirely accurate. Such phrases as 'The Doctor says you ought to have it done' may result from free interpretation of the doctor's opinion that vasectomy would be suitable as a solution of that couple's fertility problems. Before answering any questions, the doctor should attempt to obtain from the wife some idea of whether the suggestion originated from her or from her husband and whether he is keen, lukewarm or antipathetic to vasectomy. Then can be given the information about the operation, coupled with a stern warning that the wife who nags or otherwise pressurizes her husband into vasectomy is asking for trouble. Better for her to stay on the Pill for another twenty years than spend them with an antagonistic, frigid, impotent, vasectomized consort.

Once he is reasonably sure that the husband looks on the idea of vasectomy with favour, the family doctor should extend an open invitation to him to come and discuss it. Following this discussion, or in place of it if the wife can assure the doctor that her husband is keen on the idea, and that none of the information he has given her is likely to make the husband change his mind, an appointment for counselling may be made.

The importance of the husband being a volunteer rather than a conscript has been emphasized. The willing agreement of the wife to her husband's operation is of course of equal importance.

> A patient was referred by an agency outside general practice for vasectomy. The couple were interviewed at a clinic and vasectomy agreed. Some days later the wife appeared in the surgery of the GP, burst into tears and begged him to prevent the surgeon performing the operation. She claimed that her husband had overruled her timid objections, and she had not dared to voice them in the clinic as 'They all seemed to think vasectomy was the right thing.'
>
> A personal letter from the GP to the surgeon at the clinic solved the wife's problem.

In this case, thoughtlessness and insensitivity on the part of the husband was, I am sure, the reason for the near tragedy. However, sterilization may on occasions be a deliberate attempt by one partner to hurt the other, and the doctor must be careful to avoid being made the instrument of that hurt.

Requests for sterilization from female patients were once rare in general practice, and almost always from women who had more than three children. Of recent years, the publicity accorded male sterilization has been noted by the female and, presumably feeling that what was sauce for the gander must be sauce for the goose, many more women are today requesting sterilization as a means of family limitation. I have noted a great increase in the number of young women, aged less than thirty, with only two or perhaps three children, who ask for sterilization.

I feel that any request for sterilization by a female should be countered by the doctor with the suggestion that the male should undergo operation, as vasectomy is less dangerous, less complex and less expensive than even laparoscopic sterilization. Only when it has been ascertained that operation on the male is out of the question should female sterilization be considered.

Much of what has been said concerning requests for male sterilization applies equally to the female. No woman should be nagged, either by her husband or her medical attendant, into sterilization against her will. Sterilization is more acceptable to the higher social classes than the lower, but the difference between the classes is less marked in female sterilization than in male. Particularly is this so of West Indian immigrants, women accepting sterilization far more readily than their male consorts, but usually after a greater family size has been achieved than in the case of their white counterparts. West Indian men, however, often object to the sterilization of their wives, a situation rarely seen among the white native population of these islands. Ideally both partners should agree to sterilization, but where it is being performed for medical reasons rather than as permanent contraception, the written consent of the woman alone is enough.

SATISFACTION FOLLOWING STERILIZATION

Most series report a very low incidence of dissatisfaction following operation. Many women say they wish that it had been performed earlier, before their family had reached its present size. Most men proclaim themselves well satisfied after vasectomy, and almost all – providing no painful complications arose – say they would recommend it to their friends.

Regret following sterilization is seen

1. Where the operation was not wholeheartedly desired by the patient.
2. When the sterilization was requested as a solution to sexual problems other than those arising from excessive fertility. The difficulty here is to be quite certain that this is the true and only cause of the sexual problem. Fear of pregnancy may be only a secondary cause of a disorder such as frigidity in women or inability to achieve erection in men, and removal of this cause by sterilization may merely unmask the primary cause without improving the sexual disability.
3. Several authors have suggested that the existence of emotional instability or psychiatric abnormality before sterilization is associated with adverse psychiatric sequelae to the operation. Sim *et al.* (1973) pointed out that in many of these series there was a high incidence of sterilization either with abortion or during the post-partum period, whereas in a series of 151 patients, none of whom underwent post-partum or post-abortal sterilization, the incidence of adverse psychiatric sequelae was very low (3.3 per cent) even though 23 per cent of the patients had a history of depression and anxiety prior to sterilization.

Sim makes the suggestion that in order to minimize the incidence of adverse psychiatric reaction, interval sterilization should be performed after confinement or termination of pregnancy rather than at the time.

My own experience indicates that sterilization at or immediately after termination of pregnancy is rarely, if ever, followed by depression or regret provided no question of a 'package deal' arises ('You may have the abortion you want provided you submit to sterilization as well') and provided the unwanted pregnancy occurred after the patient's desired family size had been achieved.

In any event, when considering the effect of performing sterilization, one has to take into account the possible sequelae of failing to perform sterilization. Women suffering from recurrent episodes of depression or anxiety state are unlikely to use contraception either regularly or efficiently and repeated unwanted pregnancies would certainly have a greater total adverse psychiatric and physical effect than sterilization.

Adequate counselling before operation is essential in all cases, but in patients with a history of psychiatric disturbance it is important to make sure that the counselling does not take place at a time when the patient is in the throes of a depressive episode, including either post-abortal or post-partum depression. Provided counselling and operation do not take place at such a time, a previous history of emotional instability does not seem to be associated with a high incidence of psychiatric sequelae after operation.

These groups apart, patients who have been sterilized report they feel that their general health and happiness, their enjoyment of life in general and sexual activities in particular, have been unimpaired, or sometimes improved.

There is no reason for abnormalities of menstruation to follow female sterilization by interruption of tubal patency. Reports of such sequelae probably indicate poor selection of cases and poor pre-operative counselling and any symptoms are due to the undoubted influence of the emotions on the menstrual functions.

The fear that increased promiscuity will follow sterilization has not been capable of demonstration in follow-up studies. There is no doubt that the libertine, male or female, will be no less of a libertine following sterilization, but there is no evidence that normally responsible people become libertines because of it. Indeed, sexual responsibility is seated within the skull, so operations on the genital tract should not be expected to have any effect.

SHOULD THE GP SUGGEST STERILIZATION?

In practice the suggestion to sterilize in cases of maternal or inherited disease is made at the hospital and the GP usually plays a small part in the decision, although the patient may seek confirmation of the hospital advice from the family doctor. Again sterilization is usually offered to grand multiparae at hospital, but if the GP raises the matter before sending his patient for booking it allows her more time to consider it.

Patients who request the family doctor's help to obtain an abortion, especially the multiparous patient who has completed her family, may accept the suggestion of sterilization gladly. Women who have completed their family but fail to find any of the present contraceptive methods to their liking, or who persistently run the risk of unwanted pregnancy due to inefficient use of an effective method, are often grateful for the suggestion of sterilization. In addition, women who have completed their family and are faced with many years of effective contraception welcome the suggestion of sterilization instead. These women may be quite young, having had all the children they want by their early twenties. The GP may realize that the woman attending his surgery for a check-up for the Pill has been doing so for the last eight or ten years, is now only in her early thirties, and thus is faced with another two decades of oral contraception. Such women are sometimes grateful for the offer of sterilization.

All these are patients in whom sterilization should be suggested by the family doctor. The circumstances have been related to the female because it is the female who usually makes the contact with the doctor, but the sterilization offered may of course be of the male consort. Women still seem to have the idea that they may be 'allowed' sterilization and thus wait for the suggestion to be made to them by others. The male approach to the doctor is quite different. He rarely attends for contraceptive advice, but once he considers vasectomy may be a suitable solution of his problems he simply asks the doctor for it. Today many men ask for vasectomy in order to protect their wives from the necessity for long-term contraception: 'She's done it all so far, Doctor. Now it's my turn.'

SHOULD THE GP REFUSE HIS CONSENT TO STERILIZATION?

There are rare occasions when the GP should refuse his consent to sterilizing operations proposed and arranged for his patients by organizations outside general practice. Sterilization as part of an abortion deal is an obvious example. Occasionally his superior knowledge of the patients over many years may make him feel that sterilization may have disastrous results, and he should insist on discussing the matter with the surgeons.

Some men decide to undergo vasectomy during the last months of their wife's pregnancy, in order that their period of waiting for negative seminal specimens may coincide with the weeks before and after delivery. I regard this as tempting providence, and invariably advise them to wait until the baby is safely delivered and a few weeks old.

Patients requesting sterilization at an early age, with a small family, are others to whom I often suggest a postponement of operation. If after six months they are still of the same mind, then I would not stand in their way. I feel unhappy about agreeing to sterilization in such patients immediately after confinement; babies are not babies for very long and although a young mother may feel that she wants no more when she has a babe in arms, she may feel very differently when babe has toddled off to school and left her alone at home.

Of course, many such women look forward to this day, so that they can return to work and escape from their domestic prison. Such differences in patient attitudes emphasize the necessity to assess each request for sterilization on its merits and the absurdity of attempts to conform to sets of rules. Once again, the importance of counselling must be emphasized.

COUNSELLING BEFORE STERILIZATION

Counselling is a complex activity. It involves the extraction of information from the patient and the imparting of information to the patient; an assessment of the degree of understanding by the patient of the factors involved; consideration of the expressed wishes of the patient and an assessment by the counsellor as to whether the patient has made an informed decision.

Counselling should not mean making decisions on behalf of patients. It does not even mean helping patients to make the correct decision because even counsellors are human and therefore fallible. Neither does it mean persuading patients to agree with the decision of the counsellor: a patient may well wish to follow a course of action which would be the last one that the counsellor himself would choose.

On the other hand, sterilization on demand is undesirable because the patients' decision may be uninformed, based on inadequate or incorrect information. The validity of the arguments used by the patient in reaching a decision should be tested by the counsellor, armed with experience gained from counselling others, and from other counsellors.

Counselling a patient who requests sterilization means an attempt to ensure that the patient has all the information required to make a decision, and after consideration of all other possibilities and likely eventualities, has voluntarily reached an informed decision that is unlikely to be regretted in future.

In practice, the final decision reached by the patient is usually one with which the councellor readily agrees. Fortunately, there is rarely any need to reach decisions in a hurry (unlike the situation existing in abortion counselling), and in cases where the counsellor feels certain that the patient's decision is unwise, it is possible to delay. Telling the patients to think it over and return six months later also gives time for the counsellor to consider, to take further advice and marshall further argument. Except after termination of unwanted pregnancy, some element of delay should be built in to any sterilization procedure, to enable changes of mind. Interval sterilization after childbirth has already been referred to: 30 of the 1140 couples accepted for vasectomy at the Margaret Pyke Centre in 1973 changed their minds while awaiting operation.

Counselling procedure

The couple should attend for counselling together, and the counsellor should beware of the dominant partner who answers all the questions on behalf of both. Such a situation may merely indicate that the couple has agreed that one of them will do all the talking, but it may also indicate that one partner normally makes all the decisions. In the consideration of sterilization it is essential that both partners make decisions.

In cases where sterilization may be performed on eugenic grounds, or because of maternal disease, the severity of these indications may outweigh all other considerations. The remarks which follow refer to patients for whom sterilization is being considered purely as a method of fertility control.

Relevant factors in sterilization counselling

Among factors which may be relevant in a consideration of sterilization for any particular couple are the following:

Age

That there are limits beyond which sterilization should not be considered is obvious. Reports from the United States in 1973 of the sterilization of coloured girls in their early 'teens highlights this. Equally, to sterilize a woman of 49 would seem to be somewhat superfluous. But there are no age limits which apply equally to all men and to all women; the circumstances of each individual must be taken into account in any consideration of age. The attitude of society in general, and the medical profession in particular, changes also, so that sterilization might be thought unsuitable for one patient at one time, but suitable for a similar patient of the same age a few years later.

> In 1966 I referred to a consultant gynaecologist a patient of 26, deserted by her husband, who had five children, one of them mentally retarded, one an epileptic. She had requested sterilization and I strongly backed her request. Her request was refused because she was too young. It seems unlikely that any gynaecologist would refuse on such grounds today.

The relative age of the partners has significance. Faced with a husband of forty married to a wife in her early twenties, vasectomy for him would seem reasonable whereas tubal ligation for her would not.

In general, men retain their fertility longer than women, and so although sterilization after the age of fifty would not be entertained for a woman, it is a reasonable request for a man for at least a further decade.

Marriage

Whether a couple have gone through a marriage ceremony or not has little relevance as an indication for sterilization. Of far more importance is the stability and duration of the relationship.

It is of interest that most vasectomy clinics today seem to have the same attitude as contraceptive clinics of a decade ago, offering their services only to married men. There would seem to be little justification for this; the man who frequently changes sexual partners and avoids marriage being particularly likely to father unplanned and unwanted children. Should such a man request vasectomy I see no reason why his request should not be granted, providing he has passed the immature 'wild oat sowing' stage, and provided he accepts the operation as irreversible.

Parity

Couples having large families often state that the later arrivals were unplanned, and such evidence of previous failure to limit their families to the desired size is certainly evidence of their need for sterilization. Whatever the family size, however, if the couple is certain that for them it represents the ideal, then sterilization should be available. In my view this applies equally to couples whose desired family size is zero, provided they are responsible mature adults, have had adequate time to consider the matter, and accept the operation as irreversible. Professional people in particular may find their work provides complete fulfilment, and there are some couples who just do not like children.

The number and ages of any children should be recorded, as should the numbers of stillbirths or neonatal deaths, miscarriages or terminations.

In general, the presence of a long gap since the birth of the last child, or a history of one or more terminations since then, indicates that the decision to limit the family has already been taken, and sterilization is being requested to replace permanent contraception.

Previous medical and obstetric history

Details of previous operations should be recorded. A history of operations in the scrotal area which may complicate matters, and make use of local anaesthesia unwise, should be sought in all applicants for vasectomy. Adhesions due to operations in the pelvis may prevent the safe passage of the laparoscope and make Steptoe sterilization impossible.

An obstetric history, with details of any abnormalities in pregnancy or the performance of any obstetric procedures should be noted. Occasionally discussion of such details has unexpected results.

> A couple in their mid-twenties requested vasectomy. They maintained no more children were wanted, the wife in particular proclaiming that one was enough. She gave a history of prolonged and painful labour lasting 36 hours ending with a forceps delivery under (apparently inefficient) local anaesthesia. I sympathized with her and remarked that such labours were rare after the first pregnancy and today women were fortunately able to have epidural analgesia at the local maternity hospital.
>
> 'In that case,' said she, 'I want another one! Come along dear!'
>
> As he was swept out of the door, her husband was heard to say 'But I thought you wanted me to, darling.'

Contraceptive practice

Information should be obtained as to the method of contraception, if any, being used at the moment, and methods used in the past. Ignorance of available methods may in rare cases have led to the decision to request sterilization, as also may an exaggerated, ill-informed fear of oral contraception. Correction of such misinformation may result in the withdrawal of a mistaken application.

More often is the finding that the patients have tried many methods, but find fault with all, and since all methods have their faults and failings, this is not an unreasonable basis for a decision to request sterilization.

Today vasectomy may be requested as permanent contraception by a couple using an effective method efficiently – again not an unreasonable basis for their request.

Sex life

Questions should be put regarding frequency of intercourse, satisfaction obtained by both partners and the presence of any difficulties. As already mentioned, sterilization must not be regarded as a cure for difficulties in sexual relationships or performance, and the presence of such difficulties should indicate postponement of operation pending their investigation.

Religion

If the patient has got as far as attending the doctor with a request for sterilization, it is probable that they have already come to terms with their religious convictions, but it is well to ensure as far as possible that they entertain no lingering doubts or uncertainties.

Difficulties may arise where the two partners are of differing religions, sterilization requested by the one being regarded as a sin by the other.

Racial differences

Reference has already been made to the infrequent appearance of the West Indian male as an applicant for vasectomy, and the relatively more frequent request for sterilization by the female. Care must be taken, however, in agreeing to sterilization in West Indian women as fertility, to West Indian male eyes, seems to be a very desirable attribute in the female, even when the fertility has been demonstrated to excess when judged by native British standards.

Classical questions

As rumour has it, all conscientious objectors were asked the question 'What would you do if you saw one of the enemy attempting to rape your sister?' In a similar way, there are two questions which must be asked of all requesting sterilization:

1. 'Suppose your children were all killed in a car crash; would you not then regret being sterilized?' The answer, of course, is that in such an unlikely event, regret at being sterilized would be as nothing compared to the regret at the death of the children, and anyway the production of further children would merely substitute for the originals, not replace them. All women requesting sterilization find it possible to give a firm negative answer to this question.
2. 'Suppose your husband/wife dies and you marry again; would you not then regret being sterilized?' This question presupposes two events, at least one of which is unlikely. Women reply that if the first happened, then they would choose to marry a man who did not want children.

These questions, far-fetched as they are, should nevertheless be put to all applicants. They ensure that the future has received consideration as well as the past, and certainly any applicants unable to give a negative answer should be pressed to reconsider operation.

Reversible sterilization would render these questions obsolete. To my mind, the occurrence of such rare and unforseeable circumstances constitutes the only reason today for attempting to reverse sterilization in an adequately counselled person.

Information to be given to the patient

A brief explanation of the normal anatomy and the operative procedure should be given. In the female it should be emphasized that menstruation will not be affected, nor will the menopause be induced. The ovaries will remain intact, producing their hormones as usual. The egg will still be produced each month, but because the tube along which it usually progresses to the womb is to be blocked, it will be absorbed from the abdominal cavity.

In the male, it should be pointed out that the operation is not one of castration. The testis will remain and will continue to produce hormones and sperm, which, because the tube carrying them to the penis is cut, will be absorbed again. Nevertheless, because a large amount of the ejaculate consists of secretions from the prostate and elsewhere, orgasm will be accompanied by emission as usual.

In both sexes it should be emphasized that sexual feelings and performance originate in the brain, which will not be operated on, and are mediated by the nerves, which will not be cut. No effect on sex life may therefore be expected, other than a beneficial one due to release from the fear of pregnancy.

It must be made abundantly clear to the applicants that one hundred per cent success following operation is not guaranteed, and that a further operation may in rare cases be necessary. As with any operation, unexpected complications may arise, but although this should be stated honestly, it should not be dwelt upon unduly.

Men awaiting vasectomy should then be told to come to operation already shaved and to make arrangements to have a day away from work afterwards. The routine arrangements in force at the clinic with regard to the collection and examination of post-operative seminal specimens, and their timing, should be explained. The necessity to continue intercourse and the necessity to use efficient contraception during this period must be made clear to the patient. The method of contraception to be used may usefully be agreed at this interview.

Counselling—at the surgery or at the clinic?

Because he may have known the patients for years, looked after them during childhood, during pregnancy, during illness, may know their social and family circumstances, and has all their medical records to hand, the family doctor is the ideal person to counsel the couple requesting sterilization.

However, it must be admitted that some family doctors do not feel able to find the time for counselling for sterilization, or have religious or conscientious objections to the operation. Their patients must be counselled elsewhere, either by neighbouring interested GPs or at a clinic specially set up for the purpose.

Should the family doctor's permission be obtained before operation?
Ethically there is no doubt that no surgeon should operate on another doctor's patient (other than in cases where failure to operate may mean death or serious damage to health) without first obtaining the doctor's permission. Counselling agencies report that outright refusal by doctors to give permission is unusual. In such cases I feel that the doctor should be approached in order to ascertain the reason for his refusal. It may be that he is aware of circumstances of which the clinic is in ignorance, or for some other reason feels it is in the patient's interest to refuse his permission.

> I refused permission for a clinic run by a charity organization to perform vasectomy on one of my patients. I was aware (and the patient was not) that the local authority paid the cost of vasectomy for their residents, of whom my patient was one, at an equally excellent clinic elsewhere. By refusing my permission to one clinic and directing him to another my working class patient with three small children was able to spend £25 on his family instead of on vasectomy fees.

Should the family doctor be notified that his patient has requested an appointment at a vasectomy clinic?
Undoubtedly the answer should be in the affirmative and the following case history shows why.

> Mr S, aged 34, married with two children, sought my advice because of a swelling in his scrotum. The surgeon to whom I referred him put him on the waiting list for removal of the cyst of the epididymis. Meanwhile, unknown to me, Mrs S requested the advice of someone at the local authority welfare clinic regarding vasectomy for her husband. This clinic worker arranged an appointment for Mr S at the local vasectomy clinic.
>
> The genito-urinary surgeon was quicker off the mark, admitted Mr S and operated on his epididymal cyst. After his discharge from hospital Mr S happened to mention to me that he had an appointment for vasectomy counselling the following week.
>
> That the vas and the epididymis are connected was unknown to Mr S, but he was somewhat displeased to learn that had I known he wished vasectomy both operations could easily have been performed at the same time.

Legalities
There is no law regarding sterilization comparable to the Abortion Act. For some time it was feared that sterilization might be unlawful in some circumstances, for example, if performed simply for fertility control. Counsel's opinion was sought by the defence societies in 1960, and as a result there now seems no reason to believe that sterilization for such a reason would be regarded as illegal.

However, it is essential that both husband and wife give written consent to the sterilization of either before the operation is performed.

The only exceptions are in cases where the operation is to be performed to preserve the life or health of one partner, or where husband and wife are divorced or separated, when the signature of the patient undergoing operation will suffice.

REFERENCES

CRAFT, I. and McQUEEN, J. (1973). Effect of irrigation of the vas on post-vasectomy semen-counts. *Lancet,* **i,** 515.

FRANGENHEIM, H. (1964). *Geburtshilfe und Frauenheilkunde,* **24,** 470.

McEWAN, J., NEWTON, J., and ELIAS, J. (1973). Contraception today: sterilization. *Update,* May, 1459.

MEDICAL DEFENCE UNION (1973). *Annual Report,* p. 16.

PEEL, J. and POTTS, M. (1970). *Textbook of Contraceptive Practice.* Cambridge University Press.

SCHMIDT, S. S. (1966). *Fertility & Sterility,* **17.**

SIM, M., EMENS, J. M. and JORDAN, J. A. (1973). *British Medical Journal,* **3,** 220.

STEPTOE, P. C. (1970). Recent advances in surgical methods of controlling fertility and infertility. *British Medical Bulletin,* **26,** 60.

URQUHART-HAY, D. (1973). *British Medical Journal,* **3,** 378.

13

ABORTION

The Offences against the Person Act of 1861 made any attempt to procure a miscarriage a felony unless performed by a duly qualified and registered medical practitioner 'in good faith, and for the purpose only of preserving the life of the mother'.

It is worth remembering that this Act dictated the behaviour of the medical profession for over a century. Doctors were sent warning notices by the General Medical Council in which abortion was classed as one of the five deadly sins for which doctors could be struck off the register. It is not surprising that the passing of the Abortion Act in 1967, with its very much more liberal attitude to abortion, resulted in a situation that many doctors, especially older doctors who had been in practice for many years, found difficult to accept. To find that an 'illegal operation' as abortion was often called, was no longer illegal was an enormous change in itself. But associated with this change was an even greater one: where a family doctor had previously been commended by society for refusing to aid and abet a patient in obtaining an abortion unless her life was at stake, with the threat of erasure from the register if he did, the same doctor now found that it was his duty to advise and assist patients needing abortion under the Act, and society condemned him for failing to do so.

Naturally doctors who qualified during the years when Abortion was an 'illegal operation' were taught nothing of the counselling of women requesting it, and little of the indications, methods or complications of the procedure. As a result many advisory organizations came into existence, counselling women with unwanted pregnancies and arranging terminations. Some were run on a charitable basis, and some were frankly commercial. In general, the charities attacked the medical profession for their indifference, and the medical profession in turn attacked the commercial operators for their greed.

The Abortion Act 1967 became law in 1968. The major change brought about by the passing of this Act has been that in assessing a woman's need for abortion, not only the threat to her life presented by the pregnancy may be taken into account, but also the threat to the health, mental or physical, of both the patient and her existing children. The possibility that the pregnancy may result in a severely handicapped child also may be considered. In the years since 1967 a new generation of doctors has started to appear who have never known abortion as an illegal operation. Successive opinion polls have shown the development of a more liberal attitude towards abortion by all sections of society, including family doctors, gynaecologists and psychiatrists. Safer methods of abortion, more practical administrative procedures within the National Health Service, and a better understanding of the needs of the patient requesting abortion have resulted in the development of the concept of an abortion service as a community health service like any other.

THE ABORTION ACT 1967

Under the terms of this Act the legal situation regarding abortion has been clarified. The operation must be performed in a National Health Service Hospital or some other place specially approved for the purpose by the Department of Health. Regulations exist which control the certificates to be signed, the notification of the operations, and the length of time that the certificates must be preserved.

Certificate A, the 'Green Form' is the form with which general practitioners are most concerned. It must be completed before the abortion is performed, and it must not be destroyed within three years of the date of the operation. On it, two registered medical practitioners certify that they are of the opinion, formed in good faith, that in the case of this particular patient:

1. The continuance of the pregnancy would involve risk to the life of the pregnant woman greater than if the pregnancy were terminated.
2. The continuance of the pregnancy would involve risk of injury to the physical or mental health of the pregnant woman greater than if the pregnancy were terminated.
3. The continuance of the pregnancy would involve risk of injury to the physical or mental health of the pregnant woman greater than if the pregnancy were terminated.
4. There is a substantial risk that if the child were born it would suffer from such physical or mental abnormalities as to be seriously handicapped.

The practitioners are instructed to ring the appropriate number or numbers that apply in the particular case, to further certify that their signatures have been appended before starting to terminate the pregnancy, and both must sign and date the form.

Both doctors may be general practitioners, but the usual procedure is for the family doctor to sign the form and send it, with a detailed covering letter, to a gynaecologist, who, having examined the patient and confirmed the need for abortion, adds his signature to the form and retains it.

Medical practitioners who have a conscientious objection to abortion are under no legal duty to participate in the procedure. However, where a practitioner believes that, but for a conscientious objection, to advise an abortion would be legal; or where he feels that he is unable to make an unbiased decision because of his conscience, he should inform his patient so, and fulfill his legal obligations to her by arranging for her to consult an unbiased colleague. Failure to do so might result in an action for negligence against him. Under the terms of his contract with the Health Authority, a general practitioner practising within the National Health Service must see and advise any of his patients requesting abortion.

Roman Catholic family doctors and gynaecologists are thus absolved from taking part in performing abortions, but neither are absolved from the responsibility of advising their patients who request abortion, nor from ensuring that their patients who need abortion obtain help elsewhere. General practitioners should avoid referring patients who may need a pregnancy terminated to Roman Catholic gynaecologists: neither patient nor gynaecologist will appreciate it, and delay will result from the necessity to refer her to another.

If a doctor finds it necessary to refer a patient to a hospital where the gynaecologists are unknown to him - a situation that sometimes arises in London with its many hospital districts - a word on the telephone with the gynaecological out-patient appointments clerk will avoid such a mistake.

The written consent of the patient should be obtained before operation. A girl aged sixteen or over may give consent, but in younger girls the consent of the parent must be obtained. In the case of a married woman it is not necessary to obtain the consent of the husband, which is fortunate where the husband is not the originator of the pregnancy.

In an emergency, in order to save a patient's life or to prevent grave permanent injury, either physical or mental, an abortion may be performed by a registered medical practitioner without delay. Certificate B must be signed by him either before commencing the abortion or within twentyfour hours after it. No second signature is required in such a case.

INDICATIONS FOR ABORTION

There is no list of indications for abortion that will be acceptable to every doctor. At one extreme are those who maintain that any abortion, at whatever stage, and for whatever reason, is tantamount to murder. At the other extreme are those who believe that abortion should be available to all women who request it, provided the foetus has not reached legal viability at twentyeight weeks. Most family doctors will steer a course midway between these two extremes, assessing the pros and cons of an abortion in each particular patient, and it is to such doctors that this chapter is addressed.

Few would argue that the co-existence of an unwanted pregnancy and severe maternal disease is not an indication for abortion. Such conditions as severe heart disease, renal disease, hypertension, neurological or psychiatric disorder may be cited as examples. This type of problem rarely presents to the GP today, and when it does reference to his specialist colleagues is essential. Perhaps the most difficult decisions to make are those where severe disease and a wanted pregnancy co-exist. Having been referred for the most expert opinions, many women will return to ask the GP what he thinks. It will then be his duty to consult with the specialist and attempt to put the alternatives to his patient in the simplest terms possible. It is also his duty, I believe, to point out to her that abortion is never compulsory, and if she knowingly decides to risk her life to obtain a baby, then this decision will be accepted by the medical profession.

Similarly, the combination of the possibility of an abnormal baby and the fact that a pregnancy is unwanted rarely presents difficulties, both patient and GP agreeing that abortion is the wisest course.

Genetic counselling is available in most areas today, so that the patient with hereditary disease has usually embarked on the pregnancy aware of the risk, and the question of abortion does not arise. A list of Genetic Advisory Centres is included in the booklet 'Human Genetics' prepared by the Standing Medical Advisory Committee and published by Her Majesty's Stationery Office in 1972.

In general practice possible rubella infection in early pregnancy is the most worrying problem. Serial rubella antibody titres and the advice of the consultant virologist should be obtained as soon as possible after exposure to infection.

Fortunately more than 80 per cent of women of child-bearing age in metropolitan areas have been infected with rubella prior to pregnancy, so the results of the investigations usually enable the doctor to reassure the patient. Where it is confirmed that the patient has suffered the infection during early pregnancy, then any doctor who has seen children severely afflicted by rubella *in utero* would surely not hesitate to advise the mother to 'terminate and try again', unless exceptional conditions with regard to maternal age or fertility co-existed.

The vast majority of the women seeking the GP's advice about abortion will not belong to any of the groups so far discussed. They will be normally healthy women with unplanned pregnancies, and it is here that abortion counselling by the family doctor is of great importance.

NUMBERS OF ABORTIONS PERFORMED

Since the Act became law in April 1968, there has been a steady increase in the number of abortions notified annually in England and Wales.

A considerable proportion of the annual increase has been due to the influx of women from countries overseas where abortion laws are more restrictive. In 1969–70 for example, more than two thousand women came from the United States to England for abortion, while in 1969, at King's County Hospital in Brooklyn, only sixteen abortions were performed. As a result of the passing of more liberal abortion laws in New York, the same

Table XIII. Abortions notified in England and Wales annually 1968–1973 (April to March), figures adjusted to nearest thousand.

	1968–69	*1969–70*	*1970–71*	*1971–72*	*1972–73*
Total abortions notified	34,000	60,000	89,000	141,000	156,000
Rate per 100 live births	4.1	7.7	11.2	18.4	19.2
Number on foreign women	2,000	5,500	10,000	27,000	50,000

hospital recorded over six thousand abortions in 1971, and in the same year only nine hundred women from the United States came to England for abortion.

During the first quarter of 1973, almost half the abortions performed in England and Wales were on women from abroad, one-third of these coming from France.

The total number of abortions notified annually thus represents to a large extent the result of restrictive policies operating overseas, and as overseas governments amend their laws we can expect to see a reduction in the total figures.

When expressed as a rate per 100 live births, the abortion experience in England and Wales shows a fivefold increase between 1968 and 1973, but is still a very low rate when compared with other countries where abortion was liberalized. In Hungary in 1972, for example, with a population one-quarter the size of that of the United Kingdom, there were 178,000 induced abortions, and only 153,000 live births, a rate of well over 100 abortions per 100 live births. In Japan in 1972 there were one-and-a-half million abortions, a rate of 80 per 100 live births. All these figures pale into insignificance however, when compared to Rumania, where in 1965 there were four abortions to every one live birth.

AGE AND MARITAL STATUS OF WOMEN UNDERGOING ABORTION

Despite the hullabaloo concerning 'schoolgirl abortions' in some sections of the national press, the percentage of total abortions composed of patients aged less than sixteen has never exceeded two-and-a-half per cent, and has tended to decrease. There has been some increase in the abortions performed on girls aged between sixteen and nineteen, from 15 per cent in 1968–9 to 18 per cent in 1971–2, but the percentage of the total population in this country aged sixteen to nineteen has also increased. About eighty per cent of the abortions performed each year have been on women aged twenty or more.

Investigation of the marital status of women undergoing abortion has not revealed much change year by year. The percentage of single women varied from 46 per cent to 48 per cent, married women constituted 44 per cent of total abortions, 9 per cent were widowed, divorced or separated, and the marital state was not recorded in the remainder. More than half the women aborted each year had had a previous birth, stillbirth or miscarriage.

The high proportion of married and parous women undergoing abortion would seem to indicate that lack of knowledge or provision of contraceptive advice and supplies may not be the main reason for women having unwanted pregnancies.

CONTRACEPTION AND ABORTION

Every abortion may be.looked upon as a failure of contraception; sometimes a failure of the method used, but more often a failure to use any method. In a study of 155 women seeking abortion at the Royal Northern Hospital, London in 1970, three-quarters of the single women and one-quarter of the married women had never attempted birth control. In 1971, of 16,244 women consulting the British Pregnancy Advisory Service about termination of their pregnancies, four-fifths of the girls pregnant for the first time had used no birth control, and neither had one-third of the remainder. A report from King's College Hospital, London (Newton *et al.*, 1973) concerning more than 3,000 terminations performed during the three years 1970 to 1972, recorded that 45 per cent of the women had never used birth control prior to operation, and 55 per cent had used no contraception at the time of conception.

WHY NO CONTRACEPTION?

This is the vital question to which we do not know the complete answer. Several suggestions may be considered.

1. The girl may be ignorant of the existence of contraception.
2. Though aware of its existence she may not know where to get advice or supplies.
3. She may be unable to afford to purchase supplies.

It is true that the proportion using any method of contraception decreases from social Class I to social Class V, and it is tempting to equate lower social class with ignorance. That this is not the complete answer was indicated in a report by Diggory (1969) of 1000 terminations he carried out. The patients included 18 doctors, 99 nurses, 84 students at universities and polytechnics, and 29 teachers. Ignorance of contraception or lack of intelligence could certainly not be blamed in these patients.

Despite enormous publicity in all the media of mass communication during the past few years, and despite the increasing number of local authorities who supplied free contraceptive advice and/or supplies, and despite the increasing percentage of general practitioners and hospitals providing advice, the total number of abortions annually has increased. All this would seem to indicate that the three simple answers proposed above are, at least, of only minor importance.

Further evidence comes from an examination of the patients of my own practice who requested abortion.

During the years 1970–1973 inclusive, there were 94 requests for abortion from patients registered with me under the NHS. Patients already pregnant when joining my list were excluded. Not all these patients persisted in their requests for abortion, but the fact that a request was made indicated that the pregnancy was unplanned and unwanted at the time of the request (Table XIV).

Table XIV. Use of contraception among 94 women requesting abortion in one general practice in London, 1970–1973.

Contraceptive usage	*Number of women*	*Relation of pregnancy to usage*	*Number of women*
Used contraception at some time	71 (75%)	Alleged failure of method	22 (23%)
		Failure to use method, or to use it properly	49 (52%)
Never used contraception	23 (25%)	Failure to respond to advice	11 (12%)
		IGNORANCE POSSIBLE	12 (13%)

Seventyone patients, three-quarters of the total, had used some form of contraception in the past. Twentytwo of these alleged failure of the method, but the remainder admitted to improper use of a method, failure to use any method on the occasion they became pregnant, or abandonment of a method without seeking medical advice.

Of the 23 patients who had never used any form of contraception, a note on their medical record card showed that eleven had been offered contraceptive advice in the past. Only the remaining twelve girls could have pleaded ignorance of the existence of contraception, or where to obtain advice about it, and in fact all of them attempted to do so. The plea of poverty was not entered by any patient.

It would seem that few patients requesting abortion can justifiably offer the simple explanations of ignorance or poverty to explain their failure to use contraception. What other explanations can be offered?

Often there seems to be a deep-rooted psychological motive behind the achievement of the pregnancy. The young unmarried girl who manages a pregnancy may be doing so in order to punish a domineering, nagging mother. Her pregnancy is 'one in the eye for Mum', something she has achieved for herself, and a situation which Mum cannot resolve without the permission of the girl. To continue with the pregnancy is unnecessary, viewed in this light, and a request for an abortion follows.

For other girls, doubts about their own sexuality or fertility or fears that they may be homosexual, may lead them to prove themselves by achieving a pregnancy. Feelings of guilt, based on real or imaginary failings or misdemeanours, may lead some girls to punish themselves by becoming pregnant. Abortion in these circumstances is almost desirable, as it is a further punishment to expiate the guilt.

The married woman, already possessing a sensible number of children, judged by her economic and social circumstances, but bored with her domestic routine and denied her reproductive role, may find relief and excitement in the attainment of a pregnancy. To proceed to confinement and then to nappies, schools and economies would represent neither relief nor excitement, and abortion is requested.

More mundane is the girl who tries to force her lover into marriage, and when the threat fails - as it usually does today - requests termination of the then unwanted pregnancy.

There remains a number of girls who have an unplanned and unwanted pregnancy, who say 'I thought it would not happen to me'. This I call the Safety-belt Syndrome. We all know we should wear safety-belts in our cars, but how many of us do on every occasion?

A recent study (Beard *et al.*, 1974) has attempted to show a correlation between neuroticism scores, as obtained by the Eysenck Personality Inventory, and the use of contraception by patients requesting abortion. The highest mean score was found in the group of women who had used no contraception. Among users of contraception, the reliability of the method used was inversely related to the neuroticism scores. Ninetytwo per cent of the married women in the study had used contraception at some time, as had 65 per cent of the single girls. Thus neuroticism, rather than ignorance of contraception, may be the significant factor in the occurrence of unwanted pregnancy.

Contraception cannot be considered the complete answer to such a varied motivation for unwanted pregnancy. Indeed, the use of contraception itself may induce feelings of guilt and conflict, leading to its rejection.

The family doctor must do what he can to combat the effects of broken homes, unhappy family relationships, and inner conflicts leading to psychosexual disturbances and unwanted pregnancies, but the amount he can do is limited.

There remain the simple causes, the ignorance, the poverty, and the

Safety-belt Syndrome. These he can attempt to eliminate by the offer of contraceptive advice and supplies, and then attempt to motivate the patient to make use of them. He can also attempt to avoid recurrent abortion by the same means.

ABORTION COUNSELLING

Professional non-medical counselling organizations are necessary to counsel women coming from abroad, and women who do not wish to go to their own family doctor. Their reasons for avoiding him may extend from not knowing him well enough to knowing him too well, and fearing that to confess to a need for abortion will diminish themselves in his eyes. Regrettably some women may fear that their relatives will find out if they ask the family doctor about abortion. Sometimes they fear that the doctor may be cold and antagonistic. On occasions they know, or think they know, that because of his religious beliefs they will receive no help from him, and for this reason by-pass him.

In almost every instance the patient will be mistaken in her beliefs, but the GP will find it difficult to correct her views when he does not know she holds them. Certainly every family doctor must make quite certain that all the staff working in his surgery are aware of the confidential nature of the patient's notes, and are on their guard against the casual remark that may reveal a patient's secrets to others. Apart from this, he must just do his best, hoping that by his attitude during discussions of contraception with his patients, he will be able to indicate to them indirectly that he would be equally neutral and non-moralizing in any discussion on abortion.

ATTITUDES: DOCTOR'S AND PATIENT'S

There are hopeful signs that the attitudes towards abortion adopted both by doctors and patients are becoming less hostile. A National Opinion Poll in 1973 found that 52 per cent of family doctors questioned felt that the Abortion Act should remain unaltered, and a further 21 per cent thought that it should be altered to make it easier for women to obtain abortion. The same Poll reported that two-thirds of the general public, the patients, are in favour of abortion to preserve a woman's health, and three-quarters in favour of abortion where an abnormal baby is likely.

Family doctors like myself who have practised before and after the passing of the Abortion Act have noticed an enormous change in the emotional atmosphere in the surgery during interviews with patients requesting abortion for unwanted pregnancies. Formerly high drama was the rule, sometimes hysteria, and sometimes histrionics. Today quiet reason prevails, the request to the GP for his help in the removal of the unwanted pregnancy being stated in the same hopeful and polite terms as a request to remove young Willie's unwanted tonsils. This attitude is particularly noticeable in the younger patient, and the Opinion Poll referred to found that younger married people with children were the strongest supporters of the Abortion Act.

Rational discussion of the need for, and legality of abortion is thus more possible today than five years ago but even so the GP must remember that the interview, and particularly the initiation of the interview will appear markedly different viewed through the eyes of the patient. For the GP, this is one more of the fifty or more people who sit in that chair and present their problems each day. For the patient, this is a very special, hopefully unique occasion, and she is testing every action, every word, every gesture of the doctor, seeking signs, real or imaginary, of rejection.

Any hesitation on the part of a girl of reproductive age in presenting her problem should alert the doctor to the possibility that the problem may be concerned with sex, abortion, contraception or similarly personal matters. It will be helpful if, suspecting this, he can break the ice himself. The way he chooses will depend on his personality, and his estimate of the personality of the patient. My own standard response to the girl who says, 'I don't quite know how to put it, doctor', is to reply 'Well, its either sexual troubles, birth control, or abortion, so please put me out of my misery and tell me which.'

The opening made for her, the patient can start to tell me her troubles, because usually the subject does fall under these headings. Occasionally it is something quite different, like psychiatric illness in a relative, which still retains a remarkable aura of sin in the minds of some patients. Again, the complaint when it arrives may be something even the experienced GP had not foreseen.

A young married woman with a baby several months old sat in the chair in the surgery and obviously did not know how to formulate her distressing complaint into words. Catalysed by the ice-breaker, she was able to tell me that she had awoken to find her husband attempting to obtain vaginal penetration using a large cucumber.

CONFIRMATION OF PREGNANCY

Once the request for advice about abortion has been made, and the menstrual history has been obtained, the patient should be examined to confirm pregnancy. Nowadays it is not uncommon for girls who have delayed menses after stopping the Pill to present with a self-diagnosis of pregnancy. Pregnancy tests are of great value to confirm clinical impressions, but I have learnt to distrust the result of a pregnancy test as the sole evidence of cyesis. Two per cent of positive tests are incorrect, even when performed at the correct stage of pregnancy.

In one year I was visited by three patients, all requesting referral for abortion, all reporting positive pregnancy tests, all without clinical signs of pregnancy, and all proving not to be pregnant. One had come from a suburb of London, one from North Africa, and one had made the trip from Orange City, USA. She was furious with me.

A great deal can be learnt about the girl from chatting during the examination and, once the pregnancy has been confirmed, further details can be elicited, but adequate time is essential, and the best course is often to ask the girl to return by appointment at a later date. Not too much later, however, as if abortion is necessary then the earlier it is performed the greater is the safety of the procedure.

HISTORY-TAKING

The history required from a girl requesting termination of her pregnancy is partly medical and partly social. The family doctor may know the patient so well that, his memory refreshed by perusal of her NHS records, few questions are necessary.

1. Gynaecological details

The date of the last menstrual period, and, if possible, the suspected date of conception.

The previous pattern of menstruation, and past gynaecological disorders (e.g. salpingitis) or operations (e.g. myomectomy).

Contraceptive usage if any, at the time of conception on this occasion, and in the past, with particular reference to recent use of oral contraception and possible amenorrhoea following it.

The presence or absence of vaginal discharge or irritation, and, if present, any relation in time to recent acts of intercourse.

Previous pregnancies, miscarriages, or terminations of pregnancy. In immigrants there should be additional questions as to the number of children 'back home' as these are sometimes omitted.

Abnormalities during pregnancy (e.g. severe toxaemia) or at delivery (e.g. Caesarean section).

2. Medical details

Severe disease of any system, together with details of any relevant treatment, paying special attention to the ingestion of any drugs in early pregnancy that might have damaged the foetus.

Past or present psychiatric illness, its severity, duration, and type of treatment required.

The possibility of infectious disease in early pregnancy.

A history of hereditary disease, or congenital abnormality.

3. Personal details

Married or single: divorced or separated: are divorce proceedings contemplated at the moment?

If married, does the husband know of pregnancy? What is his attitude to abortion? Is it his child? If it is not, then further questions follow: is this a solitary indiscretion likely to smash a marriage, or is the marriage already beyond salvage? Is re-marriage planned? Was this pregnancy the result of a stable relationship developed over some considerable time, or is it the result of a casual encounter?

If single or divorced, is marriage planned?

4. **Economic details**

Economic details required relate to both the girl herself and her consort. Is she still a schoolgirl or a student, needing financial assistance herself? If she is at work, how much does she earn? What are the man's earnings, or is he also at school or college? Has he other responsibilities, a married man with a family, perhaps?

5. **Living accommodation**

Does the unmarried girl live in her parents' house? If so do they know of her pregnancy? Is there room for a baby, and if so are the parents likely to help? Or is there already overcrowding, with the girl sharing a bed with her sister? Does she live in a bed-sitter, on her own, or sharing with other girls? Is it likely that she will lose the roof over her head if the landlord discovers she is pregnant? What rent does she pay?

Much the same considerations apply to the married woman. Has she a place of her own, or are they living with in-laws? Will the in-laws welcome a baby? How many rooms have the couple, or are they in one room? Are they in rented accommodation, furnished or unfurnished? Will their landlord throw them out if they have children? If the local council owns the property, are they recognized tenants or have they an 'unofficial' sub-letting? If this is the case and the property is due for demolition they may have little chance of being rehoused.

Sadly, one must also ask whether the girl, married or unmarried, has any home at all.

6. **Family details**

The relationship of the single girl with her parents. How many siblings and her relationship with them? Has she children of her own already? Their number, whether living with her, adopted, in care of the local authority, or being looked after by relatives? Does she appear to love and care for children living with her?

Much the same information is needed for married women. How many children has she already? Can she cope? Are the children well cared for at the one extreme, or is 'baby battering' a factor at the other? Is the general health of the children good? Have any of them chronic or recurrent illness demanding extra care?

Does the male consort help with the children, or does he leave the burden entirely to the wife? Is he kind, gentle and considerate or is he a drunkard and a bully? How does he treat the children?

7. **Age and marital status**

Neither of these factors are of much importance, taken alone. The degree of emotional development is of far greater significance than age in years when considering the youth of the patient. At the other end of the scale, an unwanted pregnancy may bring great difficulties to a woman of fortyfive already struggling to bring up a family. Similarly, the presence of a stable relationship is of far more importance than the existence of a marriage. Certainly marriage should not be contemplated solely because of the existence of a pregnancy.

ASSESSMENT OF THE NEED FOR ABORTION

Armed with details of the patient's personal, family, economic, medical and gynaecological circumstances, together with his knowledge of her living conditions, the general practitioner is in a position to apply the overall picture thus built up to the four conditions itemized on the green form and ask himself 'Is this pregnancy, if it were allowed to continue, likely to risk the life or damage the physical or mental health of the mother, or her existing children more than if it were to be terminated? Or is there a risk of serious physical or mental abnormality in the baby?'

Each case must be considered on its merits, assessing the patient and her total environment as detailed, and the family doctor will usually be in no doubt as to the course to advise. Before voicing his advice, however, he has one more duty to fulfil, and that is to point out the alternatives to abortion.

ALTERNATIVES TO ABORTION

1. **Adoption**

Most girls reject this out of hand. Certainly, having seen the anguish and distress suffered by girls who handed over their babies for adoption in the years before 1968, I regard it as a most cruel solution. On a purely materialistic level it is also unsatisfactory as a solution, since many girls cannot afford a year out of their lives. A student, for example, would find it almost impossible to continue at her place of learning during the whole of her pregnancy, and quite impossible to regain her place after many months absence.

The long queues waiting to adopt babies demonstrate that very few girls choose adoption rather than abortion today. It is perhaps inevitable that reports are appearing of large sums of money being offered to girls who agree to continue their pregnancy and agree to adoption.

2. **Placing the child with foster parents**

This alternative may be regarded as the reversible equivalent of irreversible adoption. It is sometimes chosen by a girl who can forsee a time in the near future when her situation may be expected to change and she will be able to have the child back to live with her. Most girls in such circumstances today choose abortion now and another pregnancy later.

3. **Hostels for unmarried mothers**

Hostels existed in large numbers before the passing of the Abortion Act, where girls could stay for three months or longer before confinement, and for about six weeks afterwards. The fact that such hostels are closing all over the country due to lack of demand for their services speaks for itself.

4. **Social Security payments**

Payments of this type are available for any girl who needs financial help during pregnancy. Like most Social Security benefits they are not over-generous, and for most girls the financial difficulties of unplanned pregnancies are not their major consideration.

None of these alternatives are acceptable to most women requesting abortion, and are unthinkable as a solution to most married women. Nevertheless the GP should make sure the patient has considered them.

It is possible to sue the father of the child for maintenance. In practice the man is either willing to provide assistance on a voluntary basis, or the girl is unwilling to submit to the legal procedures to obtain it.

There remains for young unmarried girls one further source of assistance.

Help from parents

Very often the family doctor knows the parents, and it is sad to learn the unfavourable assessment made by the girl of her parents' reaction to her unwanted pregnancy. Sometimes, from his knowledge, he must agree with her estimate of their probable reaction. On occasions however he can be so certain that she is mistaken that he can say so, and offer to tell them on her behalf - with her permission of course.

The offer is in my experience very rarely accepted, because most daughters prefer to tell their mothers themselves. The family doctor can point out how hurt the mother would be if she were ever to find out that 'her little girl' had been in trouble and needed help, but did not turn to Mum. If told, no doubt Mum will be shaken, possibly even horrified, but the initial acute reaction over, she usually busies herself in every way possible to render assistance to her daughter, now and in the future. As for Dad, leave Mum to deal with him.

Occasionally the girl feels that her father is the one who should be approached first: sometimes she is sure that only one parent should be told while the other remains in ignorance. As evidence to the correctness of her view, subsequent interviews with the family doctor are with the girl and the one parent, who subscribes to the view that the other should not know.

This facet of abortion counselling, the suggestion and gentle persuasion of the young girl to confide in her parents, is possible only when the parents are known to the counsellor, and is one reason why the family doctor is superior to other agencies in this field. The support of the parents is a most valuable asset for the young girl with an unplanned pregnancy, and the support is usually ongoing, avoiding the girl making the same mistakes again.

In my experience the parents never seem to resent the fact that their daughter chose to approach the family doctor in the first place. And it usually transpires that Mum was not as unaware that problems existed as her daughter believed.

Unfortunately there are occasions when the relationship between daughter and parents is bad, or when any relationship at all no longer exists. In such a case, provided the girl is of age, the GP will agree that to keep them in ignorance is the wisest policy.

The patient as her own counsellor

The Abortion Act lays down that the decision to terminate a pregnancy must be a clinical decision made by doctors. To implement that decision, the patient's consent is necessary, but she cannot decide for herself that her pregnancy will be terminated.

This is as it should be, because with so many factors to be assessed, every woman is entitled to a consideration of her individual situation by someone with more experience of the problem than she has.

This is not to infer that the woman, unaided, usually makes an incorrect decision. After considering the problem for many worried days and sleepless nights she has usually reached a conclusion with which the GP will agree. Nevertheless there are instances where undue influence has been applied, or situations where the patient is not in possession of all the facts, especially medical facts, where the discussion with someone not personally involved can avoid the patient making a mistake.

The opportunity to discuss the problem is also therapeutic, and many patients tell of a great relief of anxiety after discussion, whether or not a decision has been reached.

> Mrs C, aged 20, married one year and on the combined Pill for eighteen months, had, she told me, missed two Pills owing to an unexpected weekend away from home and was now two weeks overdue. She couldn't possibly have a baby, she said, since they had a large mortgage, lots of hire purchase, and she and her husband had agreed that at least another year, probably two, must elapse before they started their family. She wanted a baby eventually, but meantime, 'I must have an abortion. Please help me, doctor'.
>
> Questioning her while the pregnancy test was performed, I discovered that there was no question of her husband agreeing to an abortion, nor even disagreeing. The poor chap hadn't even been told of the pregnancy, so sure was she that he would not want a baby now. He had so often castigated those of his friends who had unplanned pregnancies or started families too early, that she was certain he would be furious if he found she was pregnant.
>
> As we talked, it became increasingly obvious that her request for an abortion was based on a completely untested assumption regarding her husband, and I

refused to consider a termination of the pregnancy on that basis. Tears and entreaties followed, but happily when she returned a few days later, they had been replaced by smiles. Husband had been overjoyed to find himself a prospective father and had willingly thrown all his ideas of postponed pregnancies out of the window. Wisely, she did not see fit to mention to him that she had requested abortion from me.

In practice, 80 per cent of women consulting the family doctor because of an unplanned pregnancy will already have made a decision with which he agrees. The remaining 20 per cent comprise those few with whom he disagrees, and those who due to confusion, ignorance, or fear cannot make a firm decision without help.

The social worker or health visitor

Where it is difficult to be certain of the best course to follow, the help of a social worker or health visitor may be invaluable.

A pitfall for the unwary

One type of patient deserves special mention. There is a small but appreciable minority of girls who ask for abortion, but are in reality looking for an ally to encourage and help them to keep the pregnancy. Usually, they are young or very young girls who have been exposed to undue influence from older people, either parents or boyfriends, or even husbands, and it is essential that the GP recognizes these cases and offers his help.

A girl of 17, eight weeks pregnant, was dragged into the surgery by her very upset and voluble mother. 'She's got herself pregnant, Doctor, and wants an abortion. Tell the Doctor, Marlene.' Marlene, standing dejectedly by the couch, said, 'That's right, can I have an abortion please'. Mother then proceeded to list a large number of reasons why a baby was an unthinkable addition to the household, as far as mother was concerned, including 'What would the neighbours say.' Daughter remained sullenly silent, and eventually mother was persuaded to depart to the waiting room, so that I could talk to the daughter.

It transpired that daughter was delighted with the prospect of having a baby. She had looked after her little brother and sister from infancy onwards, regarding the time she spent at school as an interruption of her proper duties. Now she had left school, and her siblings had started there, her life seemed empty. She confessed that although she was fond of her 18-year-old boyfriend, and he had asked her to marry him, she did not want to marry. She wanted a baby to look after. But her mother did not seem to understand, and had assumed abortion was the only answer. The girl had attempted to explain, but had been overawed by her mother's very strong character.

The situation was explained to the mother, who eventually came to realize her daughter's strong maternal instinct. She confessed that her own children had been unplanned and, as their care tended to interfere with her many social commitments, they had indeed been looked after mainly by her elder daughter. On reflection, she agreed that her daughter had never suggested abortion: the doctrine of 'mother knows best' had ruled relationships with her quiet and pliable daughter for so long that she had never thought to question it herself.

The mother's request for abortion was withdrawn, and the baby duly arrived.

Not surprisingly baby had a happy and devoted mother: in addition baby had an equally devoted grandfather, who continued to defer in all things to the decisions of the females in the house. To her surprise, a somewhat confused grandmother found a fierce pride in her daughter and her new baby, and her social commitments increased rather than diminished. Two years later Marlene and baby were carried off by a young man who wanted a large family, and they disappeared from my practice, but reports of a very happy marriage continue.

It is the occasional appearance of patients similar to the two whose histories have been outlined above that makes me certain that abortion on demand has nothing to recommend it.

Relevance of previous contraceptive usage

The law makes no mention of this factor at all. Indeed, the need for abortion is often most obvious in those who have never used contraception.

However, it seems to me that where a patient has diligently practised an efficient method of contraception on the advice of the family doctor, and that method has failed, then the practitioner would be less than human if he did not regard that patient's request for abortion as one which he would not gainsay without very definite medical contra-indications.

The second signature

Certificate A requires two signatures, but lays down no requirement as to the types of duly registered medical practitioners who provide the signatures. Ideally, the first signature should be that of the patient's family doctor, and the second that of a competent gynaecologist capable of performing the termination, of dealing with any sequelae or complications, and chosen by the family doctor. Within the National Health Service this means, for practical purposes, the consultant gynaecologist at the District General Hospital. Where the area of the general practice extends across several hospital districts, then several gynaecologists may receive patients from the one practice, but this does not alter the ideal situation where patients requiring abortion are referred as part of the total gynaecological load between doctors of the two specialities, general practice and gynaecology, who know and respect each others' capabilities. Under such circumstances, the main contribution of the gynaecologist to counselling the patient is the accurate assessment of surgical risk.

For this reason the letter from the family doctor to the consultant should be detailed, giving the full medical and social history, and expressing a definite opinion as to the need for abortion. Certificate A, already signed by the GP should be enclosed. In my opinion, the consultant should then be guided by the GP, and should rarely differ from his opinion other than on purely surgical grounds.

The ideal situation exists where the consultant can rely on the GP to have counselled the patient adequately, and the GP can rely on the consultant to accept that this has been performed. The result should be that, having read the GP's letter, the consultant need only examine that patient and decide whether or not to terminate the pregnancy.

Unhappy situations will arise where the GP does no more than merely refer to hospital all patients requesting abortion. The consultant will then rightly feel deprived of the help the experienced GP can give. By the same token, where the GP offers his help, the consultant should not insist on going over the same ground again, and especially should not refer all cases to a social worker or a psychiatrist. If such a procedure is routine, then the GP will feel that his advice and opinion are being valued at zero, and will cease to play the part he undoubtedly should.

In cases where neither patient nor GP can be certain what is best, then help from others can be invaluable, but as a routine it cannot be justified.

Hospital appointments

It is essential that after counselling a patient and deciding that abortion is indicated, an appointment to see the gynaecologist may be made for her rapidly, easily and soon. Such devices as insisting on a personal approach by letter from the GP to the gynaecologist, with the possibility that the letter will be lost in the post, or limiting the number of appointments available for girls wanting abortion to a certain number each week, as though a standard number of girls get unwantedly pregnant weekly or, as already mentioned, insisting on prior referral elsewhere in the hospital; all these devices may cause delay resulting in the transformation of a safe, rapid early termination into a mid-trimester operation.

Ideally, the family doctor should be able to lift the telephone and make an appointment for his patient to be seen within a few days, certainly less than a week. The appointment should be made with the appointment clerk in out-patients. To insist that such appointments may be made only after conversation between the consultant and the GP is unsatisfactory because of the difficulty in finding busy consultants at the time suitable for them to come to the telephone.

To insist that all patients considered for abortion should live in a specified area would be a reasonable condition if abortion facilities were equal in all areas. Until they are, hospitals must accept that many patients will give false addresses, or the addresses of friends or relatives who do live in the favoured area. Once the decision to terminate has been made, arrangements for the selected procedure must follow with the minimum of delay.

THE BRITISH SITUATION

Do all general practitioners, all consultants, and indeed all patients in all areas of the United Kingdom when confronted with the unplanned unwanted pregnancy react in the way I have indicated as ideal? In evidence to the Lane Committee on the working of the abortion act, Cartwright and Waite (1972) showed that, sadly, this was not so.

Of six hundred GPs sent a postal questionnaire in late 1970, twelve per cent had a conscientious objection to termination of pregnancy in virtually all cases, but half of these could identify special circumstances in which they would recommend it. Religion was the most important factor in relation to the doctor's attitudes.

Patients attending their family doctor thus run the risk of finding that the clinical decision required by the Abortion Act may be replaced by a completely negative attitude towards abortion on the part of the doctor, resulting in an obstruction to their referral within the National Health Service. Indeed, Cartwright refers to the general practitioner as a 'hurdle' that the patient must overcome when seeking an abortion.

That he is not the only hurdle was evidenced by the fact that the GPs estimated that one-third of their referrals under the Act were refused. One-quarter of the GPs found it so difficult to arrange terminations that they sometimes failed to do so even in cases where they thought it indicated.

Examination of the figures from different hospital regions of the country showed that there were wide variations both between the proportion of doctors with conscientious objections, and the proportion of National Health referrals that were turned down.

Table XV. Numbers of live births in NHS hospital areas, and abortions in NHS hospitals; first quarter of 1973.

(The Registrar's General's Quarterly Return for England & Wales)

Area	*Live births*	*Abortions*
Newcastle	11,075	1,421
Leeds	11,948	526
Sheffield	17,864	944
East Anglian	6,999	568
N.W. Metropolitan	13,473	1,331
N.E. Metropolitan	13,030	1,058
S.E. Metropolitan	11,445	1,133
S.W. Metropolitan	12,896	649
Wessex	7,223	493
Oxford	8,843	555
South Western	11,344	1,289
Welsh	9,957	932
Birmingham	20,657	640
Manchester	17,066	1,294
Liverpool	8,809	484

Table XV allows a comparison between the number of live births in each hospital region in England and Wales in the first quarter of 1973 and the number of abortions performed in National Health Service hospitals in that area. It will be seen that enormous variations exist between areas.

Expressing the numbers of abortions as a percentage of the figures for live births for that area, the percentage obtained varies from over 11 per cent for the South Western Region, and nearly 13 per cent for the Newcastle region, to as low as 4 per cent for Leeds and 3 per cent for Birmingham.

In practice this means that a girl with an unwanted pregnancy eligible for abortion under the 1967 Act living in Newcastle has almost four times the chance of obtaining abortion under the National Health Service as her sister living in Birmingham, who will probably have to go to the private sector for abortion, if she can afford it.

Assuming that girls in Birmingham are just as likely to be eligible for abortion under the terms of the Act as girls in Newcastle - which seems to me a reasonable assumption, although I must admit that as my practice is in London I have no intimate knowledge of either - it would appear that the medical profession in different parts of the country are interpreting the Act in differing ways, and Cartwright and Waite showed that this difference in interpretation applied to GPs as much as to gynaecologists.

This has resulted in two suggestions. The first, from the protagonists of abortion, is that abortion units should be set up in those areas where abortion is difficult to obtain. The second, from the opponents of abortion, is that the Act should be altered in some way to make it a more difficult operation to obtain.

Both suggestions are wrong. The operation of termination of pregnancy should not be regarded as intrinsically different from any other operation, and should be part of total patient care practised by all GPs and all gynaecologists. Education is the answer: education of those doctors with conscientious objections to encourage them to refer patients to others; education of patients to realize that they need not take no for an answer but should seek advice elsewhere.

METHODS OF ABORTION

(a) Before diagnosis

This method, known as 'Menstrual Extraction', or 'Menstrual Regulation' has received much publicity recently due to a group of campaigners known as the Interception Group. A diagnosis of pregnancy is not awaited, the treatment being applied whenever a women who has reason to believe she may be pregnant finds that her period does not start on the day it is due to arrive.

The technique consists of the passage of a narrow bore (4 mm.) polythene canula through the undilated cervix into the uterine cavity. Vacuum aspiration is performed by means of a 100-ml plastic syringe, fitted with a side valve to prevent insufflation of the uterus with air. Endometrium and any products of conception are thus extracted from the uterus with the minimum of delay, no necessity for an anaesthetic, and the virtual elimination of anxiety on the part of the patient. The protagonists of the method maintain that it is safe, danger to the woman from perforation, infection or blood loss being minimal.

At the moment trials are being undertaken to assess these beliefs. If verified, it would seem a useful addition to the methods of fertility control now available, and particularly useful as a surgery procedure, provided back-up facilities were available from the district hospital. It would appear to be well within the competence of any general practitioner practised in the insertion of intrauterine devices, and should carry less risk to the patient than such procedures as home confinement and circumcision widely practised by family doctors today.

It is to be hoped, therefore, that, provided the safety of the procedure is established in properly conducted trials, it will not be so hedged about with regulations and conditions that its performance in the surgery by GPs will become impossible.

(b) **Up to eight weeks**

(i) *Dilatation and curettage*

In bygone years the most widely practised method of terminating early pregnancy, the disadvantages outweigh the advantages so greatly that it should never be used today. In the hands of an experienced operator retention of part of the uterine contents is unlikely to occur, but this is the sole advantage. Among the disadvantages may be listed possible perforation of the uterus, damage to the cervix during dilatation, resulting in laceration at the time, or cervical incompetence later, and a heavier blood loss than modern suction methods. General anaesthesia, with its added dangers is usually required.

(ii) *Vacuum aspiration using the Karman catheter*

The Karman catheter (Fig. 45) is a flexible polythene tube with a rounded end, below which are placed two openings. One opening is placed immediately below the top of the catheter and the other a short distance below the first on the opposite side. The placing of these openings serves two purposes, firstly to enable suction to be applied in two directions within the uterine cavity simultaneously, and secondly, by reducing the strength of the tubular section of the catheter, they ensure that bending of the end of the

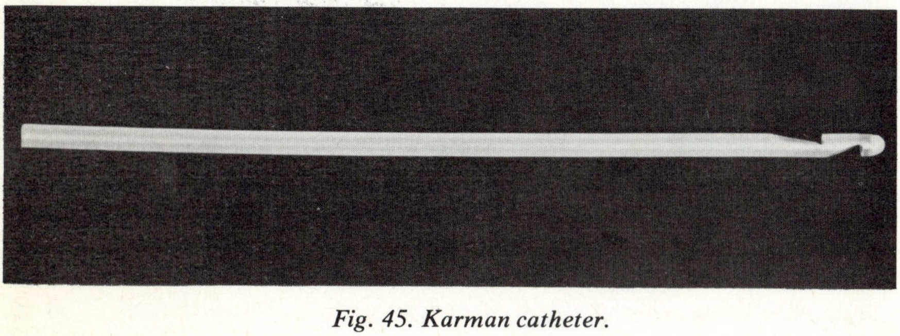

Fig. 45. Karman catheter.

catheter is more likely than perforation of the uterine wall. A suction pump is attached to the proximal end of the catheter, and considerable negative pressure induced (25–30 inches of mercury).

The diameter of the tubing is only 6, 8, or 10 mm. The 6 mm size can usually be passed through the multiparous os without further dilatation, though this may be needed in nulliparous patients. The degree of dilatation needed is much less than that needed to facilitate the passage of a curette.

Local anaesthesia is adequate, either by paracervical or intracervical block, providing the patient is instructed in the procedure beforehand and is attended by a member of the nursing staff whose duty it is to allay anxiety and provide reassurance.

The contents of the uterus can be seen passing down the tube, and should be fed into a large jar of water to facilitate visual examination at the end of the procedure. A very accurate estimate can thus be made of the completeness of the evacuation. A small Friedman curette may be used to ensure that the uterine cavity is empty.

This method has been used at King's College Hospital, London, since early 1971 (Lewis *et al.,* 1971). The suction procedure on average takes less than three minutes, the blood loss is less than 100 ml provided the pregnancy is of less than eight weeks duration, the complication rate is low, and it is unnecessary for the patient to be admitted to hospital.

(c) **Between eight and twelve weeks of gestation**

Vacuum aspiration of the contents of the uterus is again the method of choice, but the larger Biera catheter is used. Made in three sizes, 10, 12 and 14 mm in diameter, this device has one hole through which the products of conception are removed.

Dilatation of the cervix is always required. Some form of general anaesthesia is needed, either by inhalation or the intravenous administration of drugs such as diazepam (Valium) and methohexitone (Brietal, Brevital). Admission to hospital for about 48 hours is necessary.

Loung *et al.,* (1971) reported the results of 1,000 consecutive terminations of pregnancy at Lewisham Hospital, the majority being between eight and twelve weeks gestation. Ninety per cent of the patients remained in hospital 48 hours or less and few complications were encountered. Uterine perforation occurred in only five patients, and haemorrage in excess of 500 ml was seen in only 61 patients.

(d) **After fourteen weeks gestation**

(i) Intrauterine injection of some substance which will persuade the uterus to empty itself is the safest method to use after the fourteenth week of pregnancy. Unfortunately, to inject into the amniotic cavity without damaging the structures in the abdomen such as the bladder, is not easy at this stage, and it is safer to wait until the uterine size has advanced to 16–18 weeks.

Hypertonic saline or urea are the substances usually injected. Dextrose or one of the prostaglandins have also been used. Combinations of these agents, used together, have undergone trials. The delay between initiating the abortion and its completion may be reduced by the simultaneous administration of an oxytocin drip intravenously.

This procedure is distinctly unpleasant for the patient: the wait until the uterine size is adequate, the injection procedure itself, the side-effects of the substance injected (prostaglandins induce nausea, vomiting and diarrhoea as well as abortion), the fact that the injection-abortion interval may be many hours or even days, and that the abortion itself constitutes a mini-labour, with possibly a living foetus produced, all add up to an experience the patient does not enjoy. Nor do the nursing staff.

The safety of intra-amniotic injection of hypertonic saline has been questioned, severe electrolyte imbalance and even maternal death having been reported as sequelae. However Kerenyi (1973) has reported a series of 5,000 abortions using this technique, with no maternal deaths, and maintains that incorrect selection of patients, or incorrect use of the method are to be blamed for catastrophes rather than the method itself.

Complications include a high incidence of incomplete abortion, necessitating subsequent uterine evacuation, and occasional failure of the method to produce abortion. In such cases hysterotomy must follow.

(ii) Hysterotomy may be required where pregnancy exists in the presence of other uterine pathology, or where intra-amniotic injections have failed, but the mortality of the operation is greater than that associated with other methods.

(iii) Other methods which have not progressed beyond experimental investigation include intravenous and transcervical application of prostaglandins and extra-amniotic injection of various substances.

(e) **Methods of historical interest**

(i) *Utus paste.* The injection of this substance through a canula into the uterine cavity constituted a method of abortion in the past, but should today never be used. Sood (1971) reported six cases of septicaemia and one death following use of this method.

(ii) *Solid rubber bougies.* Packing solid rubber bougies or catheters into the uterus outside the membranes resulted in much discomfort for the patient and frequent failure of the method, which has nothing to recommend it.

(iii) *Laminaria tents.* Slow dilatation could be obtained by packing laminaria tents in the cervix. Abortion frequently failed to ensue.

(iv) *Hysterectomy.* The mortality of this operation when used as a method of abortion is far too high. Hysterectomy is indicated only as a method of dealing with some complication of abortion such as uterine perforation with internal haemorrhage.

DANGERS OF ABORTION

Considering these under two headings, immediate and long-term, it becomes obvious that although exact figures relating to the method of abortion and the state of pregnancy can be produced for the former, accurate information regarding long-term complications is very scanty and, very often, more a matter of opinion than fact.

(a) Risk of death

An analysis of the statistics for 1971 by the Registrar General reveals that 126,777 legal abortions were performed in England and Wales during that year. There were eleven deaths, but in only seven of these was the abortion procedure thought to be directly responsible. The death rate due to legal abortion in 1971 was thus 5.5 per 100,000 legal abortions. The maternal mortality rate for England and Wales for 1971 was 17 per 100,000 total births.

Further examination of the statistics gives grounds for hope that the risks will decrease still further in the future. In 1971 dilatation and curettage was used as the method of termination more often than vacuum aspiration. Today the reverse would be true, hopefully with a lower mortality. Six of the eleven deaths followed either hysterotomy or hysterectomy. Again these operations are less often performed today.

The age of the patient undergoing abortion is also of significance in relation to the risk of death. Table XVI demonstrates that this risk in 1970 and 1971 was greater for women aged thirty or over at the time of operation.

Table XVI. Deaths due to abortions in 1970 and 1971, and age of patient.

	Number of abortions	*Deaths due to abortion*
Aged less than 30	113,000	11
Aged 30 or more	58,000	14

There would seem little doubt that to have an abortion is safer, in terms of the risk to life of the mother, than to have a baby. However, two facts should be borne in mind. Firstly, figures from other countries, notably Hungary, Yugoslavia and the United States (New York) show an even lower mortality for legal abortion, so there must be no complacency regarding the figures for England and Wales. And secondly, there is not the slightest doubt that contraception is even safer than abortion.

(b) Risk of complications other than death

Patients remain in hospital for only a short time after operation and follow-up is scanty. All the reports of complication rates that I have seen have been published by National Health Service hospitals, despite the large number of terminations performed in other approved places. The definition of some complications is inexact. For example, infection may be reported as being present only after bacteriological proof, or it may be indicated as 'pyrexia'. If a patient returns home after twentyfour hours, especially if she is resident abroad, subsequent infection or pyrexia will be very considerably under-reported.

Differing complication rates may be expected for terminations carried out by differing methods, by operators of differing skills and at differing stages of pregnancy, and the performance of other operations such as sterilization at the same time will also affect the rates.

Apart from the purely physical sequelae, such as haemorrhage, infection or retained products, occurring soon after pregnancy, there are possible long-term physical effects such as impaired fertility or liability to subsequent spontaneous abortion to be considered.

Finally, subsequent psychological sequelae, which again may be immediate or long-term, must be taken into account. The prevalence and severity of these conditions in women aborted must be compared with the outcome in women refused abortion, and in such cases the effects on the child must also be examined.

At the moment the reporting arrangements following abortion in England and Wales are so poor that it is impossible to produce meaningful answers to any of the questions raised above. Most of the patients undergoing termination are returned to the care of general practitioners who have no obligation to report any complications they may see. Treatment may involve admission to the place where the termination was performed, or to another place in a different part of the country, or the treatment may be administered in the patient's home. The prevalence and severity of complications seen by family doctors after induced abortion must be compared with the picture they formerly saw after 'spontaneous' abortion in the days before the Abortion Act came into operation.

There is no doubt that prospective studies are needed to provide accurate answers to all these questions. Meanwhile, a survey of the literature gives some indication of the complication rates being reported under present day conditions.

(i) **Pyrexia**

Reported rates vary from 27 per cent (Sood, 1971), through 16.5 per cent (Stallworthy *et al.*, 1971), to 0.3 per cent (Beric and Kupresanin, 1971).

(ii) **Haemorrhage**

Stallworthy *et al.* (1971) reported a rate of 10 per cent in terminations of under ten weeks gestation, whereas Newton *et al.* (1973) experienced bleeding needing transfusion in only 0.7 per cent of nearly a thousand terminations performed by suction with the Karman or Biera catheter.

(iii) **Retained products**

In 1971, Sood reported re-evacuation to be necessary in 9.5 per cent of his cases, Stallworthy and his colleagues found it necessary in 10 per cent, whereas Beric and Kupresanin reported the low figure of 3.4 per cent.

Newton *et al.* in 1973 divided their cases into those treated by Karman catheter, Biera catheter and saline, with rates for re-evacuation of 3.2 per cent, 1.3 per cent and 30.4 per cent respectively.

(iv) **Perforation of the uterus**

This complication did not occur in the 1,117 terminations in 1972 reported by Newton *et al.*, but Sood (1971) found that perforation had definitely occurred in 2.7 per cent of 1543 operations.

The wide variations in these figures illustrate the influence of different methods of termination, and of duration of gestation. Sood's cases, for example, included 83 patients where Utus paste had been used as a method of termination, and 51 patients had reached between twenty and twentyeight weeks gestation. Thirteen patients had undergone hysterectomy. Only 27 per cent of the cases reported by Stallworthy's team were of less than ten weeks gestation, whereas all cases reported by Beric and Kupresanin were of less than twelve weeks.

Examination of the figures in these four series demonstrates that haemorrhage, pyrexia and retained products are least likely as complications using the Karman catheter in very early pregnancy, but their incidence rises steadily as the duration of pregnancy increases. After fourteen weeks, the likelihood of retained products increases greatly due to the necessity to use intra-amniotic injections, between one-third and one-half of these patients needing re-evacuation. Haemorrhage and retained products become less likely if hysterotomy is used, but pyrexia increases in frequency as a complication.

Methods involving forcible dilatation of the cervix increase the possibility of cervical tears, and the use of rigid instruments within the uterus, including their use during evacuation of retained products, makes perforation more likely.

Hysterotomy is followed by the possibility of endometriosis occurring in the uterine scar, or the possibility that the scar may rupture during a subsequent pregnancy. Infertility or ectopic pregnancy may follow damage to the tubes caused by infection following abortion.

More recently, the Chief Medical Officer's annual report for 1972, quoted by Arthure (1973), confirms that when pregnancies were terminated before thirteen weeks, the risk of sepsis and haemorrhage were each 2.9 per thousand notifications. After 13 weeks, the rates are roughly doubled, being 6.1 for sepsis and 5.1 for haemorrhage.

It must also be remembered that other complications, such as pulmonary embolism or chest infection, may follow any operation and the more complicated procedures required in second trimester abortion are more likely to be followed by such complications.

A recent report (Paktar *et al.*, 1973) showed that the risks for all complications after 330,000 abortions were seven times greater when abortion was performed after the first trimester.

Cervical damage following abortion

Apart from severe laceration lesser damage to the cervix resulting in incompetence with subsequent spontaneous abortion or premature labour may follow methods of abortion requiring forcible cervical dilatation.

A report in 1972 (Wright *et al.*), compared the numbers of second trimester spontaneous abortions, usually regarded as due to incompetence of the cervix, occurring in pregnancies following a vaginal termination of pregnancy, with the numbers of such abortions in all the patients delivered at Queen Charlotte's Hospital in London in 1971, and reported a tenfold increase. In addition it was noted that only one termination had been performed before ten weeks, which seemed to indicate that it was forcible dilatation of the cervix that was to blame.

From Hungary has come evidence, quoted by Klinger (1970), that premature labour is more common after abortion. The percentage of live births weighing 2,500 grammes or less showed a steady increase between the years 1960 and 1968, an increase paralleled by the increase in total abortions. The percentage of premature labours also increased relative to the number of terminations undergone by the patient.

Abortion—a 'safe' operation?

Abortion is a very good illustration of the fact that there is no such thing as a safe operation. Although the risks of death are small, the possibility of physical damage is not.

Psychiatric disturbance following abortion

One of the reasons for referring women who requested abortion to psychiatrists before 1968 was the general assumption that termination of pregnancy was often followed by pathological feelings of guilt, remorse, shame or depression. This assumption may have been based on the sequelae of criminal abortions where women, with no counselling were submitted to dangerous and degrading experiences, often in unhygienic surroundings, without anaesthetic, with no support to follow, and often even no opportunity for catharsis of their emotions by discussion with others.

The situation following legal abortion, preceded by adequate counselling and taking place in a society which accepts abortion as almost, if not entirely, respectable, is quite different. Care must also be taken to distinguish between the girl who feels regret at the necessity for abortion - which almost all do - and those who regret their decision to have an abortion, as opposed to keeping the pregnancy.

Several studies, among them those of McCoy (1968) and Pare and Raven (1970) have demonstrated that providing women want abortion, and do not have it forced upon them by others (i.e. that adequate counselling precedes the abortion), and providing no psychiatric disturbance existed before the occurrence of the unwanted pregnancy, then the likelihood of psychiatric disturbance as a sequel to abortion is extremely remote. Women with psychiatric disorders existing before pregnancy, however, may suffer an exacerbation of their condition either as a result of the pregnancy, or of the abortion, or both.

Were women after abortion likely to become genuinely psychiatrically disturbed, then general practitioners and psychiatrists should be seeing increasing numbers of such cases as the annual abortion figures rise. The attitude of psychiatrists to abortion was illustrated by the answers to questionnaires sent to members of the Society of Clinical Psychiatrists in 1967, and again in 1971. During those four years there was a 75 per cent increase in the proportion of psychiatrists who replied who were in favour of the woman having a free choice during the first trimester as to whether she wished to continue with the pregnancy or not - hardly a result to be expected if psychiatrists were seeing increasing numbers of post-abortal psychiatric disease.

There is some evidence (Kaltreider, 1973) that women seeking abortion after the end of the first trimester tend to be less mature, often have less satisfactory relationships with their parents, feel more of a sense of loss and need more care and support after abortion than those who come earlier in the pregnancy.

Little information is available from general practice as a whole, but certainly in my practice I have yet to see a patient without previous psychiatric disorder suffer severe pathological guilt or depression after abortion. Most women tell me they feel as though an enormous load has been lifted from their shoulders.

Perhaps depression after abortion is an indication of poor counselling and a lack of sympathy and understanding from her attendants (for women don't enjoy abortion), as a result of which she has been made to feel guilty and rejected.

In which case, possibly the medical attendants should be referred to the psychiatrist.

Consequences of refusal to terminate unwanted pregnancy

In the United Kingdom the woman with money who is refused abortion under the NHS will turn to the private sector. Those without money will turn to criminal abortion, possibly self-induced, with its inherent dangers, or will continue with the pregnancy.

Few studies of the consequences, to both mother and child, of refusal to abort have come from the United Kingdom, although certain obstetric conditions, notably hyperemesis, premature labour and prolonged labour, have long been said to be more common in unwanted pregnancy, and are known to have unfavourable effects on perinatal mortality and morbidity rates.

From Sweden, where abortion has been legal for over thirty years, long-term studies have been published.

Forssman and Thuwe (1966) followed-up 120 children born after their mother's application for abortion had been refused. The study lasted until the children were 21 years old, and compared these children with 120 matched control children. It was found that the children born after abortion had been refused needed more psychiatric care, showed more criminal and antisocial behaviour, were more often exempted from military service on medical grounds, showed lower educational achievement, and suffered more insecurity in their family life.

Suicide in pregnancy is uncommon but does occur as a way out of an intolerable situation. Suicide may be the way out chosen by a child in response to parental rejection. The myth that all unwanted pregnancies eventually become wanted babies must be abandoned: they are at least as likely to become neglected or battered babies, perhaps even murdered babies.

Thus in any consideration of the dangers of abortion to the mother, the dangers of refusal to abort, for both mother and child, must be borne in mind.

Recurrent requests for abortion

In some countries there is evidence that girls are having repeated abortions rather than using effective contraception. The suggestion has been made that recurrent requests for abortion are an indication of psychiatric illness, and this may well be so in a small proportion of cases.

My limited experience in one general practice, however, leads me to believe that girls requesting their second abortion (I have no experience of third or subsequent requests) show no distinguishing characteristics in any parameter.

They have merely been careless, foolish or unlucky on two occasions instead of on one. The exception, I believe, is the girl who waits, in her second unwanted pregnancy, until the first trimester has passed before seeking help from the doctor. Unless other reasons were manifest, I would suspect a desire to continue the pregnancy led to the delay in asking for termination.

The question remains as to the attitude the doctor should take when faced for the second time by the same girl with an unwanted pregnancy. I find it impossible to avoid a feeling of irritation, impatience or even fury, when I know full well that contraception was offered - nay, pressed upon her - after the last abortion. However, I attempt to suppress my impatience, since recrimination will help nobody.

Should a second abortion be refused in such circumstances? Should every patient be told at the time of the first abortion that 'under no circumstances' will a subsequent pregnancy be terminated? This type of procedure is adopted by at least one hospital in London.

I cannot believe that such an attitude is correct. Leaving aside the fact that 'under no circumstances' indicates an unjustifiable negativism in the medical assessment, to refuse to terminate a pregnancy only because it is a second or subsequent request must mean that this pregnancy will be allowed to result in a baby *as a punishment*. Surely an unsuitable punishment for the girl, for society, and not least, for the baby.

I am certain that repeat requests must be assessed and dealt with in precisely the same way as first requests. I do believe, however, that it is permissable to insist, without making conditions, that an intrauterine device will be inserted at termination in order to remove from the patient the option of failing to make use of contraception.

Infertility following abortion

There is the theoretical possibility that tubal infection following abortion may cause subsequent infertility, a possibility that would be welcomed by the mother who had completed her family.

Little evidence can be found that this risk of infertility is anything more than theoretical. Certainly in general practice, infertility following full-term delivery is a more common presentation. Pregnant women occasionally give the history that a medical attendant has told them in the past, immediately after an episode of pelvic infection, that they would probably be sterile.

> A girl in her early twenties gave a history of a therapeutic abortion in Japan. From her story I deduced that laminaria tents had been used. She had developed severe abdominal pain, profuse offensive vaginal discharge, fever and rigors. During her six days in hospital she had been taken to theatre twice for vaginal procedures. Large doses of antibiotics had been given. She had been told she had suffered severe infection of the uterus and both tubes, was lucky to be alive, but regrettably was certainly sterile as a result. She had consulted me because she feared she was again unwantedly pregnant. Her fear proved correct.

Rhesus iso-immunization following abortion

All women undergoing abortion, no matter how early the pregnancy, should have their Rhesus grouping identified before operation. 50 microgrammes of anti-D immunoglobulin should be administered within 24 hours of operation to all Rhesus-negative (D) women.

Sterilizing operations following abortion

The practice of offering abortion to only those women who will agree to sterilization as well cannot be sufficiently condemned. Such conditional operations, or 'package deals' were not uncommon before the passing of the Abortion Act, the argument being that if the termination of the existing unwanted pregnancy was genuinely indicated, then the indication would be just as strong, or stronger, in any subsequent pregnancy, and therefore sterilization was also indicated. This argument did not take into account the anxious and confused state of the mind and emotions of the patient, who would grab at any straw offered which would result in an immediate solution to her problem, without adequate consideration of the future consequences.

Under such circumstances women were deprived of the right to change their mind later, surely a recognized privilege of their sex. The result of some of these package deals, as seen by the family doctor observing the patient over many years, were indeed tragic.

> An unmarried coloured girl of eighteen found herself to be pregnant. She already had two children who were looked after by foster parents. She paid for their upkeep from her meagre earnings, and was both fond and proud of the children, visiting them as often as she could. However, the prospect of a third child seemed to her an insupportable burden, and she requested abortion. This was in the days before the Abortion Act, and before the IUD was generally available. She had used oral contraception but was incapable of taking Pills regularly.
>
> She was referred to a gynaecologist, who, armed with a psychiatric opinion that the patient had an immature personality, offered termination of the pregnancy provided she agreed to sterilization at the same time. As she said later, 'I would have agreed to having my arm cut off, if only I could get my abortion.'
>
> Four years later she formed a stable relationship with a man whom she wished to marry, and who wanted children. She bitterly regretted undergoing sterilization, and embarked on a series of operations in an attempt to reverse the effects of the operation. Unfortunately, the method of sterilization used precluded much hope of their success.

This is an extreme example, and one hopes that such a situation would not arise today. Some disquiet arises from a statement attributed to the Abortion Law Reform Society that in 1971 46 per cent of married women undergoing abortion in National Health Service hospitals were sterilized at the same time. The percentage seems a good deal higher than I would expect from experience in my own practice.

That many women, especially those with completed families, welcome sterilization if offered during abortion counselling is undoubted, and this offer should always be made by the family doctor in cases which seem suitable. It should be made clear however that the offer is unconditional: the decision is for the woman herself to make, and completely separate from the question of termination of the existing pregnancy. The subject of sterilization should be raised by the doctor, rather than waiting for the patient to raise it, since many women seem to believe that they will not be 'allowed' to have the operation unless their family size has reached enormous proportions, or severe disease co-exists.

The additional risk when sterilization is performed in addition to abortion is indicated in Table XVII.

It can be seen that the mortality rate at all ages in 1970 and 1971 following the double operation was greater than that following abortion alone. Increasing age of the patient was also associated with a further increase in the mortality rate.

Table XVII. Deaths following abortions, and abortions with sterilization: Residents of England and Wales, 1970 and 1971 (Registrar General's Returns).

	Aged less than 30	*Deaths*	*Aged 30 or over*	*Deaths*
All abortions	113,068	11	57,464	14
Abortion with sterilization	7,219	3	21,189	11

These figures on their own do not indicate that the double operation is an unsound procedure: the indications for sterilization may themselves have carried a high mortality, with or without further pregnancies or operations.

Laparascopic sterilization is today the method of choice when sterilization is to be performed at the time of abortion, and no doubt the low mortality of this operation will result in an improvement of the comparative figures in the future.

Benefits of the Abortion Act

After this rather dismal list of complications, it is a relief to find that it is possible to identify improvements that have occurred. Soskice (1973) has assessed the effect of abortion on the illegitimate birth rate, premarital conceptions, and septic abortions, all events which proponents of the Abortion Act maintained would decrease in numbers once more liberal abortion was available.

He concluded that in England and Wales between 1967 and 1970 the number of illegitimate births fell by 8 per cent, the fall being greatest (up to 15 per cent) in those areas where most abortions were performed. During the same period, the numbers of premaritally conceived births, which had been increasing year by year, started to decrease annually. Comparing the numbers of patients discharged from hospitals after septic abortions, he found an annual increase until 1969, and thereafter a marked decrease. Finally he made estimates which suggest that the increase in maternal deaths due to legal abortion is more than offset by the decrease in deaths from illegal abortion.

Certainly every general practitioner who has practised both before and after the Abortion Act sees enormous benefits, quite incapable of measurement, to the happiness of women, and their families, when released from the burden of unwanted pregnancy.

Contraception after termination

The importance of preventing further unwanted pregnancies should be impressed on the patient even before termination is performed. Afterwards there is a noticeable diminution of enthusiasm on the part of almost every girl: one-third of my patients for whom an appointment had been made to obtain contraceptive advice after termination defaulted. Some genuinely do not need it, for example those where pregnancy has followed a single occasion of intercourse in circumstances unlikely to recur. Others make extravagant assurances ('I shall never have intercourse again, Doctor.') which are most unlikely to be kept.

That there is some urgency in the provision of contraception has been demonstrated by Boyd and Holmstrom (1972) who found that in 91 post-termination patients, the earliest presumptive time of ovulation was the tenth post-operative day, and all had ovulated by the thirtyfifth day.

Insertion of an intrauterine device immediately after abortion is the ideal method, as contraception will then continue until positive action on the part of the patient results in her attendance for its removal. If oral contraception is chosen, it should be started on the seventh day post-partum, to avoid an increased liability to breakthrough bleeding, and confusion with possible bleeding due to retained products. However, many hospitals prefer to issue oral contraceptives before the patient leaves them and instruct the patient to start taking them immediately, before her contraceptive enthusiasm wanes.

This attitude is understandable, but will result in some difficulty for the family doctor confronted with a patient bleeding both after termination and after taking Pills. There is also a danger that the idea is self-defeating since the girl may cease taking the Pill because of the bleeding without consulting any doctor at all.

The requirement after termination is that the girl should be encouraged to take a firm decision to initiate contraception; she should then be offered the choice of agency to continue its supervision, either hospital, local clinic or family doctor - and it must be agreed that many girls undergoing abortion have no family doctor in the neighbourhood - and arrangements should exist, at district level, for the follow-up of non-attenders.

An area service

In 1974, the new Area Health Authority will take over responsibility for providing contraceptive services. Part of its responsibility should be the provision of an integrated abortion service. General practitioners providing contraceptive services should also supply abortion counselling services: facilities for abortions of all types should be available at each district hospital, as part of the total gynaecological care of the district. That this can be done without disrupting other types of patient care has been demonstrated by the experience at King's College Hospital in London, reported by Newton *et al.* (1973). A similar service has been provided at a non-teaching hospital in Lewisham (Buckle and Anderson, 1972).

Follow-up may be provided by general practitioners, health visitors, social workers or, on rare occasions, domiciliary family planning teams. Coordination of these activities should take place at area and district level.

Patients of other family doctors

Until all general practitioners adopt a similar attitude towards abortion it is inevitable that girls with unwanted pregnancies will be advised by their friends to visit doctors who have been found sympathetic and helpful on previous occasions. In addition, some girls will choose not to visit their own family doctor because they do not wish him to know of their unwanted pregnancy.

The general practitioner should point out to the patient that the help of her own doctor may be needed at some time in the future for some complaint connected with the abortion, or for some condition, such as infertility, where the knowledge of a previous pregnancy would be highly significant. For these reasons, and in the interest of promoting good relations between professional colleagues, the patient's permission should be requested for a letter to be written to her own doctor informing him of the findings and the proposed line of treatment.

Sadly, my own experience is that for reasons that seem good to them, most girls refuse to allow me to write to their own doctor, and I feel certain that their wishes must be respected. To do otherwise would represent a breach of the confidence which must exist between doctor and patient. However, I think it reasonable in such circumstances to ask the girl to sign a note confirming that she has refused permission, lest her own doctor should reproach me later.

Where permission is granted the letter should be written without delay, and the receipt of a kind acknowledgement from the patient's family doctor makes a satisfactory completion to the affair.

The Lane Report

Since this section was written, the Report of the Committee on the Working of the Abortion Act, under the chairmanship of Mrs Justice Lane, has been published. Its main findings, that abortion should remain the responsibility of the general practitioner and gynaecologist working within the National Health Service, that every request for abortion should indicate careful assessment and counselling, and that there should be greater equality of opportunity to obtain abortion throughout the country do not necessitate any further comment here.

Further recommendations made in the report, that abortion should not be carried out after 24 weeks of pregnancy, that foreign women should not be prevented from seeking help in the United Kingdom, and that there should be stricter control of agencies giving advice about abortion, should be welcomed by all.

REFERENCES

ARTHURE, H. (1973). *British Medical Journal*, **1**, 549.

BEARD, R. W., BELSEY, E. M., LAL, S., LEWIS, S. C. and GREER, H. S. (1974). Contraceptive practice before and after outpatient termination of pregnancy. *British Medical Journal*, **1**, 418.

BERIC, B. M. and KUPRESANIN, M. (1971). *Lancet*, **ii**, 619.

BOYD, E. F. and HOLSTROM, E. G. (1972). *American Journal of Obstetrics & Gynecology*, **113**, 469.

BUCKLE, A. E. R. and ANDERSON, M. M. (1972). Report on a year's working of abortion clinics and operating sessions. *British Medical Journal*, **3**, 381.

CARTWRIGHT, ANN and WAITE, M. (1972). Evidence to the Committee on the Working of the Abortion Act. *Journal of the Royal College of General Practitioners*, **22**, Suppl. 1.

DIGGORY, P. L. C. (1969). Some experiences of therapeutic abortion. *Lancet*, **i**, 873.

FORSSMAN, M. and THUWE, I. (1966). Survey of 120 children born after termination had been refused. *Acta Psychiat. Neurol. Scandinavica*, **42**, 71.

INGHAM, C. and SIMMS, M. (1972). Study of applicants for abortion at the Royal Northern Hospital, London. *Journal of Biosocial Science*, **4**, 351.

KALTREIDER, N. B. (1973). Emotional patterns related to delay in decision to seek legal abortion. *California Medicine*, **18**, 5, 23.

KERENYI, T. (1973). Reported in *General Practitioner*, March 2, p. 13.

KLINGER, A. (1970). Demographic consequences of the legalization of induced abortion in Eastern Europe. *International Journal of Gynaecology & Obstetrics*, **8**, 680.

LEWIS, S. C., LAL, S., BRANCH, B. and BEARD, R. W. (1971). Outpatient termination of pregnancy. *British Medical Journal*, **4**, 606.

LOUNG, K. C., BUCKLE, A. E. R. and ANDERSON, M. M. (1971). Results in 1,000 cases of therapeutic abortion managed by vacuum aspiration. *British Medical Journal*, **4**, 477.

McCOY, D. R. (1968). The emotional reaction of women to therapeutic abortion and sterilization. *Journal of Obstetrics & Gynaecology of the British Commonwealth*, **75**, 1054.

NEWTON, J., BROTMAN, M., McEWAN, J. and OWENS, C. (1973). Hospital family planning: termination of pregnancy and contraceptive use. *British Medical Journal*, **4**, 280.

PAKTAR, J., O'HARE, D., NELSON, F. and SVIGIR, M. (1973). *American Journal of Public Health*, **63**, 524.

PARE, C. M. B. and RAVEN, H. (1970). Follow-up of patients referred for termination of pregnancy. *Lancet*, **i**, 635.

Report of the Committee on the working of the Abortion Act (The Lane Report). (1974). HMSO, London.

SOSKICE, D. (1973). *British Journal of Hospital Medicine*, **9**, 299.

SOOD, S. V. (1971). Some operative and post-operative hazards of legal termination of pregnancy. *British Medical Journal*, **4**, 270.

STALLWORTHY, J. A., MOOLGAOKER, A. S. and WALSH, J. J. (1971). *Lancet*, **iv**, 1245.

WRIGHT, C. S. W., CAMPBELL, S. and BEAZLEY, J. (1972). Second trimester abortion after vaginal termination of pregnancy. *Lancet*, **i**, 1278.

14

CHOICE OF CONTRACEPTIVE METHOD

In theory, a couple would enter the doctor's surgery, sit down and - following routine enquiries after the state of the doctor's health and comments concerning the weather - say something like this:

'Doctor, we have come for your expert advice as to the most suitable method of contraception for us to use'.

In practice this rarely happens. Couples do not usually come for advice together; it is usually the female, either to request information on her own behalf or, as a result of the well-known cowardice of the male, on behalf of her consort. The exception to prove the rule is concerning requests for vasectomy, when men do appear alone on occasions.

I have already emphasized that family doctors should not wait for enquiries, but initiate discussion of contraception themselves. Where patients do open the discussion however, the request is usually for information about a particular method, rather than for contraceptive advice. Common openers are:

'Doctor, I want to go on the Pill', or 'Doctor, I'm thinking of having the Curl fitted'. (All IUDs are curls to my patients, even the Gravigard is 'the new copper curl').

Many interviews thus start with consideration of a particular method, a method suggested by the patient herself, and therefore, because acceptability is so important from the point of view of side-effects and continuation rates, a method that the doctor should advise against only in the presence of clear-cut contra-indications.

Choice of method is a combined operation, choice by the patient combined with choice by the medical adviser, and both interact with each other and are affected by outside influences and personal prejudices. Figure 46 illustrates some of the factors influencing choice.

A list of the factors influencing the patient would include whether the male has the dominant role in the relationship - in which case coitus interruptus, the condom or vasectomy would be the preferred methods, or whether the

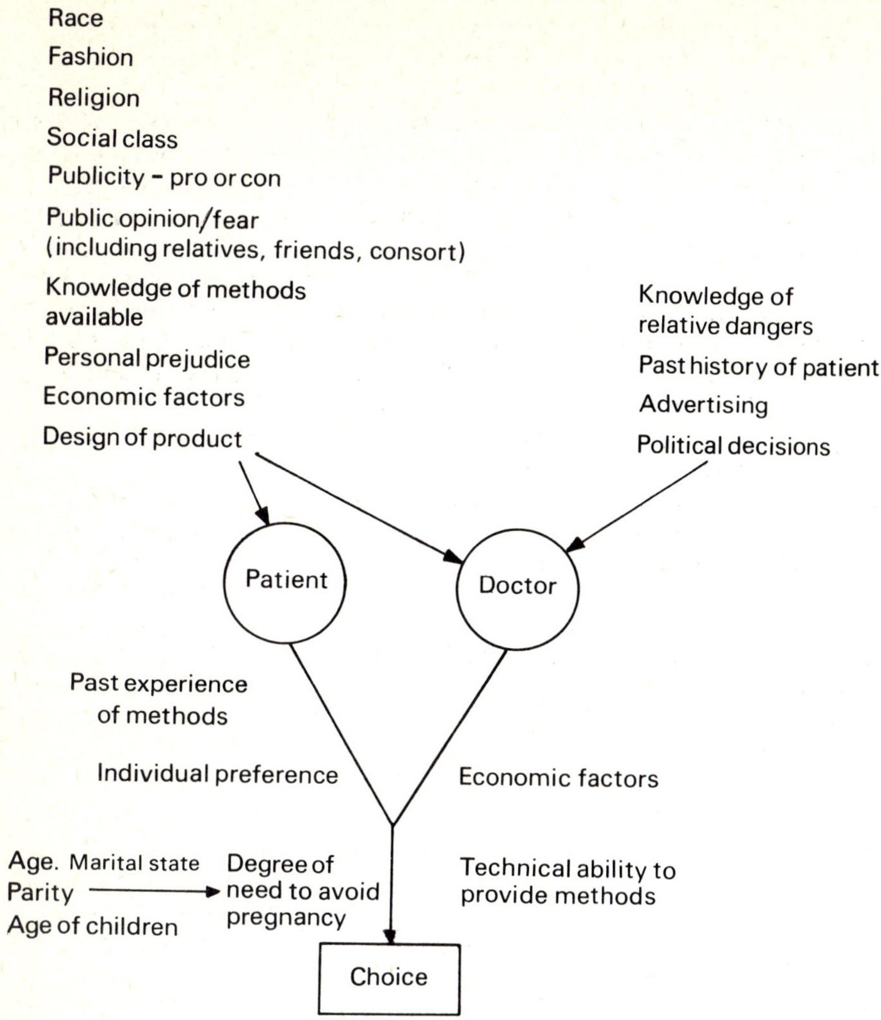

Fig. 46. Factors influencing choice of method.

female is the dominant, or at least equal, partner - in which case the cap, the Pill, the intrauterine device or tubal ligation would be preferred. Race, religion and social class also influence choice. West Indian males accept vasectomy as willingly as decapitation, caps and diaphragms are today almost the prerogative of the higher social classes, and religion may dictate the avoidance of a method likely to result in extra bleeding, such as the progestogen-only Pill or the intrauterine device, among Asian or Jewish women. Roman Catholic patients may insist on using only the rhythm method, although fear of Hell Fire in the next world tends to diminish as family size increases in this one.

Family size is indeed a most potent factor influencing choice in all women, and as family size alters, so will choice of method, those with the lowest failure rates being preferred.

Adverse publicity, justified or not, for any particular method may exert enormous influence on the acceptability of any method. The Scowen report was the classic example, and one hopes, will never be repeated. Largely as a result of this adverse publicity, women chose progestogen-only Pills in numbers unjustified by the efficiency of the product.

That fashion influences the clothes women wear is indisputable, and it is obvious to those of us involved in the trial of new methods of contraception that fashion influences choice of contraceptive method also. Produce a new Pill or a new device, or even an old Pill in a fresh wrapper or of a different colour, and women are queueing up for it in no time. Design is important. I have been asked several times for a certain Pill because of the elegant Grecian lady's head on the packet.

Related to fashion is public opinion, that is, the opinions received by patients from other patients. An extreme example was one of my patients who had decided after confinement in my District Teaching Hospital to be fitted with a copper '7'. She had the misfortune to ascend in the hospital lift with a lady who informed her 'twixt the ground and fifth floor that the obvious uterine enlargement she enjoyed contained both a foetus and a copper bearing-device. My patient changed her mind, and now takes the Pill.

A less extreme example is the well known fact that if Mrs A suffers certain side-effects from a certain Pill or IUD, then her friend Mrs B is very likely to suffer the same side-effects. I have found that this sequence of events may be interrupted by suggesting to Mrs B, obliquely, that Mrs A's side-effects occur only in neurotic women - a contention that Goldzieher's double-blind cross-over trial tends to bear out. However, I believe that side-effects are very likely to be similar in patients who are blood relatives. I base this opinion on observations made when I was carrying out trials of Pills containing the same ingredients but manufactured in different shapes and packaged in different ways. If one sister had troubles with one Pill, then the other sister was likely to have the same troubles, even if the Pill looked completely different. We know a similar state of affairs exists with antidepressant drugs.

The personal prejudices of the patient must also be taken into account in choice of method. Some women regard the idea of something inserted in their uterus as horrifying, but will cheerfully swallow Pills for years. For others, the reverse is true. Men are not immune to prejudice either, the idea of a sheath being anathema to some, 'like eating a banana with the skin on', as my patients picturesquely put it, whereas others regard sheath-wearing as agreeable. Many women are prejudiced against asking for sheaths in chemists' shops. At least one unwanted pregnancy in my practice resulted because the husband's overtime prevented him getting to the shops and the wife, asked to buy on her husband's behalf, simply could not bring herself to make the purchase. At least one ethical pharmaceutical company has realized this problem exists and markets an attractively packaged product, 'Shields', which women may ask for without embarrassment, and which look sufficiently different in their packaging from conventional sheaths to allow display on the cosmetics counter without seeming out of place.

Social class has in the past influenced contraceptive choice to a marked degree, the effectiveness of the method of contraception used tending to increase as the social class of the patient rose. Whether this really demonstrated a choice of method, or was simply the result of ignorance of methods, lack of availability of advice and the influence of economic factors is doubtful. The oral contraceptive, available from twenty thousand general practitioners and well publicized among the population at large, was willingly accepted by the lower social classes. This seems to indicate that circumstances rather than choice resulted in the use of the less effective methods by the less privileged social classes, and now that all methods of contraception will be almost equally available to all, these social class differences will largely disappear.

Similar considerations apply to the influence on choice that knowledge of available methods will have. Manifestly, no patient can choose a method he or she has never heard of. Improvements in education, in schools, of patients and of doctors themselves should ensure that all couples in the future are sufficiently well informed of the wide choice of methods now available.

Given that a couple were well informed of methods available, economic factors have in the past influenced choice. It was of little use advising vasectomy at a cost of forty pounds to a man who, with his family, was existing at almost poverty level. Once again, the inclusion of all methods of fertility control in the National Health Service should remove this barrier to free choice of method.

All these factors influence choice by the patient, and the medical adviser, as a member of the public, is also influenced by the same factors. In addition, the special knowledge that the family doctor has will also influence the advice he gives regarding choice. His expert knowledge of the relative dangers involved in various methods will be used, quite correctly, to influence the combined choice made by him and by his patient together. The past medical history of the patient, including his knowledge of her use or misuse of contraceptive methods, may indicate that one method should be chosen rather than another.

All doctors are subjected to powerful advertising campaigns promoting certain methods and individual products. Most of the information received in this way is accurate and helpful, but naturally is presented with a certain unavoidable bias in favour of the product being promoted. It is essential that other sources of information are made available, and the results of independent comparative trials should be accessible to all workers in the contraceptive field. The Family Planning Association has long published a News-Letter sent to all within its ranks. A similar information service should be available in the future to all family doctors.

Political decisions have in the past influenced the doctor in the type of contraception he could advise. The infamous medical reasons/social reasons ruling affecting the cost of oral contraceptives is one example. Choice of intrauterine device is still influenced by its availability on NHS prescription form EC10. Some political decisions have been the result of prejudice by doctors, the sad case of the condom's exclusion from methods that may be prescribed by general practitioners being the prime example.

All the factors considered above have acted or are acting on both doctor and patient before they meet to consider a choice of method. There is then an interaction proceeding during the interview which may modify or reverse the attitudes held by either at the start of the consultation.

The doctor's opinion that a certain method would be ideal for the patient, in view of her circumstances and history, may be negatived by the simple statement that the method has already been tried and found unsatisfactory, or the even simpler statement that the very idea of the method is distasteful.

The doctor may feel that tubal ligation may be ideal, but his knowledge that in that locality none of the NHS gynaecologists will perform the operation without excessively severe medical indications, together with the patient's response to the estimated cost of the operation as a private patient, may indicate the abandonment of that choice.

The technical ability of the family doctor to provide only a limited range of contraceptive methods may influence the patient's choice. For example, she may feel that an intrauterine device would be most suitable, but when she discovers that to use that method she will have to travel some miles to a clinic and see a different doctor she may change her mind.

Many patients bring to the interview ideas of the dangers, or of the safety, or of the efficiency of a method that are quite wrong. The dangers of combined oral contraceptives, for example, are frequently overrated, the possibility of pregnancy with the intrauterine device commonly underrated. Correction of misbeliefs may result in an alteration of choice.

The method chosen by any couple will vary from year to year according to their need to avoid pregnancy at that time. A method with a relatively high failure rate may be acceptable in the early years of marriage while spacing a family, but may be quite unacceptable before marriage or after the desired family size is attained. The need to avoid pregnancy will thus vary in degree for the same couple from year to year, and age, parity, marital status and the age of existing children will all influence the degree of need.

The decrease in fertility which occurs as men and women age is to some extent balanced by the dismay they would feel were they to start increasing their family at the end of reproductive life, especially if their children had already started their own reproductive careers. On the other hand, the most effective reversible method of all, the Pill, carries increased dangers as age advances, but to balance this is the increased danger both of pregnancy and abortion with increasing age.

In general, an unplanned pregnancy in an unmarried woman would be a greater catastrophe than an unplanned pregnancy within marriage, but this simple statement needs qualification. The importance of marriage prior to childbirth varies according to social class, race and religion. Again the unplanned pregnancy within marriage will seem a much greater catastrophe to the mother with five children already than to the woman with only one child.

What of the influence of the source of contraceptive advice on the choice of method used? If we examine the published records of choices made by women obtaining advice from different sources within the space of a very few years we find remarkable variations in the proportion of women choosing one of the two most effective methods (Table XVIII).

Table XVIII.

Source of advice	*Year of consultation*	*Pill*	*IUD*
General practitioners (Cartwright & Waite, 1972)	1970–71 Method most often advised	90%	0%
	Method next most often advised	5%	35%
FPA Clinics 1973	1973 First attenders chose	60%	11%
All sources (Hull Family Survey, Peel, 1972)	1970 Methods ever used	51%	3%
General practitioner and patient's choice? (Barley, 1971–72)	1971–72 Attenders chose	48.4%	41.7%
Hospital and patient's choice? (King's College Hospital, Newton *et al.*, 1973)	1972 Choice immediately after termination	255 patients	271 patients

BARLEY, N. H. (1973). A family planning clinic in general practice. *Journal of the Royal College of General Practitioners,* **23,** 663.

CARTWRIGHT, ANN and WAITE, M. (1972). General practitioners and contraception in 1970–1. *Journal of the Royal College of General Practitioners,* **22,** Suppl. 2.

NEWTON, J., BROTMAN, M., McEWAN, J. and OWENS, C. (1973). Hospital family planning, termination of pregnancy and contraceptive use. *British Medical Journal,* **4,** 280.

PEEL, J. (1972). Hull Family Survey II. *Journal of Biosocial Science,* **4,** 333.

Women attending the general practitioners sampled by Carter would most often be advised to use the Pill, rarely the IUD. On the other hand women attending one GP's clinic (Barley, 1973) chose the Pill only slightly more often than the IUD. Of the patients attending FPA clinics in 1973, and the young married couples surveyed in Hull in 1970, rather more than half chose the Pill, and a much smaller proportion the IUD. The difference between the proportion choosing intrauterine contraception from those two sources probably relates to the increasing general popularity of this method between the years 1970 and 1973. Finally, women immediately after termination at King's College Hospital in 1972 demonstrated a quite different pattern of choice, for more of them chose intrauterine contraception than oral contraception.

At first sight it may appear that choice of contraceptive method will be influenced by the source of advice chosen by the patient. In fact, the same factors will be operating on both patient and doctor, irrespective of source of advice. Self-selection by patients is a factor very difficult to assess, which will undoubtedly influence choice relative to source of advice. Women who want the Pill will tend to go to their GP, those who want the diaphragm or intrauterine device will tend to go to a clinic, and those who wish to use the sheath will go to the chemist's shops, unless sheaths are provided free of charge at certain clinics.

The figures quoted from King's College Hospital are remarkable, however, in that they indicate a complete reversal of the pattern shown elsewhere. In the very special situation existing after a termination of pregnancy, more women chose intrauterine than oral contraception. This may have indicated that the patients, aware of the possibility that they might fail to use a method under their own control, chose a method not under their control. They may already have experienced failure of a method, or failure to use a method, and so chose intrauterine contraception because of its low failure rate in use, and the need to take active steps to cease using it. The fact that a device could be inserted at termination would certainly influence some girls in their choice.

Another possibility is that in this very special situation, after termination of pregnancy, the choice of method was dictated by the medical attendant. There is no evidence that such dictation took place, but assuming that it did, would this be an undesirable situation? I think not. In such circumstances it seems to me that the patient often needs protection, not only against pregnancy, but also against herself. To insist on the use of a reliable, reversible method of contraception after abortion, seems to me reasonable, and if a patient of mine would not agree to use such a method, I would question my estimate of her need for abortion. To insist that the method used is one which the patient cannot fail to use seems a logical extension. To make such a condition prior to termination is not analogous to the infamous package deal of abortion plus sterilization, the vital difference being of course the reversibility of the method.

THE CLINICAL INTERVIEW

To identify and consider all the factors mentioned at each initial interview with each patient is quite impossible. But there must be some basic plan for the conduct of the consultation, sufficiently simple to occupy little time, yet capable of modification to suit the patient's preferences and prejudices.

Let us assume that the relative cost to the patient and availability of the various methods need not be considered, now that contraception is at last within sight of being wholly available as part of the National Health Service. Let us also assume that the identification of medical contra-indications to the use of any method will take place, and be acted upon at some time during the interview.

The most important factor to be considered in the choice of contraceptive method by any patient is the degree of need to avoid pregnancy at that moment in time. The method chosen should therefore be the most effective method that the patient finds acceptable. The plan to be adopted during the interview should be to evaluate the degree of need, to suggest methods suiting that degree of need, and then, in concert with the patient, accept or reject the method guided by the patient's preferences and prejudices. The doctor's preferences and prejudices must be sternly suppressed, except, as I have already suggested, where it is felt that the patient needs protection against herself as well as against pregnancy.

Even where the patient presents a request for a particular method at the beginning of the consultation, the plan to fit the method to the degree of need to avoid pregnancy should still be followed. The patient's request may be based on misapprehension, or be made in ignorance of the full variety of methods available.

Assuming the patient to be female, which is usually the case, either she wishes maximal protection against pregnancy, or she does not.

If she does, then it may be required for the rest of reproductive life, when sterilization, preferably of the male, but otherwise of the female, will be needed. If operation is refused, then only combined oral contraception provides the required degree of protection against pregnancy.

If she does not require complete protection, as is the case with patients spacing their families, especially between the first and second child, then any method of birth control, excluding sterilization, would be suitable, judged solely by the need to avoid pregnancy.

On to this simple plan must now be grafted the likes and dislikes of the patient, medical contra-indications, and the assessment between patient and doctor, of the likelihood of the particular patient continuing regular use of the method, all influenced by the factors already discussed.

Thus I do not think it very helpful to talk of indications for a method of contraception. Any list of indications must be so hedged about with 'ifs and buts and except fors' as to be almost valueless.

More useful is to look at the sort of people within the community who do use a method, together with the sort of patients in whom that method should be avoided. A profile could be constructed identifying those types of patient characteristically found in large numbers in any large group of patients using a particular method, but not, of course, to the total exclusion of those usually found in profiles of other methods.

PROFILE OF PATIENTS CHOOSING COMBINED ORAL CONTRACEPTION

1. Likely to be young or very young - aged 15–25 years.
2. Likely to have had no children.
3. Likely to be unmarried, divorced or separated.
4. Likely to have had one or more unwanted pregnancy.
5. May be using the Pill for its therapeutic effect.
6. May be awaiting a sterilizing operation.

Avoid this method where:

1. Medical contra-indications exist.
2. Fear of oestrogens.
3. Individual distaste.
4. 'Feckless females'.
5. Previous failures.
6. Lactating mothers.
7. Older patient.
8. Infrequent intercourse.

Most of the factors influencing the items in this profile have already been discussed in the chapter on oral contraception. Apart from those choosing the combined Pill for its therapeutic effect, the efficiency of the method at preventing pregnancy is the attraction for these groups of women.

The reasons for avoiding the method in certain groups are mostly self-explanatory and have also been discussed elsewhere. 'Feckless females' is a generic term used to cover the type of woman all GPs know very well. Of inadequate personality, low intelligence and prone to anxiety, they are bound to miss Pills, or stop taking Pills without seeking medical advice.

Side-effects can be guaranteed to be severe and multitudinous. Recurrent unwanted pregnancies and pitiful pleas for abortion will result.

To summarize, the factors influencing choice of contraceptive method are many: some will affect only the patient, some will affect only the doctor, but many will affect both patient and doctor. The influence of such factors will vary according to the timing of the interview, in relation to events occurring in the life of the patient, the attitude of the community, and of the medical attendant. Finally the likelihood of making a particular choice of method will appear to vary according to the source from which advice is requested.

Patients who have previously failed to avoid pregnancy while using oral contraception as their chosen method are likely to fail again, and a method beyond their control is to be preferred.

PROFILE OF PATIENTS CHOOSING THE PROGESTOGEN-ONLY PILL

1. Unable to use the combined Pill for medical reasons.
2. Likely to be nulliparous or have only one child.
3. Very likely to exhibit fear of oestrogens.
4. Many will be in the age group 20–25.
5. They may find the risk of pregnancy desirable.
6. Very unlikely to have had a termination of pregnancy.

Avoid this method where:

1. Periods are a source of worry.
2. Pregnancy would mean a request for abortion.

Again this is a summary of much written in preceding chapters, and needs little elaboration. The two main factors influencing choice of this method are the fear of oestrogens, and the lack of fear of pregnancy. Many will be young married women spacing their families. The possibility of pregnancy while using this form of oral contraception make it the ideal method for use in those who regard intercourse without risk of conception as an empty charade.

PROFILE OF PATIENTS CHOOSING THE INTRAUTERINE DEVICE

1. Unable to use the Pill for medical reasons.
2. Have suffered side-effects on the Pill.
3. Are simply ‘fed up’ with taking Pills.
4. Are likely to have had two children.
5. Exhibit fear of oestrogens.
6. Few will be in the age group 15–20.
7. May have had one or more terminations.

Avoid this method where:

1. Medical contra-indications exist.
2. Pregnancy would result in a request for abortion.

Readers may care to exercise themselves by constructing similar profiles for the users of other methods. Roman Catholics would figure almost exclusively among rhythm users, and a failure to seek medical advice at all would be a characteristic of those using either the sheath or coitus interruptus.

Choice within methods

Turning to the choice of varieties available within each method, provided caps and sheaths fit, sensitivity to rubber is not a factor, and the colour suits aesthetically, there is not much to choose between them.

Choice of the various types of intrauterine device has been considered in some detail in the appropriate chapter.

Choosing the right Pill is a subject dear to the heart of all manufacturers of Pills, all of whom, as we know, manufacture the right Pill.

There is in my view nothing to choose between the various types of progestogen-only Pills available today. For the combined Pill, the idea of constructing a 'hormonal profile' for each woman is attractive. A list of items such as character of periods, size of breasts, type of skin, etc. is constructed. and a Pill chosen to suit the profile. Unfortunately, in practice this idea just does not work.

However, the normal menstrual pattern of the candidate for combined oral contraception does give some indication of the type of Pill most likely to suit her. If bleeding is heavy, or frequent, or both, then a Pill containing a relatively higher dosage of progestogen is needed. If bleeding is light, then a Pill containing a relatively low dosage of oestrogen should be chosen. If bleeding is very scanty and infrequent, then avoid the combined Pill altogether.

Even then, low-dosage Pills such as Minovlar or Minilyn may be associated with breakthrough bleeding in early cycles but, after a year or so, absence of withdrawal bleed becomes common.

Three negative instructions may be listed:

1. DO NOT give Pills containing more than 50 microgrammes of oestrogen.
2. DO NOT give high-dose progestogen Pills - notably Anovlar - as a first choice. They are invaluable to suppress dysmenorrhoea and ovulation pain, often not relieved by modern low-dosage Pills, and to suppress persistent breakthrough bleeding on Pills of lower dosage.
3. DO NOT give high-progestogen or low-oestrogen dosage Pills to girls with acne.

It would seem good medical practice to give the lowest dose of any substance which will produce the desired effect. Thus to start with a Pill containing only 30 microgrammes of oestrogen, especially in young girls of low weight, would seem a sensible sugrestion. The enormous differences in potency of the available progestogens makes it difficult to apply the same advice to them, but certainly the lowest effective dose of any particular progestogen should be used. The new micro-dosage Pills (Microgynon and Ovranette) are as yet so new that one must await further evidence of their efficacy in all types and weights of women.

Finally, it would appear that the advice on contraception given by doctors may be an example of the 'Do as I say, not as I do' syndrome.

The *American Journal of Obstetrics and Gynecology* in 1973 reported that of the wives of American gynaecologists who declared their contraceptive usage (and only 43 per cent of 800 questioned responded) only 27 per cent of the wives took the Pill, whereas 64 per cent of their husbands recommended the method.

Twentythree per cent used the intrauterine device, 14 per cent the diaphragm, 12 per cent the condom; either husband or wife had been sterilized in 9 per cent, and 15 per cent used douching, chemicals, withdrawal or rhythm.

15

DOMICILIARY FAMILY PLANNING

No matter how many family planning clinics are provided, how well advertised they are, and how cheap advice and supplies are made, there will always be some families who do not make use of the service. For some, this will be a conscious decision, a refusal to make any effort to limit their families because they want a large family. There are women who are never happy unless they have a baby to look after. Providing they are rich and well housed, no problems ensue. If they are poor and badly housed then social problems do ensue, but it is a mistake to think that contraception is the answer for such families. The offer must be made, but it will either be refused or used in an inefficient way until the desired family size is reached. Care must be taken not to force sterilization on such families, since regret and unhappiness will certainly follow.

There are other families where recurrent pregnancies and the demands of a large family make it impossible for the mother to attend a clinic to obtain the contraceptive help she wants. Her difficulties are increased by poverty, lack of education, poor housing conditions, low intelligence or frank mental handicap, perhaps with associated disease such as recurrent bronchitis. Inadequate in coping with her own problems, each additional child increases her inadequacy. Such women usually pair with inadequate men, bringing the problems of unemployment, alcoholism and debt to plague the family. Criminal activities may contribute to, and stem from these difficulties, and may involve the adults, when prison will remove them from the family circle and make matters even worse; or may involve the children, resulting in visits to police and probation officers, and difficulties with the 'school board man'.

Once imprisoned in such a vicious downwards spiral a family will need help from society in order to escape. Finance, rehousing, and the support of the social services will certainly be necessary, but without contraception to halt or at least delay the increase in the family, such help will be insufficient. It is unrealistic to expect such parents who have so notably failed to organize their lives, to be able to organize appointments at clinics or hospitals, or even to attend their family doctor with any degree of regularity.

Domiciliary Family Planning

A family planning service brought into the home is the only way of getting the advice and supplies so urgently needed to these patients. Peberdy in 1965 described such a service, and showed that the very high pregnancy rate existing among such families before the service began could be markedly reduced. Since then many authorities throughout the country have started domiciliary services, and at the time of the new Health Service Organization in April 1974, about fifty such schemes were in operation in England and Wales.

Identification of patients in need of such a service is the first consideration, and in areas with a high rate of hospital confinement the hospital is undoubtedly of vital importance in this respect. In some areas in London, for example, 95 per cent of babies are born in hospital and thus the mothers can be offered contraceptive assistance at that time. Sterilization or the insertion of an intrauterine device may be carried out before the mother leaves hospital. Where the mother chooses to use another method, and the hospital fear that she is unlikely to persevere with it or unlikely to use it correctly, they can enlist the aid of the domiciliary family planning service to follow up the patient after her return home. Those mothers who have their babies at home will need to be identified by domiciliary midwives, health visitors, social workers and welfare workers of all kinds.

General practitioners have, of course, a most important part to play in the provision of contraceptive advice to such patients. Indeed, if the GP offers it to his patients in the way described earlier in this book, and the hospital offers sterilization to all who feel their family size is complete, the need for a domiciliary family planning service greatly diminishes. It can be argued that the sort of patient needing the service is also the sort of patient who is always in and out of the doctor's surgery - usually without an appointment - either needing treatment for illness of the mother or children, or needing the bits of paper so necessary to obtain Health Insurance payments on the part of the husband. If any motivation to use contraception exists at all, it is as easy for the patient to get it from the GP while visiting the surgery as to wait at home for the visit of the domiciliary family planning team.

Under such circumstances, domiciliary family planning becomes necessary only for those of very low intelligence, or who are psychiatrically disturbed, and who have refused the offer of sterilization or intrauterine contraception. For them, a degree of care may be necessary that no general practitioner could contemplate. For example, it may be necessary to visit every month in perpetuity - or at least until the menopause - in order to do the calculations necessary for the rhythm method, or to ensure that the supply of condoms has not run out. I have been told of nightly visits to place Pills in patients' mouths, but for all I know such stories may be apocryphal.

The cost of such a service may be high, when calculated against the small number of patients involved. When set against the cost of a child in care, presently about £2,000, it is cheap at the price.

Unfortunately, once set up, a domiciliary family planning service tends to extend its activities to patients perfectly well able to make use of more normal types of service.

Supply tends to create increasing demand, as any Casualty Department open 24 hours a day will demonstrate. In addition, the members of a domiciliary team soon find a need for deputies and assistants. The tendency to expansion, both as regards staff and types of patients, must be monitored by those responsible for the organization of the service lest the praiseworthy image of the scheme when initially promoted falls into disrepute.

> A patient of mine, recently delivered, told me that she had accepted the proffered domiciliary service to check her IUD. She also told me that she intended to leave the baby with a child-minder and return to work as soon as possible. Her occupation? A ward orderly at the hospital where the device was inserted.

Where the circumstances described above, with contraceptively-conscious GPs and co-operative gynaecologists, do not exist, then domiciliary family planning assumes greater importance. Wilson (1971) describing such a service in Glasgow recorded that of sixty patients, not one had been referred by the family doctor. A considerable proportion of these doctors were Roman Catholics, whose conscientious objections presumably must have prevented them playing a full part in the contraceptive care of their patients. One may imagine that in an area served by a majority of Roman Catholic consultant gynaecologists sterilization may not be easily obtainable.

Under such circumstances it might be justifiable to expand domiciliary services, but even then the provision of child-minding services and transport for the patient to the source of contraceptive advice may prove just as efficient and far less expensive.

Where more normal circumstances obtain it is to be hoped that the inclusion of sterilization, vasectomy and most methods of contraception within the reorganized Health Service will lead almost to the disappearance of the need for domiciliary family planning.

REFERENCES

PEBERDY, M. (1965). In *Biological Aspects of Social Problems,* ed. Meade, J. E. and Parks, A. S. Oliver & Boyd, Edinburgh.

WILSON, E. (1971). Domiciliary family planning service in Glasgow. *British Medical Journal,* **4,** 731.

16

SEXUAL PROBLEMS, INFERTILITY, AND VENEREAL DISEASE

It is traditional that any book dealing with contraception should include chapters devoted to these subjects. In reality their only connection with contraception is that sexual activity is associated with each. None of the three is more likely, nor less likely to arise in contraceptors, than in non-contraceptors. All three subjects are a part of general practice and a basic knowledge of each should be part of the equipment of every general practitioner.

SEXUAL PROBLEMS

The family doctor supervising his patient's contraception will already be discussing intimate personal matters, and it is a short and easy step to the discussion of the degree of sexual satisfaction and any difficulties experienced. Many women do take this step and discuss their own or their consort's problems. The male is not so willing, usually sending the female to break the ice.

The GP must always be ready to listen to the patient with problems, and although it may be necessary to postpone full discussion to a more convenient time, his willingness must be made apparent. He must also develop a sixth sense that there is a sexual problem awaiting discussion. Patients often hint that all is not well, and then wait for the doctor to follow up the hint. If the hint is ignored the patient may feel unable to go any further, may feel that the doctor is uninterested or actively hostile, and will feel rejected. That this does on occasion happen is evidenced by the growing demand for counselling from agencies outside general practice. It would be a tragedy if the traditional role of the family doctor as the counsellor and friend should be usurped. Advice should be available from the GP at all stages of the patient's sexual career, both within and without marriage, and before and after marriage, recent or long gone.

The family doctor must also be able to deal with the patient's sexual queries. No sexual disability may exist, but an authoritative opinion may be sought as to the wisdom of indulging in a particular sexual activity, and whether any harm may be expected from so doing.

It is not uncommon for women to ask the doctor's opinion about fellatio. Knowledge that the Kinsey report revealed that oral sex was widely practised, especially among the higher social classes, is often reassuring for the patient. Masturbation is a sexual practice so hedged about with myth and fable that enquiries about its effects are common. Patients may be reassured that almost every male and very many females masturbate, and the practice is not a cause of blindness - nor even short-sightedness.

In order to be able to deal with such queries and to diagnose and treat sexual disorders such as impotence, premature ejaculation, vaginismus and failure to attain orgasm - all far from uncommon ailments - the family doctor must (to use a phrase beloved of the psychiatrists) adopt a positive attitude towards sex. He must not close his eyes to its problems, but must make efforts to find out about them. To assume that his or her own sexual experience and innate wisdom are adequate to enable informed advice to be given is a mistake.

As medical students most doctors received no training in sexual matters. The situation is today vastly improved, but it was sad to see a news item in 1974 stating that a course of lectures on contemporary sexual issues and marital problems at a famous London teaching hospital was to be given by the Family Planning Association because there was allegedly no doctor on the staff of the hospital capable of giving such lectures.

Medical students of the future should insist that education about sexual activity and the diagnosis and treatment of sexual problems should form part of their curriculum, if necessary taking the place of education concerning the more exotic and unusual medical and surgical conditions they will probably never see in a lifetime of non-specialist practice. Family doctors should stimulate and if necessary aggravate those arranging postgraduate education in their regions to include sex in the list of subjects about which they should receive instruction. For those doctors who wish to find out more about this subject a short bibliography follows.

The Anxiety Makers, Alex Comfort, Panther Books.
Patterns of Sexual Behaviour, C. S. Ford and F. A Beach, Methuen.
Sexual Deviations, A. Storr, Penguin.
The Sensuous Woman, 'J', Mayflower Publications.
Human Sexual Response, W. H. Masters and V. E. Johnson, Churchill.
Human Sexual Inadequacy, W. H. Masters and V. E. Johnson, Churchill.
Understanding Human Sexual Inadequacy, Edited by F. Belliveau and L. Richter, Coronet Books.

All these books are highly recommended. The price of the two classic works by Masters and Johnson leads me to advise readers to borrow them from the library, but the others are within range of the pocket even of general practitioners. 'Understanding Human Sexual Inadequacy' a paperback explanatory version of the original work by Masters and Johnson is, at the time of writing, only 35p.

For those doctors who are unable to find educational facilities in their region, the Family Planning Association organizes courses on Sex Education and Personal Relationships. Application should be made to the Education Officer of the Association at its head office, 27-35 Mortimer Street, London W1A 4QW.

More orientated to the problems of clinical and general practice are courses on Sex and Human Relations organized by the Department of Obstetrics and Gynaecology at King's College Hospital, London SE5 9RS. Application should be made to the Lecturer in Family Planning in that department.

INFERTILITY

Although the attempt to improve a patient's fertility is the very antithesis of contraception, it is quite logical that after several years of supervising the avoidance of pregnancy the family doctor should interest himself in attempting to ensure that the patient starts her family when she wishes to do so.

None of the reversible methods of contraception influence subsequent fertility with the exception of the Pill and the intrauterine device, which, together with the possible influence of a previous termination of pregnancy, have been discussed elsewhere. The general practitioner is in an ideal position to identify patients whose history indicates that they may have difficulty in conceiving and can take appropriate action with minimal delay.

It is important to remember that in approximately one-third of patients the cause of the infertility relates to the female, in another third to the male, and in the final third both male and female are contributing to the difficulty.

Family doctors often receive warning in advance that the patient intends to abandon contraception and start a family. The opportunity then exists to tell the patient that if she has not conceived within a reasonable time, then she must return for further advice. Which leads to the question, 'How long is a reasonable time?'. To some extent this varies with the age of the patient. At 35 available time may be very limited. The length of time considered reasonable also varies from adviser to adviser, figures of one year or even two years being suggested by some authors.

I would suggest that a wait of six months after giving up any method of contraception other than the Pill is reasonable, since about 65 per cent of women manage to conceive by then without any medical interference. Whether the patient has previously been pregnant or not has no bearing on the length of time that should be waited before investigation, since complications of the previous delivery may be the cause of the present infertility. The girl who has been taking the Pill should be warned not to rush out and buy a pram because her period is delayed immediately after the withdrawal bleed at the end of her last pack. For her, the six months should start from the time she resumes normal menstruation.

If pregnancy has not occurred after six months the couple should be questioned to make certain that intercourse is taking place at the correct time in the cycle, and physical examination of both partners should be performed to exclude obvious gross abnormality. The female will probably have undergone regular checks during her time using contraception, but the male may never have put in an appearance at all. It is as well to ascertain early on that he has testicles in his scrotum. Assuming no abnormality is revealed, the woman should be told to keep a basal temperature chart, as outlined in the chapter on the rhythm method. A biphasic chart usually means that ovulation is taking place, but is not incontrovertible evidence. The couple may be instructed to have intercourse immediately the chart shows the mid-cycle rise. Ideally they should time it to take place immediately before the rise, of course, but this is impossible until they have kept the chart for a month or two, and timing at the rise seems to work equally satisfactorily.

If after two months a biphasic chart is produced, then a post-coital test should be performed during the immediate pre-ovulatory phase. A satisfactory test indicates that the male is probably playing his part satisfactorily; absence of spermatozoa indicates that investigation should start with the male.

Further investigation and treatment should be carried out in a consultant unit. Thus the patient will reach the consultant after about one year of infertility, and from the consultant viewpoint this is about the correct length of time to wait before investigating, but the family doctor should be showing interest and carrying out simple investigations long before. Experience shows that patients much appreciate the fact that ‘something is being done’, and the simple activities outlined above do a great deal towards warding off the inevitable unhappiness and depression that result from the regular and unwelcome appearance of the period as month follows month. In addition, since it has been calculated that *any* form of treatment for infertility will be successful in 10 per cent of cases, the family doctor will stand to gain his small share of kudos.

Drugs to induce ovulation are now available. In my opinion there is no place for their use in general practice. Both multiple pregnancies and ovarian cysts may be induced by their administration, and treatment with such drugs should be reserved for specialist units with proper facilities for supervising the therapy.

Experience shows that the standard of investigation and treatment of infertility tends to vary from hospital to hospital. The standard of communication with the family doctor as investigation proceeds tends to vary from the mediocre to the absent altogether. GPs should not hesitate to interfere if investigation seems to have become bogged down, the patient having descended from the consultant to the registrar and finally to the houseman as time passes. Neither should he hesitate to refer the patient elsewhere if he is not satisfied with the care his patient is receiving.

Unfortunately, some patients will be found to be suffering from irreversible infertility, and it is then the family doctor's duty to tell them so. Either adoption or, in the case of the infertile husband, artificial insemination by donor (AID) may be a satisfactory solution. At the moment few NHS hospitals offer AID but one hopes that more will do so in the future.

Meanwhile general practitioners should inform themselves of the facilities outside the NHS available in their area so that they may advise their patients.

VENEREAL DISEASE AND CONTRACEPTION

'The accumulation of cases of long term individual misery and venereal disease as a direct result of its (the Pill's) use is more calamitous than anything precipitated by thalidomide.' R. S. Morton in 'Sexual Freedom and Venereal Disease', 1971.

True or false?

That there has during the last decade been an enormous worldwide increase in the incidence of veneral disease is undoubted. The World Health Organization reports that between 1957 and 1971 the annual number of new cases of syphilis in some countries has increased fourfold, and of gonorrhoea fivefold. In the United States of America, gonorrhoea is now considered a more common disease than measles. The increasing use of contraception has been blamed for promoting promiscuity, and because of this, a consequent increase in venereal disease. The Pill in particular has been blamed.

Before going any further it is necessary to define the meaning of some of the words used. There has been a tendency recently to include under the label of sexually transmitted disease everything from scabies to syphilis: even molluscum contagiosum, undoubtedly spread on occasions in a venereal manner, has been suggested as a candidate for the venereal portfolio. Doctors are today well aware of the dangers of inadequate treatment of venereal disease, and are therefore more willing to refer possible cases to VD clinics. Patients are similarly more willing to be referred than formerly. To look at clinic attendances as an index of any increase or decrease in the prevalence of venereal disease is a mistake: attendances are increasing because resistance to referral is decreasing. Diseases such as candidiasis often result in referral to VD clinics, but in many instances are not contracted venereally, and often are recurrences rather than new infections. The most helpful figures to examine are therefore the number of new cases of syphilis and gonorrhoea reported from the clinics, where almost all new cases are treated today. Even then, homosexual intercourse, in which contraception plays no part, is responsible for a proportion of these new cases.

Promiscuity must not be equated with premarital intercourse, probably no commoner today than in the past, but happily, because of contraception, less likely to result in pregnancy. Nor must it be equated with illegitimate pregnancy. West Indian girls, for example, are expected, and themselves expect, to demonstrate their suitability for marriage by the production of one or two healthy babies before deciding to tie the bonds of matrimony. Indeed, these bonds are being eschewed by more and more of the native population of these islands, who prefer their personal and sexual relationships to be unencumbered by legal ties until time has tested their possibilities for endurance. I do not define promiscuity as the possession by one person of several sexual partners, since if each partner is retained for several years, the condition is one of a succession of stable relationships rather than a promiscuous association. True promiscuity must involve shallow and meaningless sexual and personal relationships with many partners in rapid succession.

Accepting this definition, there is little relationship between promiscuity and contraception. The origins of promiscuity are psycho-social and are to be found in broken homes, poverty, lack of education, immaturity, inadequacy of personality and an unsatisfied craving for affection, all leading to an inability to make lasting and meaningful personal relationships. True, the use of contraception by such people would avoid the unsuitable punishment of pregnancy, but most family doctors know that such patients make very poor contraceptors. Their lives are so disorganized that no method of contraception - with the exception of the intrauterine device - is used regularly or for long. Except for doctors practising in localities where such emotional cripples tend to congregate, few meet many such patients.

The vast majority of patients attending either clinics or family doctors are enjoying stable regular sexual relationships with one partner, either a regular boy-friend or fiancé, or their husband. Very few have a rapid succession of partners.

I reject the contention that contraception leads to promiscuity: the two are in no way related. Further evidence comes from the histories of unmarried girls attending family planning clinics in the United Kingdom, and the United States. More than 95 per cent are already having sexual intercourse before seeking contraceptive advice, a situation difficult to reconcile with the theory that the advice encourages the intercourse.

One particular method, the Pill, has been singled out for blame. It has been suggested that increasing use of the Pill has been paralleled by the increase in new cases of syphilis and gonorrhoea. In fact the worldwide increase in the number of cases began several years before the introduction of the Pill, and several more years before Pill-users reached a significant proportion of the population. Once again it is difficult to believe that an event which took place later could be a cause.

The Family Planning Association have recently pointed out that one of the difficulties in comparing rates of Pill-usage and new cases of venereal disease in the United Kingdom is the very different scale by which each must be measured. There are two million women using the Pill, but only 53,000 cases of gonorrhoea annually. To minimize this difficulty statisticians advising the Association have suggested that semi-logarithmic graph paper should be used, where the intervals between each power (i.e. 10, 100, 1000) are the same. This eliminates distortion at either the high or low end of the scale, which would be present on an ordinary graph, and reduces the enormous size of graph that would be necessary to show relatively small changes annually.

Graph 1 shows the number of cases of syphilis and gonorrhoea per 10,000 population, and Pill-users per 10,000 population, plotted in semi-logarithmic form. It demonstrates that although the incidence of both diseases reached a peak after the war, that for syphilis has dropped steadily, and the rise in cases of gonorrhoea began in 1954, long before the Pill became available.

Graph 2 uses only the population aged between 15 and 45, its most

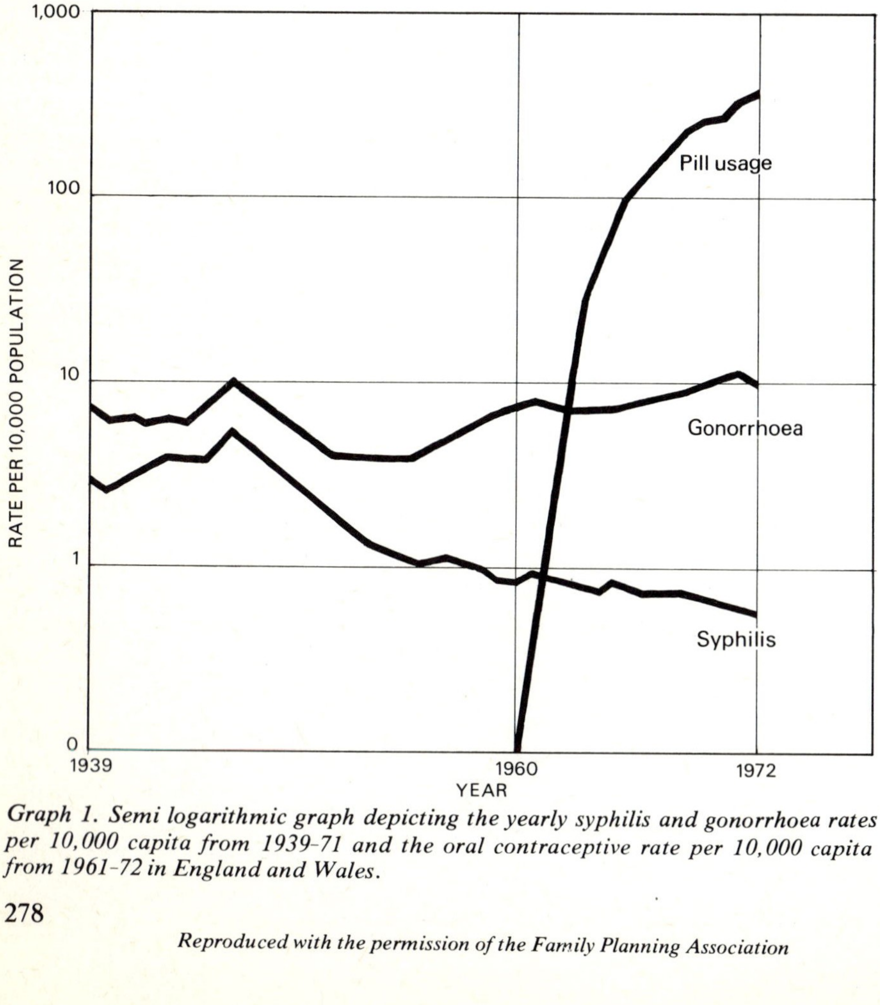

Graph 1. Semi logarithmic graph depicting the yearly syphilis and gonorrhoea rates per 10,000 capita from 1939-71 and the oral contraceptive rate per 10,000 capita from 1961-72 in England and Wales.

Reproduced with the permission of the Family Planning Association

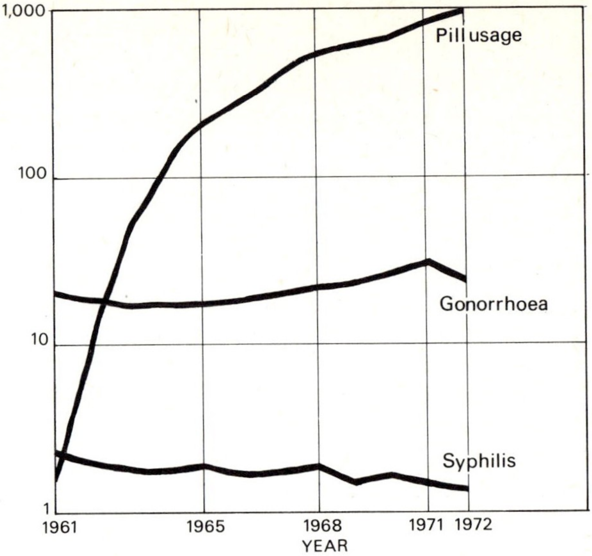

Graph 2. Semi logarithmic graph depicting the yearly syphillis, gonorrhoea and pill usage rates from 1961–72 (pop: 15–44 years old)

Reproduced with the permission of the Family Planning Association

sexually active members, and the rates as would be expected are higher, but the increase in rates is lower.

There would seem to be no statistically valid causal relationship between Pill-usage and the increase in incidence of gonorrhoea or the decrease in incidence of syphilis.

Studies of the number of sexual partners among Pill-users, as compared with those not using it, have shown little difference between the two groups. Pill-users have been shown to be more sexually active than other groups, but their high level of sexual activity is more likely to have dictated their choice of method rather than be a result of it. Pill-users are accustomed to seeking medical advice, and for reasons already discussed are likely to be referred, or refer themselves to VD clinics if they have any appropriate symptoms. The number of cases of syphilis or gonorrhoea found among clinic attenders using the Pill seems to be no greater than among attenders using other methods.

Although contraceptive usage, and Pill-usage in particular, are not the causes of venereal disease, nevertheless those using contraception are the sexually active members of the population, and as such are capable of contracting venereal disease. For this reason, those who work in family planning clinics, who know little of the patient's family and social background, should be alert to the possibility. Family doctors will know rather more about their patient's background, and will be able to assess probabilities rather better.

If any suspicion exists that a patient may be suffering from one of the major venereal diseases, referral to a special clinic is necessary. To send a high vaginal swab to the average laboratory is not an adequate procedure to exclude gonorrhoea. Better is to take a cervical swab, and place it immediately in Stewart's transport medium, but even then laboratories seem to vary enormously in their ability to culture the gonococcus successfully. Neither gonorrhoea nor syphilis may be satisfactorily diagnosed in general practice, and the treatment, follow-up and contact tracing necessary in the proved cases are virtually impossible.

Screening for VD of all patients attending contraceptive clinics has been suggested. In the United States 'pick-up' rates of between two and seven per cent have been reported, but it must be remembered that VD is five times more common in that country than in the United Kingdom. Screening trials are proceeding in this country, and may show themselves to be worthwhile in areas such as bed-sitter land in London where conditions encouraging promiscuity and venereal disease exist. Results from such areas must not be presumed to apply to more conventional areas however, and certainly not to contraceptive clinics operated within general practice in conventional areas.

The questionable protection afforded against VD by condom, spermicides and the copper intrauterine device has been considered in the appropriate sections. Certainly the condom seemed of little value in preventing the epidemic of VD which occurred in this country after World War II.

INDEX

Index